THE ENDOTHELIUM

An Introduction to Current Research

THE ENDOTHELIUM

An Introduction to Current Research

Editor

John B. Warren

Department of Clinical Pharmacology
Royal Postgraduate Medical School
London

WILEY-LISS

A JOHN WILEY & SONS, INC., PUBLICATION
New York • Chichester • Brisbane • Toronto • Singapore

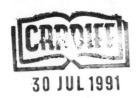
**Address all Inquiries to the Publisher
Wiley-Liss, Inc., 41 East 11th Street, New York, NY 10003**

Library of Congress Cataloging-in-Publication Data

The Endothelium : an introduction to current research / editor, John
   B. Warren.
      p. cm.
   Includes bibliographical references and index.
   ISBN 0-471-56828-7
     1. Endothelium—Physiology.   2. Endothelium—Pathophysiology.
I. Warren, John B.
QP88.45.E54   1990
612.7'9-dc20   90-43759
                                         CIP

Contents

Contributors

Ann Ager, Immunology Group, Department of Cell and Structural Biology, University of Manchester, Manchester M13 9PT, England [229,273]

Erik E. Änggård, The William Harvey Research Institute, St. Bartholomew's Hospital Medical College, London EC1M 6BQ, England [7]

H.L.C. Beynon, Rheumatology Unit, Department of Medicine, Royal Postgraduate Medical School, Hammersmith Hospital, London W12 ONN, England [209]

J.M. Boeynaems, Institute of Interdisciplinary Research, School of Medicine, Free University of Brussels, B-1070 Brussels, Belgium [53]

Renia M. Botting, The William Harvey Research Institute, St. Bartholomew's Hospital Medical College, London EC1M 6BQ, England [7]

A.J.B. Brady, Department of Medicine (Division of Cardiology), Royal Postgraduate Medical School, Hammersmith Hospital, London W12 OHS, England [157]

G. Burnstock, Department of Anatomy and Developmental Biology and Centre for Neuroscience, University College London, London WC1E 6BT, England [21]

John Clarke, Department of Medicine, Cardiovascular Division, Hammersmith Hospital, London W12 ONN, England [107]

John R. Cockcroft, Department of Clinical Pharmacology, Royal Postgraduate Medical School, Hammersmith Hospital, London W12 ONN, England; Present Address: Department of Clinical Pharmacology, Guy's Hospital, London Bridge SE1 9RT, England [65]

The numbers in brackets are the opening page numbers of the contributors' articles.

D.C. Crossman, Haemostasis Research Group, Clinical Research Centre, Harrow, Middlesex HA1 3UJ, England; Present Address: Department of Cardiology, Hammersmith Hospital, London W12 OHS, England [119]

Graham Davies, Department of Medicine, Cardiovascular Division, Hammersmith Hospital, London W12 ONN, England [107]

D. Demolle, Institute of Interdisciplinary Research, School of Medicine, Free University of Brussels, B-1070 Brussels, Belgium [53]

Victor J. Dzau, Division of Vascular Medicine, Department of Medicine, Molecular and Cellular Vascular Research Laboratory, Brigham & Women's Hospital, Harvard Medical School, Boston, MA 02115 [81]

Gary H. Gibbons, Division of Vascular Medicine, Department of Medicine, Molecular and Cellular Vascular Research Laboratory, Brigham & Women's Hospital, Harvard Medical School, Boston, MA 02115 [81]

J.C. Giddings, Haematology Department, University of Wales College of Medicine, Cardiff CF4 4XN, Wales [141]

Lee Gordon, Department of Histochemistry, Royal Postgraduate Medical School, London W12 ONN, England [253]

C. Haslett, Department of Medicine (Respiratory Division), Royal Postgraduate Medical School, London W12 ONN, England; Present Address: Department of Respiratory Medicine, City Hospital, Edinburgh EH10 5SB, Scotland [187]

D.G. Hassall, Wellcome Research Laboratories, Beckenham, Kent BR3 3BS, England [95]

E.A. Higgs, The Wellcome Research Laboratories, Beckenham, Kent BR3 3BS, England [1]

R. Jacob, SmithKline Beecham Pharmaceuticals UK Ltd., Welwyn, Hertfordshire AL6 9AR, England [33]

C. Kluft, Gaubius Institute TNO, 2313 AD Leiden, The Netherlands [129]

Simon Larkin, Department of Medicine, Cardiovascular Division, Hammersmith Hospital, London W12 ONN, England; Present Address: Department of Applied Pharmacology, National Heart and Lung Institute, London SW3 6LY, England [107]

D.C. Lefroy, Department of Clinical Pharmacology, Royal Postgraduate Medical School, London W12 ONN, England [45]

J. Lincoln, Department of Anatomy and Developmental Biology and Centre for Neuroscience, University College London, London WC1E 6BT, England [21]

J. MacDermot, Department of Clinical Pharmacology, Royal Postgraduate Medical School, London W12 ONN, England [45]

J.F. Martin, Wellcome Research Laboratories, Beckenham, Kent BR3 3BS and King's College School of Medicine and Dentistry, London, England [95]

Attilio Maseri, Department of Medicine, Cardiovascular Division, Hammersmith Hospital, London W12 ONN, England [107]

J.R. McEwan, Department of Clinical Pharmacology, Royal Postgraduate Medical School, London W12 ONN, England [45]

S. Moncada, The Wellcome Research Laboratories, Beckenham, Kent BR3 3BS, England [1]

G.H. Neild, Renal Unit, St. Philip's Hospital, London WC2A 2EX, England [209]

S. Nourshargh, Department of Applied Pharmacology, National Heart and Lung Institute, London SW3 6LY, England [171]

R.M.J. Palmer, The Wellcome Research Laboratories, Beckenham, Kent BR3 3BS, England [1]

H. Parsaee, Department of Clinical Pharmacology, Royal Postgraduate Medical School, London W12 ONN, England [45]

J.D. Pearson, Section of Vascular Biology, MRC Clinical Research Centre, Harrow, Middlesex HA1 3UJ, England [295]

S. Pirotton, Institute of Interdisciplinary Research, School of Medicine, Free University of Brussels, B-1070 Brussels, Belgium [53]

Julia M. Polak, Department of Histochemistry, Royal Postgraduate Medical School, London W12 ONN, England [253]

Robert F. Power, Department of Histochemistry, Royal Postgraduate Medical School, London W12 ONN, England [253]

C.D. Pusey, Renal Unit, Department of Medicine, Royal Postgraduate Medical School, Hammersmith Hospital, London W12 ONN, England [209]

T.J. Rink, Amylin Corporation, San Diego, CA 92121 [33]

S.O. Sage, The Physiological Laboratory, University of Cambridge, Cambridge CB2 3EG, England [33]

E.D.G. Tuddenham, Haemostasis Research Group, Clinical Research Centre, Harrow, Middlesex HA1 3UJ, England [119]

A. Van Coevorden, Institute of Interdisciplinary Research, School of Medicine, Free University of Brussels, B-1070 Brussels, Belgium [53]

John R. Vane, The William Harvey Research Institute, St. Bartholomew's Hospital Medical College, London EC1M 6BQ, England [7]

M.J. Walport, Rheumatology Unit, Department of Medicine, Royal Postgraduate Medical School, Hammersmith Hospital, London W12 ONN, England [209]

John B. Warren, Department of Clinical Pharmacology, Royal Postgraduate Medical School, Hammersmith Hospital, London W12 ONN, England; Present Address: Department of Applied Pharmacology, National Heart and Lung Institute, London SW3 6LY, England [xi,157,187,263]

David J. Webb, Department of Pharmacology and Clinical Pharmacology, St. George's Hospital Medical School, London SW17 ORE, England; Present Address: University Department of Medicine, Western General Hospital, University of Edinburgh, Edinburgh EH4 2XU, Scotland [65]

John Wharton, Department of Histochemistry, Royal Postgraduate Medical School, London W12 ONN, England [253]

T.J. Williams, Department of Applied Pharmacology, National Heart and Lung Institute, London SW3 6LY, England [171]

Introduction

The relevance of the endothelium to all aspects of human physiology and pathology is reflected by the remarkably diverse backgrounds of the authors who have kindly contributed to this book. The advances in endothelial research over the past decade have revolutionized ideas about the control of blood flow, blood pressure, and clotting, as well as the pathogenesis of conditions as varied as atheroma, vasculitis, adult respiratory distress syndrome (ARDS), and the growth rate of tumours. The aim of this book is to provide a concise review of some of the main areas of current research.

The endothelium is classified morphologically as a tissue. To some extent, this has hindered the recognition of its importance because medical research is generally subdivided into organ based specialties. The lung is a prime example of how this classification has, until recently, limited the investigation of the endothelium. As yet, few respiratory specialists study the pulmonary endothelium. The lung, however, contains about 500 g of this tissue and the majority of its functions involve these cells.

Advances in cardiovascular research suggest endothelial injury is the first step in the development of atheroma and is thus key to the etiology of heart attacks and strokes. That blood clots in a tube and not normally in vivo, indicates that the endothelium has a fundamental influence on the coagulation cascade, although this is still not fully characterized.

The site of the endothelium as a barrier between blood and tissue makes it necessarily a key cell not only in the control of coagulation but also the permeability of the vessel wall to molecules and cells. The endothelium attracts leukocytes and controls their migration through the vessel walls both in health and in inflammation. Much of this takes place at the site of the highly specialised venular endothelium.

Few foresaw how limited the sympathetic and parasympathetic nervous system is when explaining the control of blood flow and blood pressure. The extent of the influence of the endothelium on vessel calibre is remarkable. Many factors are produced, the most important of which appears to be nitric oxide. The future investigation of the control of blood flow will continue to emphasise the local influence of the endothelium.

Time-lapse photography of cultured endothelial cells has given some measure of their intelligence. Not only are they able to organise rapidly and maintain a monolayer, they are also capable of searching out relatively inert particles and phagocytosing them. They can coordinate to form tubes, the basis of neovascularisation, a phenomenon requiring considerable intercellular signalling. These complex functions highlight the limitations of our knowledge of both inter- and intracellular mechanisms.

A better understanding of endothelial function will lead to advances in the treatment of atheroma, inflammation, tumours, and disorders of coagulation. I hope this book will help increase awareness of the great potential for endothelial research.

John B. Warren
London, January 1990

The Endothelium: An Introduction to Current Research, pages 1–6
© 1990 Wiley-Liss, Inc.

1
Nitric Oxide: The Endogenous Regulator of Vascular Tone

S. MONCADA, R.M.J. PALMER, AND E.A. HIGGS

The Wellcome Research Laboratories, Beckenham, Kent BR3 3BS, England

FROM EDRF TO NITRIC OXIDE

In 1980 Furchgott and Zawadzki (1) demonstrated the phenomenon of endothelium-dependent relaxation in vascular tissue and its mediation by a humoral factor, which later became known as endothelium-derived relaxing factor (EDRF). Bioassay studies revealed the ephemeral nature of this newly recognized mediator, which is protected from breakdown by superoxide dismutase (SOD), indicating that it is inactivated by superoxide anions (O_2^-). EDRF was also found to inhibit platelet aggregation and adhesion; these actions, together with its vasodilator effects, were shown to be mediated by activation of the soluble guanylate cyclase, leading to increases in cyclic guanosine monophosphate (cGMP) within the platelet or smooth muscle cell (2–4).

In mid-1986 Furchgott and Ignarro independently suggested that EDRF may be nitric oxide (NO) or a closely related species (5,6). We examined this hypothesis by comparing the pharmacological properties of EDRF and NO on vascular smooth muscle and on platelets and found them to be identical (7). Furthermore, using a chemiluminescence method for measuring NO, we went on to demonstrate that vascular endothelial cells in culture release sufficient NO to account for the effects of EDRF on vascular strips and on platelet aggregation and adhesion (7,8). These findings have subsequently been confirmed using a spectrophotometric assay based on the reaction between NO and haemoglobin (9). Other workers have used a diazotization reaction to show that NO or a labile nitroso species was released from perfused bovine pulmonary artery in a similar manner (10). These biological and chemical data, considered together, demonstrate that EDRF is NO.

Organic nitrates, long used to treat hypertension, have been known for about 12 years to activate the soluble guanylate cyclase. More recently, these compounds were shown to generate NO in vitro by a nonenzymatic reaction, and the activation of the soluble guanylate cyclase by these compounds was found to be inhibited by haemoglobin, which binds to NO. The demonstration that vascular endothelial cells release NO strongly indicates that this is the endogenous vasodilator mechanism whose actions are imitated by the nitrovasodilators [for review, see Moncada et al. (11)].

BIOCHEMICAL PATHWAY TO NITRIC OXIDE

Evidence showing that activated macrophages form NO_2^- and NO_3^- from L-arginine (12, 13) led us to examine this amino acid as a potential precursor of NO. We found that when endothelial cells were cultured in the absence of L-arginine for 24 hr prior to the experiment, L-arginine, but not D-arginine, caused significant enhancement of NO release induced by bradykinin and by A23187 (14). Definitive experiments using mass spectrometry and ^{15}N-L-arginine demonstrated the formation of ^{15}NO from the terminal guanidino nitrogen atom(s) of L-arginine (14). The formation of ^{15}NO and ^{15}NO$_2^-$ from ^{15}N-L-arginine under basal conditions was subsequently observed using bovine aortic endothelial cells in culture (15).

We have recently demonstrated the arginine-induced stimulation of soluble guanylate cyclase in the soluble fraction of endothelial cell homogenates. This is both NADPH$^-$ and Ca^{2+} dependent, and citrulline is formed as a co-product (16). This action is inhibited by N^G-monomethyl-L-arginine (L-NMMA), an inhibitor of the generation of NO_2^- and NO_3^- in macrophages (13), but not by its D-enantiomer.

L-NMMA inhibits the stimulated release of NO from endothelial cells in culture (17) and from perfused vascular tissue (18). It also causes an endothelium-dependent increase in the tone of vascular tissue (18) and inhibits endothelium-dependent relaxation induced by various agents (17–19). These actions are enantiomerically specific and reversed by L- but not by D-arginine. All these data indicate that L-NMMA is a specific inhibitor of the endothelial NO synthase, and its effects on basal tone and on endothelium-dependent relaxation are mediated by direct inhibition of this enzyme.

BIOLOGICAL IMPORTANCE OF NITRIC OXIDE IN THE CARDIOVASCULAR SYSTEM

The identification and characterization of L-NMMA as a specific inhibitor of the endothelial NO synthase have allowed the importance of the formation of NO from L-arginine to be established in vitro. In the isolated perfused rabbit heart, we found that L-NMMA causes a rise in coronary perfusion pressure and inhibition of the fall in coronary perfusion pressure induced by acetylcholine (ACh), accompanied by inhibition of the release of NO into the coronary effluent (20). Interestingly, L-NMMA revealed the vasoconstrictor action of ACh and therefore produced what could be termed a transient *biochemical denudation* of the endothelium.

In vivo studies on the effect of L-NMMA on the blood pressure of anaesthetised rabbits revealed that intravenous administration of L-NMMA, but not D-NMMA, induced an increase in blood pressure that was associated with a reduced release of NO from the perfused aorta of treated animals ex vivo (21). Furthermore, the fall in blood pressure induced by ACh was also inhibited by L-NMMA. All these effects were enantiomerically specific and were reversed or abolished by L-arginine. These data indicate that NO derived from L-arginine plays an important role in regulating blood pressure and mediating the vasodilator response to endothelium-dependent vasodilators in vivo. L-NMMA has subsequently been shown to cause a substantial rise in blood pressure in anaesthetised guinea pigs (22) and rats (23).

The effects of L-NMMA on regional blood flow have been studied in conscious, chronically instrumented rats (24). Vascular conductance was reduced to a similar extent ($\leq 60\%$) in the renal, mesenteric, internal carotid, and hindquarters by L-NMMA, indicating the critical role of NO formation from L-arginine in the maintenance of blood pressure and flow.

Studies using L-NMMA in the brachial artery (25) and in the dorsal hand vein (26) of human subjects revealed that there is a basal formation of NO from L-arginine that contributes to the resting tone in the arterial circulation, but not in the venous circulation. This observation indicates differences in the importance of the L-arginine: NO pathway in regulating tone in different parts of the circulation and possibly explains why arterial grafts retain patency better than venous grafts. In both the arterial and the venous circulation, however, mediator-induced vasodilatation was dependent on the formation of NO from L-arginine (25,26).

At the moment it is not clear which is the major physiological stimulus for the release of NO. It is likely that NO is the mediator in the vasodilation induced by many vasodilator autacoids; it is also possible that it acts to modulate the action of vasoconstrictors that are either present in the circulation (e.g., angiotensin) or released by nerve endings (e.g., noradrenaline). Furthermore, mechanical factors such as shear stress and pulsatile flow are likely to be major stimuli for its release. In this context, it has been shown that the activity of NO (EDRF) is highest in large arterioles in which hydraulic resistance and shear stress are also highest (27).

PATHOPHYSIOLOGICAL AND THERAPEUTIC IMPLICATIONS

The ability of the endothelium to generate constantly a powerful vasodilator that controls vessel wall diameter and consequently plays a decisive role as a determinant of blood flow and blood pressure must now be considered in relationship to phenomena such as hyperaemia, autoregulation, flow-dependent dilation, blood pressure regulation, and mechanisms for oedema formation in the cardiovascular system.

A diminished endothelium-dependent vasodilator response has been reported in animal models of hypertension (11), hyperlipidaemia (11), and diabetes (28) and in human atherosclerosis and coronary artery disease (29,30). Decreased production of NO by the endothelium could account for these observations. Furthermore, reduced NO production could lead to the enhanced adhesion of platelets to the vessel wall observed in these conditions, and lack of NO may also be involved in the development of vasospasm and restenosis after angioplasty.

Nitric oxide is also cytoprotective, an action it shares with prostacyclin (31). It is not known whether NO and prostacyclin act synergistically as cytoprotectors, as in aggregation. Furthermore, neither the precise biochemical mechanism of this effect nor its biological significance is understood. It also remains to be investigated whether NO in the vessel wall modulates white cell activation or controls smooth muscle proliferation. Nitric oxide, unlike prostacyclin, is a good inhibitor of platelet adhesion via an effect on cGMP. Since the small effect of prostacyclin on adhesion is related to an effect on cGMP, it has been suggested that cGMP levels regulate membrane properties responsible for cell adhesion in general (8). Further studies on the effects and the interactions between NO and prostacyclin will help clarify the thromboresistant properties of vascular endothelium as well as its changes during pathological phenomena.

The discovery of NO as the endogenous nitrovasodilator must surely give new impetus to the search for compounds that either imitate its actions or boost its production in the cardiovascular system. As other biological actions of NO or NO-generating compounds become understood, it will be important to find compounds with selective "NO-like" activities in some systems, such as the platelets or the leukocytes, or compounds that will selectively block the synthesis of NO in other tissues.

REFERENCES

1. Furchgott RF, Zawadzki JV. The obligatory role of endothelial cells in the relaxation of arterial smooth muscle by acetylcholine. Nature (Lond) 1980;288: 373–376.
2. Furchgott RF. The role of endothelium in the responses of vascular smooth muscle to drugs. Annu Rev Pharmacol Toxicol 1984;24:175–197.
3. Griffith TM, Edwards DH, Lewis MJ, Newby AC, Henderson AH. The nature of endothelium-derived vascular relaxant factor. Nature (Lond) 1984;308:645–647.
4. Moncada S, Palmer RMJ, Higgs EA. Prostacyclin and endothelium-derived relaxing factor: Biological interactions and significance. In: Verstraete M, Vermylen J, Lijnen HR, Arnout J, eds. Thrombosis and Haemostasis. Leuven, Belgium: Leuven University Press, 1987;587–618.

5. Furchgott RF. Studies on relaxation of rabbit aorta by sodium nitrite: The basis for the proposal that the acid-activatable inhibitory factor from retractor penis is inorganic nitrite and the endothelium-derived relaxing factor is nitric oxide. In: Vanhoutte PM, ed. Vasodilatation: Vascular Smooth Muscle, Peptides, Autonomic Nerves and Endothelium. New York: Raven Press, 1988;401–414.

6. Ignarro LJ, Byrns RE, Wood KS. Biochemical and pharmacological properties of endothelium-derived relaxing factor and its similarity to nitric oxide radicals. In: Vanhoutte PM, ed. Vasodilatation: Vascular Smooth Muscle, Peptides, Autonomic Nerves and Endothelium. New York: Raven Press, 1988; 427–436.

7. Palmer RMJ, Ferrige AG, Moncada S. Nitric oxide release accounts for the biological activity of endothelium-derived relaxing factor. Nature (Lond) 1987; 327:524–526.

8. Moncada S, Radomski MW, Palmer, RMJ. Endothelium-derived relaxing factor: Identification as nitric oxide and role in the control of vascular tone and platelet function. Biochem Pharmacol 1988;37:2495–2501.

9. Kelm M, Feelisch M, Spahr R, Piper H-M, Noack E, Schrader J. Quantitative and kinetic characterization of nitric oxide and EDRF released from cultured endothelial cells. Biochem Biophys Res Commun 1988;154:236–244.

10. Ignarro LJ, Buga GM, Wood KS, Byrns RE, Chaudhuri G. Endothelium-derived relaxing factor produced and released from artery and vein is nitric oxide. Proc Natl Acad Sci USA 1987;84:9265–9269.

11. Moncada S, Palmer RMJ, Higgs EA. The discovery of nitric oxide as the endogenous nitrovasodilator. Hypertension 1988;12:365–372.

12. Iyengar R, Stuehr DJ, Marletta MA. Macrophage synthesis of nitrite, nitrate and N-nitrosamines: Precursors and role of the respiratory burst. Proc Natl Acad Sci USA 1987;84:6369–6373.

13. Hibbs JB Jr, Vavrin Z, Taintor RR. L-Arginine is required for expression of the activated macrophage effector mechanism causing selective metabolic inhibition in target cells. J Immunol 1987;138:550–565.

14. Palmer, RMJ, Ashton DS, Moncada S. Vascular endothelial cells synthesize nitric oxide from L-arginine. Nature (Lond) 1988;333:664–666.

15. Schmidt HHHW, Nau H, Wittfoht W, Gerlach J, Prescher K-E, Klein MM, Niroomand F, Bohme E. Arginine is a physiological precursor of endothelium-derived nitric oxide. Eur J Pharmacol 1988;154:213–216.

16. Palmer RMJ, Moncada S. A novel citrulline-forming enzyme implicated in the formation of nitric oxide by vascular endothelial cells. Biochem Biophys Res Commun 1989;158:358–352.

17. Palmer RMJ, Rees DD, Ashton DS, Moncada S. L-Arginine is the physiological precursor for the formation of nitric oxide in endothelium-dependent relaxation. Biochem Biophys Res Commun 1988;153:1251–1256.

18. Rees DD, Palmer RMJ, Hodson HF, Moncada S. A specific inhibitor of nitric oxide formation from L-arginine attenuates endothelium-dependent relaxation. Br J Pharmacol 1989;96:418–424.

19. Sakuma I, Stuehr DJ, Gross SS, Nathan C, Levi R. Identification of arginine as a precursor of endothelium-derived relaxing factor. Proc Natl Acad Sci USA 1988;85:8664–8667.

20. Amezcua J-L, de Souza BM, Palmer RMJ, Moncada S. Inhibition of nitric oxide synthesis inhibits endothelium-dependent vasodilatation in the rabbit isolated heart. Br J Pharmacol 1989;97:1119–1124.
21. Rees DD, Palmer RMJ, Moncada S. Role of endothelium-derived nitric oxide in the regulation of blood pressure. Proc Natl Acad Sci USA 1989;86:3375–3378.
22. Aisaka K, Gross SS, Griffith OW, Levi R. N^G-methylarginine, an inhibitor of endothelium-derived nitric oxide synthesis, is a potent pressor agent in the guinea pig: Does nitric oxide regulate blood pressure in vivo? Biochem Biophys Res Commun 1989;160:881–886.
23. Whittle BJR, Lopez-Belmonte J, Rees DD. Modulation of the vasodepressor actions of acetylcholine, bradykinin, substance P and endothelium in the rat by a specific inhibitor of nitric oxide formation. Br J Pharmacol 1989;98:646–652.
24. Gardiner SM, Compton AM, Bennett T, Palmer RMJ, Moncada S. Control of regional blood flow by endothelium-derived nitric oxide. Hypertension 1990;15:486–492.
25. Vallance P, Collier J, Moncada S. Effects of endothelium-derived nitric oxide on peripheral arteriolar tone in man. Lancet 1989;2:997–1000.
26. Vallance P, Collier J, Moncada S. Nitric oxide synthesised from L-arginine mediates endothelium-dependent dilatation in human veins in vivo. Cardiovasc Res 1989;23:1053–1057.
27. Griffith TM, Lewis MJ, Newby AC, Henderson AH. Endothelium-derived relaxing factor. J Am Coll Cardiol 1988;12:797–806.
28. Durante W, Sen AK, Sunahara FA. Impairment of endothelium-dependent relaxation in aortae from spontaneously diabetic rats. Br J Pharmacol 1988;94:463–468.
29. Ludmer PL, Selwyn AP, Shook TL, Wayne RR, Mudge GH, Alexander RW, Ganz P. Paradoxical vasoconstriction induced by acetylcholine in atherosclerotic coronary arteries. N Engl J Med 1986;315:1046–1051.
30. Bossaller C, Habib GB, Yamamoto H, Williams C, Wells S, Henry PD. Impaired muscarinic endothelium-dependent relaxation and cyclic guanosine 5'-monophosphate formation in atherosclerotic human coronary artery and rabbit aorta. J Clin Invest 1987;79:170–174.
31. Radomski MW, Palmer RMJ, Read NG, Moncada S. Isolation and washing of human platelets with nitric oxide. Thromb Res 1988;50:537–546.

The Endothelium: An Introduction to Current Research, pages 7–20
© 1990 Wiley-Liss, Inc.

2
Endothelium-Derived Vasoconstricting Factors

ERIK E. ÄNGGÅRD, RENIA M. BOTTING, AND JOHN R. VANE
The William Harvey Research Institute, St. Bartholomew's Hospital Medical College, London EC1M 6BQ, England

ENDOTHELIUM-DERIVED CONTRACTING FACTORS

In addition to the production of relaxing factors such as prostacyclin and nitric oxide, the vascular endothelium can also release vasoconstrictor substances (1). For many years, we have known that hypoxia causes pulmonary vasoconstriction (2); Vanhoutte and co-workers showed that hypoxia produces endothelium-dependent contractions of peripheral arteries (3,4). Other work suggested that the removal of the endothelium decreased the contractile responses of various isolated blood vessels to acetylcholine (ACh) or norepinephrine (noradrenaline) (1,4). Thus, it seemed possible that endogenous vasoconstrictor substances could be released from the endothelium.

At least three types of endothelium-derived contracting factors have been described (1,4). One is produced by stretch, increased transmural pressure, high potassium, calcium ionophore A23187, and arachidonic acid. Inhibitors of cyclo-oxygenase abolish or reduce this activity in canine arteries. It is therefore likely that it is a prostaglandin or related factor. In canine veins, however, a lipoxygenase inhibitor and leukotriene antagonist reduce the endothelium-dependent contractions to arachidonic acid. Thus, leukotrienes may contribute to vasoconstriction in veins.

Other constricting factors are released from the anoxic endothelium. One such factor may be the superoxide anion or a closely related free radical species (5). Superoxide anions cause contractions of canine basilar arteries, which are rapid and readily reversible. In the same preparation, endothelium-dependent contractions to the calcium ionophore A23187 are inhibited by superoxide dismutase.

A third contracting factor originating in the endothelium was present in media from cultured endothelial cells. This factor was purified and characterised as a peptide (6,7). The contractions it produced were slower in onset and were more difficult to reverse as compared with those elicited by anoxia.

Thus, although at least three different types of chemical substances have been proposed as endothelium-dependent vasoconstrictors, none was previously isolated and characterised until the discovery in 1988 of endothelins by the group of Professor Masaki at Tsukuba University (8).

DISCOVERY OF ENDOTHELIN

On the basis of the earlier observations of a protease-sensitive vasoconstrictor activity in the supernatants of cultured endothelial cells (6,7), Yanagisawa et al. (8) isolated and determined the structure of a new vasoconstrictor peptide, which they called endothelin (ET-1). The peptide had 21 amino acids bound together by two disulfide bridges (Fig. 1) at the amino-terminal end of the molecule so that the three-dimensional structure formed a conical spiral. Synthetic ET was prepared and the structure confirmed by comparing the biological activities and chromatographic properties of the natural and synthetic ET (9,10).

The structure of ET-1 is quite unusual in mammalian species. Interestingly, ET-1 seems related evolutionarily to a group of snake venoms (i.e., sarafotoxins) from the Israeli burrowing asp (11,12). Although both ET-1 and sarafotoxin S6B have strong, long-lasting vasoconstrictor properties (8,12), the messenger RNA (mRNA) for ET-1 has so far been found only in endothelial cells, whereas sarafotoxin S6B is produced only in the exocrine venom gland, which has no relationship to endothelial cells.

ET-1 is the most active pressor substance yet discovered, with a potency some 10 times that of angiotensin II (8). ET-1, like many other biologically

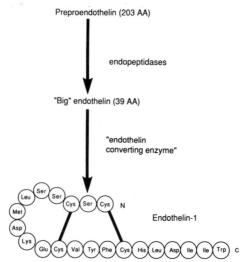

Fig. 1. Suggested pathway of synthesis for endothelin. Reproduced from Yanagisawa et al. (8), with permission of the publisher.

active peptides, is produced from a prepropeptide. The production of the active peptide involves the formation of a 38- or 39-residue, "big endothelin," and then an unusual proteolytic cleavage between a Trp and Val residue (Fig. 1) by a putative endopeptidase called *endothelin converting enzyme*. Although the production of ET-1 seems to be regulated mainly at the mRNA transcription level, the converting enzyme may well prove an important target for pharmacological control of ET-1 release, especially if ET-1 is shown to be involved in hypertension or vasospastic disorders.

The first endothelin (ET-1) was originally called porcine ET and was identical to human ET (8–10). Further work indicated the presence of an isopeptide in the rat (13). It is now clear that there are no species differences. In the human, and presumably in other mammalian species as well, three structurally and pharmacologically separate isopeptides have been predicted by three different genes (14): endothelin-1 (formerly porcine/human endothelin), endothelin-2 (ET-2), and endothelin-3 (ET-3; formerly rat endothelin). Their structures are shown in Figure 2. It should be pointed out that multiple forms of biologically active peptides are commonly found (e.g., the endogenous opiate peptides and brain/atrial natriuretic peptides). A review on the endothelins has recently appeared (15).

ET-1 is the only endothelin to be made by endothelial cells. We do not yet know where ET-2 is made, unless it is in the kidneys (see later). ET-3 seems to be associated with nervous tissue (15).

ACTIVATION/RELEASE OF ET

This is an area in which more information is needed. Clearly, ET-1 is produced by endothelial cells (EC) in culture. So far no dynamic release has been demonstrated from cells or organs although the mRNA encoding for prepro ET-1 increased after 2–4 hr when cultured endothelial cells were exposed to thrombin, adrenaline, and calcium ionophore A23187, sub-

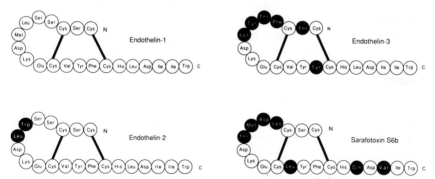

Fig. 2. Amino acid sequences of the endothelins and sarafotoxin 6B. Amino acids different from those in ET-1 are denoted by shaded circles. Reproduced from Yanagisawa and Masaki (15), with permission of the publisher.

stances known to release both vasoconstrictors as well as vasodilators (EDRF, prostacyclin) from the vascular endothelium (8,16–20).

PLASMA LEVELS OF ENDOTHELIN-1

Plasma levels of ET-1 in healthy subjects as measured by radioimmunoassay (RIA) have been estimated at 0.26–5 pg/ml (21–24). In patients undergoing haemodialysis or kidney transplantation (27,28) or suffering from cardiogenic shock (29), myocardial infarction (30), or pulmonary hypertension, the plasma levels are higher, reaching as high as 35 pg/ml during haemodialysis (27,28). The plasma levels should, however, only be regarded as an indicator of ET release, for they are far below the levels expected to produce an effect. The concentration at the endothelium–smooth muscle interface, where the ET might be released, is probably much higher than in the bloodstream. ET-1 is therefore more likely to be a local rather than systemic regulating factor.

Concentrations of "big" ET-1 were about 3 pg/ml in plasma from normal subjects and were increased to 6 pg/ml in acute myocardial infarction (30). It was unexpected to find "big" ET-1 in the circulation for, although it has only 10% of the activity of ET-1, its release by the EC may have effects on the underlying vascular smooth muscle. Furthermore, it raises the possibility, as already pointed out by Yanagisawa et al. (8), that big ET-1 could be converted to ET-1 in the bloodstream or, for that matter, in cells other than endothelial cells. This is supported by the finding that although big ET-1 exhibits only 10% of the activity of ET-1, on isolated vascular smooth muscle it is equipotent in elevating blood pressure (31).

The highest plasma levels of ET-1 reported so far have been in haemodialysis or kidney transplant patients (27,28). This may reflect reduced elimination of the peptide or increased synthesis by diseased kidney tissues. Cultured kidney cells of monkey, dog, rabbit, hamster, and pig secrete immunoreactive ET-1 and ET-2 into the culture medium (32). Immunoreactive ET has also been reported in the urine of healthy human volunteers (25). The mean concentration in urine of 33.1 pg/ml was six times higher than that detected in plasma (25). Thus, endothelins, like prostaglandins, may be synthesised by the human kidney and continuously excreted in the urine. The measurement of endothelin in urine may turn out to be a useful indicator of the activity of the renal endothelin system.

FATE/BINDING OF ET

Intravenously injected labelled ET-1 or ET-3 was quickly eliminated from the bloodstream of the rat, more than 60% being removed after 1 min (33,34). This was in contrast to its long-lasting effect on blood pressure (Fig. 3) and indicates that any ET released was rapidly taken up and bound. No labelled metabolites were found in rat blood (34). High uptake of labelled ET-1 and ET-3 was found in the lung, kidney, and liver.

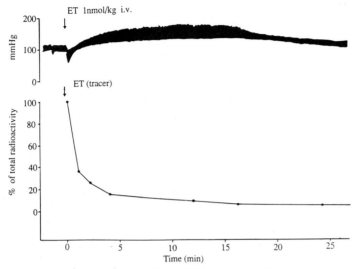

Fig. 3. Comparison between the effect of ET-1 on the rat blood pressure and the disappearance of radioiodinated ET-1 from the circulation. Reproduced from Änggård et al. (33), with permission of the publisher.

Autoradiographic studies have demonstrated specific high-affinity binding sites for ET-1 in peripheral tissues (35–38). The binding was localised to arteries and veins of all sizes and also in brain, lung, kidney, adrenal, spleen, and intestine. The widespread distribution of ET binding sites suggests a wider role for ETs than in the regulation of cardiovascular tone.

Detailed studies of ET-1 binding sites have been performed, particularly on vascular smooth muscle. A specific, single class, high-affinity binding site has been confirmed with an apparent dissociation constant of about $2–6 \times 10^{-10}$ M (39–41)—comparable to the EC_{50} values for ET-1 on vascular strips (26). The binding was not affected by catecholamines, vasoactive peptides, neurotoxins, or calcium-channel antagonists. Dissociation of the ET from its binding site is very slow. This may explain the characteristically long-lasting response to ET seen both in in vitro preparations and in vivo.

Evidence for several subtypes of endothelin and sarafotoxin receptors have been presented using competition binding (41). It is possible, therefore, that each isopeptide interacts with a specific receptor. The emerging evidence would support this concept. Thus, although a much weaker vasoconstrictor than ET-1, ET-3 produces a more profound initial vasodepressor and antiaggregating effect in vivo and is a more powerful vasodilator in the perfused rat mesentery in vitro (42–44). Furthermore, the two peptides are equipotent at contracting rat stomach strips, but ET-3 is 10 times less potent in contracting the guinea pig ileum (26).

CARDIOVASCULAR ACTIONS

The most striking property of ET-1 is the long duration of the hypertensive action, as demonstrated on the blood pressure of a pithed or chemically denervated rat (8). After a single intravenous injection, the blood pressure is elevated for more than 1 hr (14,15).

Intravenous infusions of endothelins in rats, dogs, and pigs resulted in intense vasoconstriction and a rise in mean arterial blood pressure (45–47). The constriction was more marked in the gastrointestinal, renal, and skeletal muscle vascular beds (45–47).

The endothelin peptides caused slowly developing and prolonged contractions of isolated smooth muscle from both arteries and veins. In a survey of the actions of ET-1 on vascular smooth muscle, venous tissue was more sensitive to ET-1 than was arterial smooth muscle (26). The effective concentration was in the range 10 pM to 10 nM of ET-1. The relative potency of the endothelins on vascular smooth muscle was ET-2 > ET-1 > ET-3. Contractions of veins were less effectively reversed by prostacyclin or sodium nitroprusside than were contractions induced by noradrenaline. This could indicate an interaction between ET and muscle relaxations mediated by cyclic adenosine monophosphate (cAMP) and cyclic guanosine monophosphate (cGMP). The sensitivity of renal artery segments to ET was greater in spontaneously hypertensive than in Wistar Kyoto rats (48).

In the human, infusions of 10 pmol to 10 nmol/min of ET-1 into the brachial artery decreased forearm blood flow in a dose-related manner (49). Intradermal injections of 1–100 pmol of ET-1 into the forearms caused intense long-lasting vasoconstrictions at the injection site and also a surrounding flare, most likely due to an axon reflex (50). The central pallor was sometimes still present the following day.

ETs also have positive inotropic and chronotropic effects on the heart. On isolated, electrically driven guinea pig, rabbit or human atria ET-1 exerted a dose-dependent positive inotropic effect (51–53). The maximum response was only 30–40% of that of isoprotenerol, but the EC_{50} was as low as 10^{-9} M. The effect was not antagonised by blockers of α-adrenergic, β-adrenergic, histamine, or serotonin receptors, indicating a direct effect on the myocardium. Whereas the positive inotropic effect on guinea pig atria was antagonised by nicardipine (51), studies on isolated rabbit papillary muscle have failed to confirm this finding (53). In this species, ET-1 produced the opposite effect to the calcium channel agonist BAY K 8644 and unlike the effect of the agonist was resistant to nicardipine. In spontaneously beating guinea pig atria, ET-1 at about 10^{-9} M induced a dose-dependent positive chronotropic effect (54).

RENAL EFFECTS

Infusion of ET-1 increased renal vascular resistance in the rat, dog, and pig (45–47). The kidney is about 10 times more sensitive than other vascular regions (55). The glomerular filtration rate (GFR) and urine volume were substantially reduced following infusion. ET-1 is about five times more active than angiotensin II on the renal circulation. The large fall in GFR was due to an increased arterial resistance as well as to a contraction of mesangial cells (61).

In rat isolated glomerular preparations or cortical slices, ET-1 inhibits both the basal and β-adrenoceptor agonist-induced renin release (56–58). However, in anesthetized or conscious dogs, infusion of ET-1 led to an elevation of plasma renin activity (59,60). It is therefore possible that ET-1 could influence renin release by several mechanisms, either directly or indirectly by a change in sodium concentration at the macula densa or by a change in glomerular arterial pressure.

It has been suggested that ET-1 has a role in acute renal failure (62), for ET-1 is a powerful renal vasoconstrictor and plasma levels of ET-1 are elevated in renal failure. Further work is necessary to establish whether the elevated plasma levels of ET-1 seen in uremia are the cause or consequence of the renal failure.

RELEASE OF PROSTACYCLIN, EDRF, AND ATRIAL NATRIURETIC PEPTIDE

Some of the effects of ET could be due to the release of other factors. When given intravenously into rats, the pressor activity appears to be strongly limited by the release of vasodilators (63,64). Indeed, when the basal blood pressure is high, intravenous ET unexpectedly causes a fall rather than a rise in the blood pressure. This is due to the release of both prostacyclin and EDRF (64).

In perfused isolated organs such as the guinea pig or rat lung or the rabbit kidney or spleen, ET-1 released prostacyclin, PGE_2 and sometimes thromboxane A_2 (64). This release also appeared to occur in vivo, for an antiaggregatory prostaglandin, most likely prostacyclin, was released into the circulation after injections of ET-1 or ET-3 into rabbits (65). ET-3 also released fibrinolytic activity, as measured by euglobulin clot lysis time ex vivo in anaesthetised rabbits (66). This activity was in part caused by the release of eicosanoids as it could be partly antagonised by indomethacin. It should also be mentioned that the rise in blood pressure after injection of ET-1 appears to be limited by a cyclo-oxygenase-dependent mechanism, as it can be strongly potentiated by indomethacin (64).

ET-1 also releases immunoreactive atrial natriuretic peptide (ANP) from cultured rat atrial myocytes (67). Release of ANP has also been seen in vivo

(59). The release of this potent vasodilator and natriuretic hormone could act to limit the pressor and renal actions of ET-1. However, ET-1 is probably a local factor and is most likely not released into the circulation, at least not in the concentrations achieved in the pharmacological experiments described above. The release of EDRF, prostacyclin, and fibrinolytic activity could represent the activation of defence mechanisms to overcome the intense vasoconstriction induced by pharmacological concentrations of ET-1.

OTHER ACTIONS OF ET

In a relatively short time many reports have appeared on effects of ET-1 in several biological systems. Introduced into the central nervous system (CNS), it produces an increase in blood pressure, an action which in part appears to be mediated by catecholamine release (68). In conscious rats, injection of ET into the lateral ventricle starts a bizarre behavioral change called *barrel-rolling* (69). ET-1, ET-3, and other ET-related peptides are present in porcine spinal cord (70), and ET-1 binding sites are found in numerous brain areas (71–73). The possibility therefore exists that ETs could be a new class of neuromodulators. Several reports have shown inhibition by ET-1 of adrenergic neuroeffector transmission (74, 75), whereas other authors have suggested the effect could be secondary to changes in blood flow (76).

ET-1 has potent bronchoconstrictor effects both on the isolated smooth muscle of the airways of rats and guinea pigs and in guinea pigs in vivo (77–80).

Several groups have reported endothelin-induced gastric mucosal damage in the rat (81,82). This effect was potentiated by indomethacin indicating a protective effect of a cyclo-oxygenase product.

One of the most interesting findings so far is the mitogenic effect of ET-1. This has been shown in cardiovascular smooth muscle cells (83–85), in fibroblasts (86), and in mesangial cells (87). ET also enhanced transcription of the c-fos and c-myc proto-oncogene (83,87), biochemical signals that are closely linked to proliferation. These effects suggest that ET-1 could have a trophic effect related to the development of the lesions seen in hypertension and atherosclerosis.

MECHANISM OF ACTION

The first paper from the Masaki group (8) suggested that ET-1 acted directly on membrane calcium ion channels, as extracellular calcium was needed for contraction and the action of ET was inhibited by nicardipine. According to this hypothesis, ET-1 would be implicated as an endogenous agonist to the dihydropyridine-sensitive calcium channel and provide a rationale for the mechanism of action of calcium channel blockers in cardiovascular diseases such as angina and hypertension.

Later work has confirmed the importance of extracellular calcium but failed to find inhibition of ET-1 by the dihydropridine class of calcium channel antagonists. The current view (15) is that ET-1 binds to a specific membrane receptor leading to intracellular biochemical signals involving activation of phospholipase C with the release of inositol phosphates and diacylglycerol and elevation of calcium from intracellular stores. This would in turn activate protein kinase C. Inhibition of protein kinase C reversed contractions of rabbit aortic strips induced by ET-1. ET-1 thus appears to have a specific mode of intracellular action involving phosphoinositide breakdown but not dihydropyridine-sensitive calcium channels.

SPECULATION ON THE PHYSIOLOGICAL ROLE OF ET

The wide distribution of specific ET-binding sites and the relationship to sarafotoxins point to an ancient evolutionary origin of this class of peptides. However, the fact that these structures have been conserved for so long point to a current role in mammalian physiology.

In their recent review on ET, Yanagisawa and Masaki (15) proposed two modes of ET-1 regulation in vivo in relationship to a possible role in cardiovascular control. In the first mode, ET-1 could be a signalling molecule maintaining cardiovascular homeostasis under healthy conditions, like other vasoactive hormones such as catecholamines, angiotensin and natriuretic peptides. In such a case, it is likely that ET-1 would be involved in the long-term (hours to days) regulation of the cardiovascular system. In this respect, it is of interest to note the possibilities of interaction with the release of catecholamines (inhibition), of renin (inhibition), and of atrial-natriuretic peptides (stimulation).

The other proposed mode of action would be in a defensive role. In this case, ET-1 would be produced locally in an emergency or in defensive events such as haemostastis or wound repair. The indications that mRNA for preproendothelin is induced by factors such as thrombin and transforming growth factor-1β, known to be produced at the site of injury, would lend support to this idea.

There is obviously a great deal of speculation that ET-1 might have a role in a variety of cardiovascular disorders, such as hypertension, atherosclerosis, and cerebral/coronary vasospasm. The next few years will be interesting. It may either prove that the ETs are "redundant peptides," a biochemical relic from earlier evolutionary periods, or that ET-1 and related peptides have a role in healthy conditions or as defensive factors playing a role in cardiovascular pathophysiology. Clearly, the development of inhibitors of the putative ET converting enzyme as well as receptor antagonists and/or specific antibodies will be of fundamental importance in unravelling the role of the ETs.

ACKNOWLEDGMENT

The William Harvey Research Institute is supported by a grant from Glaxo Group Research Ltd.

REFERENCES

1. Rubanyi GM. Endothelium-derived vasoconstrictor factors. In: Ryan US, ed. Endothelial Cells. Vol. 3. Boca Raton, Florida: CRC Press, 1988;61–74.
2. Fishman AP. Respiratory gases in the regulation of the pulmonary circulation. Physiol Rev 1961;41:214.
3. Rubanyi GM, Vanhoutte PM. Hypoxia releases a vasoconstrictor substance from the canine vascular endothelium. J Physiol (Lond) 1985;364:45–46.
4. Vanhoutte PM, Rubanyi GM, Miller VM, et al. Modulation of vascular smooth muscle contraction by the endothelium. Ann Rev Physiol 1986;48: 307–320.
5. Vanhoutte PM, Katusic, ZS. Endothelium derived contracting factor, endothelin and/or superoxide anion? Trends Pharmacol Sci 1988;9:229–230.
6. Hickey KA, Rubanyi GM, Paul RJ, et al. Characterization of a coronary vasoconstrictor produced by cultured endothelial cells. Am J Physiol 1985; 248:C550–556.
7. Gillespie MN, Owasoyo JO, McMurtry IF, et al. Sustained coronary vasoconstriction provoked by a peptidergic substance released from endothelial cells in culture. J Pharmacol Exp Ther 1986;239:339–343.
8. Yanagisawa M, Kurihara H, Kimura S, Tomobe Y, et al. A novel potent vasoconstrictor peptide produced by vascular endothelial cells. Nature (Lond) 1988; 332:411–415.
9. Kumagaye S, Kuroda H, Nakajima K, et al. Synthesis and secondary structure determination of porcine endothelin: An endothelium-derived vasoconstricting peptide. Int J Pept Protein Res 1988;32:519–526.
10. Itoh Y, Yanagisawa M, Ohkubo S, et al. Cloning and sequence analysis of cDNA encoding the precursor of a human endothelium derived vasoconstrictor peptide, endothelin: Identity of human and porcine endothelin. FEBS Lett 1988; 231:440–444.
11. Takasaki C, Yanagisawa M, Kimura S, et al. Similarity of endothelin to snake venom toxin. Nature (Lond) 1988;335:303.
12. Kloog Y, Ambar I, Sokolovsky M, et al. A novel vasoconstrictor peptide: Phosphoinositide hydrolysis in rat heart and brain. Science 1988;242:268–270.
13. Yanagisawa M, Inoue A, Ishikawa T, et al. Primary structure, synthesis and biological activity of rat endothelin, an endothelium-derived vasoconstrictor peptide. Proc Natl Acad Sci USA 1988;85:6964–6967.
14. Inoue A, Yanagisawa M, Kimura S, et al. The human endothelin family: Three structurally and pharmacologically distinct isopeptides predicted by three separate genes. Proc Natl Acad of Sci USA 1989;86:2863–2867.
15. Yanagisawa M, Masaki T. Endothelin, a novel endothelium-derived peptide. Biochem Pharmacol 1989;38:1877–1883.
16. Yanagisawa M, Inoue A, Takuwa, Y, et al. The human preproendothelin-1 gene: Possible regulation by endothelial phosphoinositide turnover signaling. J Cardiovasc Pharmacol 1989;13 (suppl 5):S13–517.

17. Kurihara H, Yoshizumi M, Sugiyama T, et al. Transforming growth factor-β stimulates the expression of endothelin mRNA by vascular endothelial cells. Biochem Biophys Res Commun 1989;159:1435–1440.
18. Schini VB, Hendrickson, H, Heublein DM, et al. Thrombin enhances the release of endothelin from cultured porcine aortic endothelial cells. Eur J Pharmacol 1989;165:333–334.
19. Sugiura M, Inagami T, Kon V. Endotoxin stimulates endothelin release in vivo and in vitro as determined by radioimmunoassay. Biochem Biophys Res Commun 1989;161:1220–1227.
20. Yoshizumi M, Kurihara H, Sugiyama T, et al. Hemodynamic shear stress stimulates endothelin production by cultured endothelial cells. Biochem Biophys Res Commun 1989;161:859–864.
21. Suzuki N, Matsumoto H, Kitada C, et al. A sensitive sandwich-enzyme immunoassay for human endothelin. J Immunol Methods 1989;118:245–250.
22. Ando K, Hirata Y, Shichiri H, et al. Presence of immunoreactive endothelin in human plasma. FEBS Lett 1989;245:164–166.
23. Harter E, Woloszczuk W. Radio-immunoassay of endothelin. Lancet 1989;2:909.
24. Saito Y, Nakao K, Itoh H, et al. Endothelin in human plasma and culture medium of aortic endothelial cells—Detection and characterization with radioimmunoassay using monoclonal antibody. Biochem Biophys Res Commun 1989;161:320–326.
25. Berbinschi A, Ketelslegers JM. Endothelin in urine. Lancet 1989;2:46.
26. D'Orleans—Juste P, Finet M, et al. Pharmacology of endothelin-1 in isolated vessels: effect of nicardipine, methylene blue, hemoglobin, and gossypol. J Cardiovasc Pharmacol 1989;13 (suppl 5):S46–S49.
27. Koyama H, Nishzawa Y, Morii H, et al. Plasma endothelin levels in patients with uraemia. Lancet 1989;2:991–992.
28. Totsune K, Mouri T, Takahashi K, et al. Detection of immunoreactive endothelin in plasma of hemodialysis patients. FEBS Lett 1989;249:239–242.
29. Cernacek P, Stewart D. Immunoreactive endothelin in human plasma: Marked elevations in patients with cardiogenic shock. Biochem Biophys Res Commun 1989;161:562–567.
30. Miyauchi T, Yanagisawa M, Tomizawa T, et al. Increased plasma concentrations of endothelin-1 and big endothelin-1 in acute myocardial infarction. Lancet 1989;2:53–54.
31. Kashiwabara T, Inagaki Y, Ohta H, et al. Putative precursors of endothelin have less vasoconstrictor activity in vitro but a potent pressor effect in vivo. FEBS Let 1989;247:73–76.
32. Kosaka T, Suzuki N, Matsumoto H, et al. Synthesis of vasoconstrictor peptide endothelin in kidney cells. FEBS Lett 1989;249:42–46.
33. Änggård E, Galton S, Rae G, et al. The fate of radio-iodinated endothelin-1 and endothelin-3 in the rat. J Cardiovasc Pharmacol 1989;13 (suppl 5):S46–S49.
34. Shiba R, Yanagisawa M, Miyauchi T, et al. Elimination of intravenously injected endothelin-1 from the circulation of the rat. J Cardiovasc Pharmacol 1989;13 (suppl 5):S98–S101.
35. Power RF, Wharton J, Zhao Y, et al. Autoradiographic localisation of endothelin-1 binding sites in the cardiovascular and respiratory systems. J Cardiovasc Pharmacol 1989;13 (suppl 5):S50–S56.

36. Neuser D, Steinke W, Theiss G, et al. Autoradiographic localization of (^{125}I) Endothelin 1 and (^{125}I) atrial natriuretic peptide in rat tissue: A comparative study. J Cardiovasc Pharmacol 1989;13 (suppl 5):S67–S73.

37. Koseki C, Imai M, Hirata Y, et al. Binding sites for endothelin-1 in rat tissues: An autoradiographic study. J Cardiovasc Pharmacol 1989;13 (suppl 5):S153–S154.

38. Davenport AP, Nunez DJ, Hall JA, et al. Autoradiographical localization of binding sites for porcine (^{125}I) endothelin-1 in humans, pigs and rats: Functional relevance in humans. J Cardiovasc Pharmacol 1989;13 (suppl 5):S166–S170.

39. Hirata Y. Endothelin 1 receptors in cultured vascular smooth muscle cells and cardiocytes of rats. J Cardiovasc Pharmacol 1989;13 (suppl 5):S157–S158.

40. Gu XH, Casley DJ, Nayler WG. Characterization of (^{125}-I) endothelin-1 binding sites in rat cardiac membrane fragments. J Cardiovasc Pharmacol 1989;13 (suppl 5):S171–S173.

41. Kloog Y, Bousso-Mittler D, Bdolah A, et al. Three apparent receptor sub-types for the endothelin/sarafotoxin family. FEBS Lett 1989;253:199–202.

42. Lidbury PS, Thiemermann C, Thomas GR, Vane JR. Endothelin-3, selectivity as anti-aggregatory peptide in vivo. Eur J Pharmacol 1989;166:335–338.

43. Warner TD, Mitchell JA, de Nucci G, Vane JR. Endothelin-1 and endothelin-3 release from isolated perfused arterial vessels of the rat and rabbit. J Cardiovasc Pharmacol 1989;13 (suppl 5):S85–S88.

44. Spokes RA, Ghatei MA, Bloom SR. Studies with endothelin-3 and endothelin 1 on rat blood pressure and isolated tissues: Evidence for multiple endothelin receptor sub-types. J Cardiovasc Pharmacol 1989;13 (suppl 5):S191–S192.

45. Walder CE, Thomas GR, Thiemermann C, Vane JR. The hemodynamic effects of endothelin 1 in the pithed rat. J Cardiovasc Pharmacol 13 (suppl):1989;S93–S97.

46. Gardiner SM, Compton A, Bennett T. Regional hemodynamic effects of endothelin-1 in conscious unrestrained Wistar rats. J Cardiovasc Pharmacol 1989;13 (suppl 5):S202–S204.

47. Pernow J, Franco-Cereceda A, Matran R, et al. Effect of endothelin-1 on regional vascular resistances in the pig. J Cardiovasc Pharmacol 1989;13 (suppl 5):S205–S206.

48. Tomobe Y, Miyauchi T, Saito A, et al. Effects of endothelin on the renal artery from spontaneously hypertensive and Wistar Kyoto rats. Eur J Pharmacol 1988;152:373–374.

49. Hughes AD, Thoms AM, Woodall N, et al. Human vascular responses to endothelin-1: Observations in vivo and in vitro. J Cardiovasc Pharmacol 1989;13 (suppl 5):S225–S228.

50. Brain SD, Crossman DC, Buckley TL, et al. Endothelin 1: Demonstration of potent effects on the microcirculations of humans and other species. J Cardiovasc Pharmacol 1989;13 (suppl 5):S147–S149.

51. Ishikawa T, Yanagisawa M, Kimura S, et al. Positive inotropic action of novel vasoconstrictor peptide endothelin on guinea pig atria. Am J Physiol 1988;225:H970–H973.

52. Moravec CS, Reynolds ER, Stewart RW, et al. Endothelin is a positive inotropic agent in human and rat heart in vitro. Biochem Biophys Res Commun 1989;-159:14–18. .

53. Fung AYP, Warner TD, Thomas GR, Vane JR. Endothelin-1 modulates the inotropic effects of isoprenaline in rabbit isolated papillary muscle. Br J Pharmacol 1989;98:627P.
54. Ishikawa T, Yanagisawa M, Kimura S, et al. Positive chronotrophic effects of endothelin, a novel endothelium-derived vasoconstrictor peptide. Pflugers Arch 1988;413:108–110.
55. Pernow J, Boutier JF, Franco-Cereceda A, et al. Potent selective vasoconstrictor effects of endothelin in the pig kidney in vivo. Acta Physiol Scand 1989;134:573–574.
56. Rakugi H, Nakamaru M, Saito H, et al. Endothelin inhibits renin release from isolated rat glomeruli. Biochem Biophys Res Commun 1988;155:1244–1247.
57. Matsumura Y, Nakase K, Ikegawa RI, et al. The endothelium derived vasoconstrictor peptide endothelin inhibits renin release in vitro. Life Sci 1989;44:149–157.
58. Takagi M, Matsuoka H, Atarashi K, et al. Endothelin: A new inhibitor of renin release. Biochem Biophys Res Commun 1988;157:1164–1168.
59. Goetz KL, Wang BC, Madwed JB, et al. Cardiovascular, renal and endocrine responses to intravenous endothelin in conscious dogs. Am J Physiol 1988;255:R1064–R1068.
60. Miller WL, Redfield MM, Burnett JC. Integrated cardiac, renal and endocrine actions of endothelin. J Clin Invest 1989;83:317–320.
61. Badr KF, Murray JJ, Breyer MD, et al. Mesangial cell, glomerular and renal vascular responses to endothelin in the rat kidney. J Clin Invest 1989;83:336–342.
62. Firth JD, Raine AEG, Ratcliffe PJ, et al. Endothelin: An important factor in acute renal failure? Lancet 1988;2:1179–1182.
63. Wright CE, Fozard JR. Regional vasodilation is a prominent feature of the haemodynamic response to endothelin in anaethetised, spontaneously hypertensive rats. Eur J Pharmcol 1988;155:201–203.
64. De Nucci G, Thomas R, D'Orleans-Juste P, et al. Pressor effects of circulating endothelin are limited by its removal in the pulmonary circulation and by the release of prostacyclin and endothelium-derived relaxing factor. Proc Natl Acad Sci USA 1988;85:9797–9800.
65. Thiemermann C, Lidbury P, Thomas R, Vane J. Endothelin inhibits ex vivo platelet aggregation in the rabbit. Eur J Pharmacol 1988;158:181–182.
66. Korbut R, Lidbury P, Thomas R, et al. Fibrinolytic activity of endothelin-3. Thromb Res 1989;55:797–799.
67. Fukuda Y, Hirata Y, Yoshimi H, et al. Endothelin is a potent secretagogue for atrial natriuretic peptide in cultured rat atrial myocytes. Biochem Biophys Res Commun 1988;155:167–172.
68. Ouchi Y, Kim S, Souza AC, et al. Central effect of endothelin on blood pressure in conscious rats. Am J Physiol 1989;256:H1747–H1751.
69. Moser PC, Pelton JT. Behavioural effects of centrally administered endothelin in the rat. Br J Pharmacol 1989;96:347P.
70. Shinmi O, Kimura S, Yoshizawa T, et al. Presence of endothelin 1 in porcine spinal cord: Biochem Biophys Res Commun 1989;162:340–346.
71. Koseki C, Imai M, Hirata Y, et al. Binding sites for endothelin-1 in rat tissues: An autoradiographic study. J Cardiovasc Pharmacol 1989;13 (suppl 5):S153–S154.

72. Fuxe K, Änggård E, Lundgren A, et al. Localization of (^{125}I)-endothelin-1 and (^{125}I)-endothelin-3 binding sites in the rat brain. Acta Physiol Scand 1989;137: 563–564.

73. Jones CR, Hiley CR, Pelton JT, et al. Autoradiographic localisation of the binding sites for (^{125}I) endothelin in rat and human brain. Neurosci Lett 1989; 97:276–279.

74. Wiklund NP, Ohlen A, Cederqvist B. Inhibition of adrenergic neuroeffector transmission by endothelin in the guinea-pig femoral artery. Acta Physiol Scand 1988;134:311–312.

75. Tabuchi Y, Nakamaru M, Rakugi H, et al. Endothelin inhibits presyncaptic adrenergic neurotransmission in rat mesenteric artery. Biochem Biophys Res Commun 1989;161:803–808.

76. Wennmalm Å, Karwatowska-Prokopczuk E, Wennmalm M. Role of the coronary endothelium in the regulation of sympathetic transmitter release in isolated rabbit hearts. Acta Physiol Scand 1989;136:81–87.

77. Payne AN, Whittle BJR. Potent cyclo-oxygenase mediated bronchoconstrictor effects of endothelin in the guinea pig in vivo. Eur J Pharmacol 1988;158:303–304.

78. Maggi CA, Patacchini R, Giuliani S, et al. Potent contractile effect of endothelin in isolated guinea-pig airways. Eur J Pharmacol 1989;160:179–182.

79. Uchida Y, Ninomiya H, Saotome M, et al. Endothelin, a novel vasoconstrictor peptide, as potent bronchoconstrictor. Eur J Pharmacol 1988;154:227–228.

80. Lagente V, Chabrier PE, Mencia Huerta JM, et al. Pharmacological modulation of the bronchopulmonary action of the vasoactive peptide, endothelin, administered by aerosol in the guinea-pig. Biochem Biophys Res Commun 1989;158: 625–632.

81. Wallace JL, Cirino G, de Nucci G, McKnight W, et al. Endothelin has potent ulcerogenic and vasoconstrictor actions in the stomach. Am J Physiol 1989;256:G661–G666.

82. Whittle BJ, Payne AN, Espluges JV, et al. Cardiopulmonary and gastric ulcerogenic actions of endothelin-1 in the guinea-pig and rat. J Cardiovasc Pharmacol 1989;13 (suppl 5):S103–S107.

83. Komuro I, Kurihara H, Sugiyama T, et al. Endothelin stimulates c-fos and c-myc expression and proliferation of vascular smooth muscle cells. FEBS Lett 1989;238:249–252.

84. Nakaki T, Nakayama M, Yamamoto S, et al. Endothelin-mediated stimulation of DNA synthesis in vascular smooth muscle cells. Biochem Biophys Res Commun 1989;158:880–883.

85. Hirata Y, Takagi Y, Fukuda Y, Marumo F. Endothelin is a potent mitogen for rat vascular smooth muscle cells. Atherosclerosis, 1989;78:225–228.

86. Takuwa N, Takuwa Y, Yanagisawa M, et al. A novel vasoactive peptide endothelin stimulates mitogenesis through inositol lipid turnover in Swiss 3T3 fibroblasts. J Biol Chem 1989;264:7856–7861.

87. Simonson MS, Wann S, Mene P, et al. Endothelin stimulates phospholipase C, Na^+/H^+ exchange, c-fos expression, and mitogenesis in rat mesangial cells. J Clin Invest 1989;83:708–712.

The Endothelium: An Introduction to Current Research, pages 21–32

3

Neural–Endothelial Interactions in Control of Local Blood Flow

J. LINCOLN AND G. BURNSTOCK
Department of Anatomy and Developmental Biology and Centre for Neuroscience, University College London, London WC1E 6BT, England

INTRODUCTION

The control of blood flow is a rapidly expanding field of research. It incorporates new concepts in autonomic neuroeffector mechanisms and in the role of the endothelium in modifying vascular tone, which have profound implications for the study of basic mechanisms and cardiovascular disease. Its investigation uses a wide range of different approaches, including immunocytochemical studies at the light and electron microscopic level, autoradiographic localization of receptors, pharmacological analysis of responses to vasoactive agents, biochemical analysis of the release of such agents and their mechanisms of action, and tissue culture studies of cell interactions. This chapter provides a brief outline of some recent developments in our knowledge of the contributions of perivascular nerves and the endothelium to the control of vascular tone and how they may interact to provide physiological and pathophysiological regulation of blood flow.

RELATIONSHIP OF NERVES TO VASCULAR SMOOTH MUSCLE AND ENDOTHELIAL CELLS

Ultrastructural studies have examined the nature of the relationship between perivascular nerves and the medial muscle coat of blood vessels. Characteristically, the autonomic vascular neuroeffector junction is formed by extensive terminal branching of the autonomic nerve to give a perivascular *autonomic ground plexus* confined to the adventitial–medial border (1). Smooth muscle bundles constitute the effectors, unlike the neuroeffector junction in skeletal muscle, where single muscle cells respond individually. Within the terminal plexus, there are regions free or partially free of Schwann cell covering, which form varicosities 1–2 μm in diameter. These varicosities are separated by narrow, intervaricose strands (0.1–0.3 μm). Low-resistance pathways, known as nexuses or gap junctions, interconnect and couple smooth muscle cells. This enables electrotonic spread of activity to occur following the receptor-mediated change in smooth muscle cell membrane potential induced by the release of neurotransmitters from varicosities during the conduction of nerve impulses. In contrast to skeletal neuromuscular junctions and ganglionic synapses, postjunctional specializations do not occur in vascular neuroeffector junctions, although prejunctional specializations are often seen (2).

In arteries, the width of the vascular nerve–muscle junctional cleft varies considerably with the diameter of the vessel. In densely innervated small muscular arteries, it can be 50–100 nm, whereas in some large elastic arteries it can be as wide as 2,000 nm. In veins, cleft width appears to be independent of vessel diameter. In addition, the density of the perivascular nerve plexus and frequency of nexuses is inversely proportional to the size of the vessel (2). Connective tissue has been demonstrated between perivascular nerve varicosities and the vascular smooth muscle of the guinea pig renal artery (3). This is believed to account for the finding that, in the guinea pig, the renal artery does not respond to nerve stimulation despite the fact that a sympathetic perivascular plexus can readily be demonstrated. It is not known why nonfunctional vascular neuromuscular junctions occur.

The relationship between nerves and endothelial cells is less well characterized. Unmyelinated axons, surrounded by a Schwann cell sheath, have been described in the subendothelial layer near the elastic lamina of the endocardium (4). It is still a matter for debate whether capillaries are innervated. Studies of the cerebral microvasculature have indicated the possibility of extrinsic neural regulation of capillary function with regard to both haemodynamic and transport processes (2). Terminal varicosities have been observed in apposition to capillary endothelial cells separated only by basal lamina material. In this case, the space between the varicosities and endothelial cell membranes was on the order of 400 nm (4). However, morphological proximity alone does not necessarily mean that functional neurotransmission between nerves and endothelial cells takes place. It is probable that circulating and locally produced agents are of more significance in the control of circulatory mechanisms in the microvasculature than are the perivascular nerves.

CONTROL OF BLOOD FLOW BY PERIVASCULAR NERVES
Transmitter Candidates

Until recently, nervous control of the vasculature has been considered predominantly in terms of noradrenaline (NA) released from perivascular sympathetic nerves and a variable involvement of acetylcholine (ACh) released from cholinergic nerves. During the past few years, however, it has been established that there are nonadrenergic, noncholinergic components of the autonomic nervous system (5). In addition to the classical transmitters NA and ACh, other transmitter candidates include adenosine 5'-triphosphate (ATP), vasoactive intestinal polypeptide (VIP), substance P (SP), 5-hydroxytryptamine (5-HT), neuropeptide Y (NPY), and calcitonin gene-related peptide (CGRP). All these substances have been demonstrated in perivascular nerves using fluorescence histochemical and immunohisto-chemical techniques (5–7).

Colocalization, Cotransmission, and Neuromodulation

Immunocytochemical studies at the light and electron microscopical levels have shown that more than one transmitter or putative transmitter may be colocalized in the same nerve. The most common combinations of transmitters in perivascular nerves are NA, ATP, and NPY in sympathetic nerves; ACh and VIP in parasympathetic nerves; and SP, CGRP, and ATP in sensory-motor nerves (8). The concepts of cotransmission and neuromodulation have also now become accepted mechanisms in autonomic nervous control. In order to establish that transmitters coexisting in the same nerves act as cotransmitters, it is necessary to demonstrate that, on release, each substance acts postjunctionally on its own specific receptor to produce a response. Neuromodulators modify the process of neurotransmission. They may be circulating neurohormones, local agents, or neurotransmitter substances released from the same nerves or from others close to the site at which neuromodulation takes place. Neuromodulation can occur either prejunctionally, by decreasing or increasing the amount of transmitter released during transmission, or postjunctionally, in which case the extent of action or time course of the neurotransmitter is modified. In the case of many, but not all, perivascular sympathetic nerves there is evidence that NA and ATP act as cotransmitters, being released from the same nerves but acting on α_1-adrenoceptors and P_2-purinoceptors, respectively, to produce vasoconstriction. NPY is also colocalized with NA and ATP. However, in many vessels, NPY has little, if any, direct action; rather, NPY acts as a prejunctional neuromodulator by inhibiting the release of NA from the nerve and/or postjunctionally to enhance the action of NA (7) (Fig. 1). In other vessels, notably in the spleen, skeletal muscle, and the cerebral and coronary vasculature, NPY has direct vasoconstrictor actions. In the heart and brain, this is probably because of the presence of local intrinsic (nonsympathetic) neurons that use NPY as the principal transmitter. In the spleen, NPY appears to act as a genuine cotransmitter with NA in perivascular sympathetic nerves (7) (Fig. 1).

It has been suggested that, during an axon reflex, antidromic activation of sensory collaterals can lead to the release of SP, ATP, and possibly CGRP to produce dilatation of the blood vessels. SP, ATP, and CGRP have been shown to be colocalized in the same perivascular sensory-motor nerves, and SP and ATP have been proposed to act as cotransmitters (5,7).

SYMPATHETIC NEUROTRANSMISSION

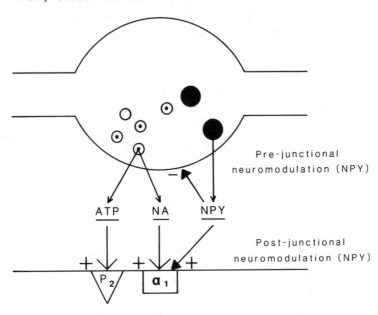

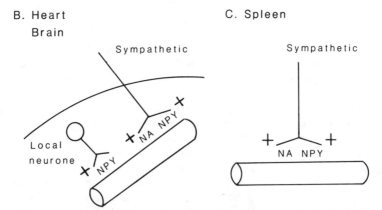

Fig. 1. Schematic representation of different interactions that occur between NPY and ATP and NA released from single sympathetic nerve varicosities. **A:** Diagram showing what occurs in the vas deferens and many blood vessels, where NA and ATP, probably released from small granular vesicles, act synergistically to contract (+) the smooth muscle via α_1-adrenoceptors and P_2-purinoceptors, respectively.

VIP and ACh have been shown to be released as cotransmitters from parasympathetic nerves supplying the salivary glands and interact in producing vasodilatation of vessels in the gland (9,10).

CONTROL OF BLOOD FLOW BY ENDOTHELIAL FACTORS
Endothelium-Dependent Responses

Since 1980, when Furchgott and Zawadzki (11) first reported that the vasodilatation response to ACh requires the presence of an intact endothelium, the role of the endothelium in the regulation of vascular tone has attracted considerable interest. Substances that have been shown to produce endothelium-dependent responses include ACh, ATP, 5-HT, SP, angiotensin II (AgII), vasopressin (VP), histamine, and bradykinin (12–14). Action on endothelial receptors by such vasoactive substances stimulates the production of endothelium-derived relaxing (EDRF) or constricting (EDCF) factors or prostaglandins. These subsequently modify vascular tone by causing contraction or relaxation of the vascular smooth muscle. Much of the current research has centred on the characterization of the endothelial factors. EDRF has been identified as nitric oxide (15,16), while the peptide endothelin is considered one of the constricting factors (17). It should be noted that there is considerable heterogeneity in the endothelium-dependent responses of mammalian blood vessels, with variations between arteries and veins and between different vascular beds. It has been suggested that this heterogeneity could reflect variations in sensitivity of either endothelial or vascular smooth muscle cells of different embryological origin. It is likely that such variations would be useful physiologically, particularly with regard to ensuring that the blood supply to the heart and brain are protected under a variety of different conditions (18).

Endothelial and Smooth Muscle Receptors

Many of the vasoactive substances that require the endothelium to produce vasodilatation are also neurotransmitters which, on release from perivascular nerves, cause vasoconstriction. Pharmacological studies have therefore investigated the receptors involved in mediating the two opposing responses. In many cases, they have demonstrated that different sub-

---

NPY, which is also released from the nerve, has little, if any, direct action on the muscle cell, but exerts potent neuromodulatory actions, both prejunctional inhibition (−) of the release of NA and postjunctional enhancement (+) of the action of NA. **B:** Diagram showing how NPY has potent direct neurotransmitter actions on the vessels in the heart and brain. This is probably because local intrinsic (nonsympathetic) neurons are using NPY as a principal transmitter. **C:** Diagram showing that in some vessels (e.g., those in spleen), NPY appears to have been used as a genuine cotransmitter with NA. Reproduced from Burnstock (7), with permission of the publisher.

types of the receptors to such vasoactive substances occur on the endothelium and on the vascular smooth muscle. An example of this is ATP, which acts on P_2-purinoceptors. Studies of the rank order of potency of the agonists ATP, α, β-methylene ATP, and 2-methylthio-ATP, together with the effects of antagonism by reactive blue 2 and densitization by α, β-methylene ATP, have resulted in the subclassification of P_2-purinoceptors. Thus, P_{2X}-purinoceptors are present on the vascular smooth muscle and are acted on by ATP released from perivascular nerves to produce vasoconstrictor, while ATP can cause vasodilatation via P_{2Y}-purinoceptors on the endothelial cells (19,20).

The Source of Substances Producing Endothelium-Dependent Responses

It is clear that neurotransmitters released from perivascular nerves have direct access to vascular smooth muscle cell receptors to produce a response. It is neither likely nor desirable that the same neurotransmitter can diffuse through the media and basal lamina of a blood vessel (without degradation) to act on endothelial receptors and produce the opposite effect. In order to establish that endothelium-dependent responses have a role to play in the control of vascular tone in the intact organism, it is necessary to identify the source of the vasoactive substances that act on the endothelial receptors. For some substances, a readily available source is the blood. Indeed, it has been suggested that the endothelium may have a protective role against vasoconstriction, which substances released from aggregating platelets, such as 5-HT and adenosine 5'-diphosphate, would otherwise cause. Furthermore, platelet aggregation at sites of endothelial cell damage could provide a mechanism for vasospasm in coronary vessel disease (12,21). In the case of ACh and SP, however, circulating levels are low because of their rapid breakdown. The possibility that endothelial cells themselves may be the source of such substances was first proposed in 1985, when Parnavelas et al. (22) reported that choline acetyltransferase (ChAT), the enzyme responsible for the synthesis of ACh, could be localized in endothelial cells lining capillaries and small vessels in the rat cortex. Since this time, using the same technique of immunocytochemical staining combined with electron microscopy, ChAT, SP, 5-HT, VP, and AgII have all been localized in endothelial cells from a variety of blood vessels (23–26). In addition, SP levels have been measured in endothelium isolated from cerebral arteries and aorta (27). Other workers have also demonstrated that endothelial cells have the capability of synthesizing AgII and histamine (28,29).

Release of Vasoactive Substances from Endothelial Cells

Currently, work is being carried out to investigate whether certain stimuli can cause the release of vasoactive substances from their endothelial stores, thus providing evidence for a physiological mechanism for the endothelium-dependent responses to such stimuli to occur. 5-HT, ATP, SP, and ACh, all of which are present in coronary endothelial cells, have been shown to be released following hypoxic perfusion of the Langendorf heart preparation from the rat (24,25,30). Hypoxic vasodilatation has been shown to be endothelium dependent. Unfortunately, it has proved difficult to find a method to remove the endothelial cells and still retain a viable perfused heart preparation (31). In the perfused rat hindlimb, increased flow causes the release of SP. After removal of the endothelium by perfusion with air bubbles (32), increased flow no longer induced the release of SP. SP has been localized in the endothelial cells of the rat femoral artery (23). Furthermore, denervation of the hindlimb vasculature of SP-containing nerves by capsaicin had no effect on flow-induced SP release (Ralevic V, Milner P: unpublished observations). SP has also been shown to be released from columns of endothelial cells grown on microcarrier beads following increased flow (Milner P, Pearson JD, Toothill VJ: unpublished observations). This supports the view that the source of the SP is the endothelial cells. It is reasonable to suggest that SP and other vasoactive substances within endothelial cells, by their release, contribute to flow-induced vasodilatation, which is known to be an endothelium-dependent response. Similarly, removal of the endothelium from the isolated rat mesenteric bed prevents the induction of ATP release by increased flow (Ralevic V, Kirkpatrick KA: unpublished observations). Studies are being extended to investigate the effects of pH and hypercapnia on release of these and other vasoactive substances in endothelial cell cultures.

LONG-TERM (TROPHIC) INTERACTIONS BETWEEN PERIVASCULAR NERVES AND ENDOTHELIAL CELLS

In view of the fact that the perivascular nerves of arteries and veins are separated from the endothelial cells by the vascular smooth muscle, the possibility of trophic interactions between perivascular nerves and endothelial cells has received little direct investigation. However, findings in studies of the vasculature in disease and following denervation or mechanical injury do provide some indication that such interactions may exist.

It has been shown that 2–8 weeks after adrenergic and sensory denervation of the rabbit ear artery, endothelium-dependent relaxation responses to methacholine are significantly depressed (33). The reduction in response was not due to any impairment of the ability of the muscle to relax, since the maximal relaxation to sodium nitroprusside (an endothelium-independent agent) was unaffected by denervation. Long-term sympathetic denervation in rabbits results in an increase in the sensitivity of cerebral arteries to hypercapnia, hypoxia, and 5-HT (34). Although morphological changes in the endothelial cells were not detected under these conditions

(35), it has not been excluded that alterations in the endothelial control of the cerebral vasculature after sympathetic denervation contributed to this effect. Conversely, in another study, the endothelium of the dog coronary artery was injured mechanically without disruption of the elastic lamina and the distribution of the vasomotor nerves were examined 1 and 3 months after injury (36). Mechanical injury resulted in intimal thickening. While adrenergic and cholinergic nerves were not altered after injury, neuron-specific enolase-positive nerve fibres were increased in number at both 1 and 3 months. An increased density of SP-containing nerve fibres was also observed in the dog coronary artery 3 months after mechanical injury to the endothelium. Endothelial cell damage or dysfunction is widely regarded as a critical initiating factor in the development of atherosclerosis. Epidemiological evidence suggests that psychosocial factors contribute to the presence of coronary artery disease, and it has been hypothesized that these behavioural influences are mediated through the sympathetic nervous system. It has been shown that stress exacerbates the development of atherosclerosis in monkeys fed an atherogenic diet (37). Furthermore, surgical sympathectomy or long-term adrenoceptor blockade by propranolol prevents or reduces the induction of atherosclerosis by diet with or without exacerbation by stress (37,38). It has been proposed that NPY and NA in cerebral perivascular nerves, which increase during the development of hypertension in rats, are involved in protection against disruption of the blood–brain barrier (BBB) and cerebral haemorrhage caused by hypertension. Sympathetic denervation before the development of hypertension results in increased incidence of stroke and increased permeability of the BBB (39).

Since perivascular nerve varicosities have been demonstrated in close apposition to endothelial cells in capillaries, this raises the possibility of direct trophic interactions between nerves and endothelial cells in the microvasculature. Adenosine can be formed from the extracellular breakdown of ATP released from nerves. Chronic inhibition of adenosine uptake with dipyridamole has been shown to cause proliferation of capillary endothelium and increased capillary density in skeletal muscle and heart (40). Furthermore, it has been suggested that neuropeptides may have a role in controlling neurochemical differentiation, cell proliferation, hypertrophy, and regeneration (6). Such interactions require further investigation in the context of endothelial cell biology.

Thus, it appears that there are trophic interactions between endothelial cells and perivascular nerves and that changes in these interactions may be involved in the progression of some cardiovascular diseases. Clearly, the vascular smooth muscle is likely to form an integral part of these processes, since trophic influences between endothelial and smooth muscle cells and between perivascular nerves and vascular smooth muscle have already been demonstrated (35,41).

CONCLUSIONS

It is evident that these recent developments in our knowledge of both perivascular nerves and endothelial cells have profound implications on the control of blood flow. It can be envisaged that the status of vascular tone will be the resultant of interactions between the neural and endothelial control mechanisms. At any one time, which mechanism has more

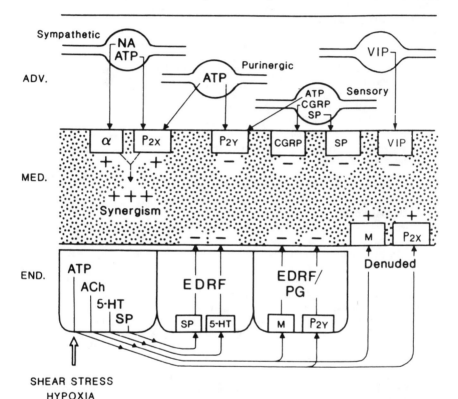

Fig. 2. Schematic representation of potential modes of regulation of vascular tone by endothelial-related mechanisms. Noradrenaline (NA), ATP, CGRP, SP, and VIP can be released from nerves in the adventitia (ADV.) to act on their respective receptors in the media (MED.) to cause vasoconstriction or vasodilatation. ATP, ACh, 5-HT, and SP released from endothelial cells (END.) by shear stress or hypoxia act on their receptors on endothelial cells to cause release of EDRF or prostaglandins (PG), which in turn act on the smooth muscle to cause relaxation. In areas denuded of endothelial cells, opposite effects may be produced by receptors on the smooth muscle. α, noradrenaline receptor; P_{2X}, P_{2X}-purinoceptor; P_{2Y}, P_{2Y}-purinoceptor; M, muscarinic receptor. Modified from Burnstock (42) with permission of the publisher.

influence is probably dependent on the prevailing conditions. It seems likely that endothelial release of vasoactive substances may be of greater significance in the response of blood vessels to local changes in their environment, such as hypoxia and increased flow. By contrast, perivascular nerves integrate the control of blood flow in the organism as a whole (Fig. 2). Disturbances in the balance of long-term interactions between perivascular nerves and endothelial cells may be of significance in the development of cardiovascular disease.

REFERENCES

1. Burnstock G, Iwayama T. Fine structural identification of autonomic nerves and their relation to smooth muscle. Prog Brain Res 1971;34:389–404.
2. Dhital K K, Burnstock G. Adrenergic and non-adrenergic neural control of the arterial wall. In: Camilleri J-P, Berry CL, Fiessinger J-N, Bariéty J, eds. Diseases of the Arterial Wall. London: Springer, 1989;97–126.
3. Cowen T. An ultrastructural comparison of neuromuscular relationships in blood vessels with functional and non-functional neuromuscular transmission. J Neurocytol 1984;13:369–392.
4. Wharton J, Gulbenkian S, Merighi A, Kuhn DM, Jahn R, Taylor KM, Polak JM. Immunohistochemical and ultrastructural localisation of peptide-containing nerves and myocardial cells in the human atrial appendage. Cell Tissue Res 1988;254:155–166.
5. Burnstock G. Nonadrenergic innervation of blood vessels—Some historical perspectives and future directions. In: Burnstock G, Griffith SG, eds. Nonadrenergic Innervation of Blood Vessels. Vol. I. Putative Neurotransmitters. Boca Raton, Florida: CRC Press, 1988;1–14.
6. Burnstock G. Neurohumoral control of blood vessels: Some future directions. J Cardiovasc Pharmacol 1985;7(suppl 3):S137–S146.
7. Burnstock G. Mechanisms of interaction of peptide and nonpeptide vascular neurotransmitter systems. J Cardiovasc Pharmacol 1987;10(suppl 12):S74–S81.
8. Burnstock G. Regulation of local blood flow by neurohumoral substances released from perivascular nerves and endothelial cells. Acta Physiol Scand 1987;133(suppl 571):53–59.
9. Bloom SR, Edwards AV. Vasoactive intestinal peptide in relation to atropine resistant vasodilatation in the submaxillary gland of the cat. J Physiol (Lond) 1980;300:41–53.
10. Lundberg J M. Evidence for coexistence of vasoactive intestinal polypeptide (VIP) and acetylcholine in neurons of cat exocrine glands. Morphological, biochemical and functional studies. Acta Physiol Scand 1981;suppl 496:1–57.
11. Furchgott RF, Zawadzki JV. The obligatory role of endothelial cells in the relaxation of arterial smooth muscle by acetylcholine. Nature (Lond) 1980;288:373–376.
12. Vanhoutte PM, Rimele TJ. Role of the endothelium in the control of vascular smooth muscle function. J Physiol (Paris) 1983;78:681–686.
13. Furchgott RF. Role of endothelium in responses of vascular smooth muscle. In: Garlick DG, Korner PI, eds. Frontiers in Physiological Research. Cambridge: Cambridge University Press, 1984;116–133.

14. Toda N. Endothelium-dependent relaxation induced by angiotensin II and histamine in isolated arteries of dog. Br J Pharmacol 1984;81:301–307.
15. Ignarro LJ, Byrns RE, Wood KS. Pharmacological and biochemical properties of endothelium-derived relaxing factor (EDRF): Evidence that it is closely related to nitric oxide (NO) radical. Circulation 1986;74(suppl II):287.
16. Palmer RMJ, Ferrige AG, Moncada S. Nitric oxide release accounts for the biological activity of endothelium-derived relaxing factor. Nature (Lond) 1987; 327:524–526.
17. Yanagisawa M, Kurihara H, Kimura S, et al. A novel potent vasoconstrictor peptide produced by vascular endothelial cells. Nature (London) 1988;332:411–415.
18. Vanhoutte PM, Miller VM. Heterogeneity of endothelium-dependent responses in mammalian blood vessels. J Cardiovasc Pharmacol 1985;7(suppl 3):S12–S23.
19. Burnstock G, Kennedy C. Is there a basis for distinguishing two types of P_2-purinoceptor? Gen Pharmacol 1985;16:433–440.
20. Burnstock G. Dual control of blood pressure by purines. In: Rand MJ, Raper C, eds. Pharmacology. Proceedings of the Tenth international Congress of Pharmacology. Amsterdam: Elsevier, 1987;245–254.
21. Houston DS, Shepherd JT, Vanhoutte PM. Adenine nucleotides, serotonin and endothelium-dependent relaxations to platelets. Am J Physiol 1985;248:H389–H395.
22. Parnavelas JG, Kelly W, Burnstock G. Ultrastructural localization of choline acetyltransferase in vascular endothelial cells in rat brain. Nature (Lond) 1985; 31:724–725.
23. Loesch A, Burnstock G. Ultrastructural localization of serotonin and substance P in vascular endothelial cells of rat femoral and mesenteric arteries. Anat Embryol 1988;178:137–142.
24. Burnstock G, Lincoln J, Fehér E, et al. Serotonin is localized in endothelial cells of coronary arteries and released during hypoxia: A possible new mechanism for hypoxia-induced vasodilatation of the rat heart. Experientia 1988;44:705–707.
25. Milner P, Ralevic V, Hopwood AM, et al. Ultrastructural localisation of substance P and choline acetyltransferase in endothelial cells of rat coronary artery and release of substance P and acetylcholine during hypoxia. Experientia 1989;45:121–125.
26. Lincoln J, Loesch A, Burnstock G. Localization of vasopressin, serotonin and angiotensin II in endothelial cells of the renal and mesenteric arteries of the rat. Cell Tissue Res 1990;259:341–344.
27. Linnik MD, Moskowitz MA. Identification of immunoreactive substance P in human and other mammalian endothelial cells. Peptides 1989;10:957–962.
28. Kifor I, Dzau VJ. Endothelial renin-angiotensin pathway: Evidence for intracellular synthesis and secretion of angiotensin. Circ Res 1987;60:422–428.
29. Hollis TM, Rosen LA. Histidine decarboxylase activities of bovine aortic endothelium and intima-media. Proc Soc Exp Biol Med 1972;141:978–981.
30. Paddle BM, Burnstock G. Release of ATP from perfused heart during coronary vasodilatation. Blood Vessels 1974;11:110–119.
31. Hopwood AM, Lincoln J, Kirkpatrick KA, Burnstock G. Adenosine 5'-triphosphate, adenosine and endothelium-derived relaxing factor in hypoxic vasodilatation of the heart. Eur J Pharmacol 1989;165:323–326.

32. Ralevic V, Kristek F, Hudlická O, Burnstock G. A new protocol for removal of the endothelium from the perfused rat hind-limb preparation. Circ Res 1989;-64:1190–1196.

33. Mangiarua EI, Bevan RD. Altered endothelium-mediated relaxation after denervation of growing rabbit ear artery. Eur J Pharmacol 1986;122:149–152.

34. Aubinea P, Pearce W, Reynier-Rebuffel AM, Cuevas J, Issertial O. Long-term sympathetic denervation increases sensitivity of cerebral arteries to CO_2 and 5-HT in vitro. J Cerebral Blood Flow Metab 1989;9(suppl 1):S506.

35. Dimitriadou V, Aubineau P, Taxi J, Seylaz J. Ultrastructural changes in the cerebral artery wall induced by long-term sympathetic denervation. Blood Vessels 1988;25:122–143.

36. Taguchi T, Ishii Y, Matsubara F, Tenaka K. Intimal thickening and the distribution of vasomotor nerves in the mechanically injured dog coronary artery. Ex Mol Pathol 1986;44:138–146.

37. Manuck SB, Kaplan JR, Adams MR, Clarkson TB. Effects of stress and the sympathetic nervous system on coronary artery atherosclerosis in the cynomolgus macaque. Am Heart J 1988;116:328–333.

38. Lichtor T, Davies HR, Johns L, Vesselinovitch D, Wissler RW, Mullan S. The sympathetic nervous system and atherosclerosis. J Neurosurg 1987;67:906–914.

39. Dhital KK, Gerli R, Lincoln J, et al. Increased density of perivascular nerves to the major cerebral vessels of the spontaneously hypertensive rat: Differential changes in noradrenaline and neuropeptide Y during development. Brain Res 1988;444:33–45.

40. Hudlická O. Development of microcirculation: capillary growth and adaptation. In: Handbook of Physiology—The Cardiovascular System. Vol. IV. Bethesda: American Physiological Society, 1984;165–216.

41. Karnovsky MJ. Endothelial-vascular smooth muscle cell interaction. Am J Pathol 1981;105:200–206.

42. Burnstock G. Vascular control by purines with emphasis on the coronary system. Eur Heart J 1989;10 (suppl F):15–21.

The Endothelium: An Introduction to Current Research, pages 33–44

4

Aspects of Calcium Signalling in Endothelium

R. JACOB, S.O. SAGE, AND T.J. RINK

SmithKline Beecham Pharmaceuticals UK Ltd., Welwyn, Hertfordshire AL6 9AR, England (R.J.); The Physiological Laboratory, University of Cambridge, Cambridge CB2 3EG, England (S.O.S.); Amylin Corporation, San Diego, California 92121 (T.J.R.)

INTRODUCTION

The endothelium is a smooth, nonthrombogenic lining to the vasculature and a carefully designed barrier between plasma and interstitium that permits ready permeation of solutes and messenger molecules while restraining the passage of large proteins. This latter property permits perfusion of capillaries at positive hydrostatic pressure without massive loss of circulating fluid due to the *colloid osmotic pressure*. Endothelial cells are also responsive to numerous biological mediators acting at membrane receptors. These mediators control the complex biochemical factory of the cell, which produces agents that act on blood vessel tone and growth. These mediators also regulate the permeability of the endothelium by influencing cell shape, transcellular transport, and intercellular connections. In many cases, the cytosolic free calcium ion concentration, $[Ca^{2+}]_i$, is an important factor in these processes; in this chapter, we shall consider aspects of Ca^{2+} in endothelial signal transduction, focusing on Ca^{2+} entry, $[Ca^{2+}]_i$ spikes, and electrophysiological studies.

Morphologically, antigenically, and biochemically, the endothelium is heterogeneous in that different properties are found in endothelium from different regions and different types of blood vessels. Thus far, relatively little variation in Ca^{2+} signalling in endothelial cells from different sources has been seen, although there has been little systematic investigation. This may be because there are relatively few Ca^{2+} mobilising processes, compared with the myriad of surface receptors and antigens. The investigation of Ca^{2+} handling by endothelium started little more than a decade ago and has served two main purposes: (i) to gain insight into stimulus–response coupling and regulation in the endothelium, and (ii) to provide a valuable model of Ca^{2+} signalling in nonexcitable cells. Nearly all the work to date has been done with endothelial cells dissociated from the vasculature and grown in primary culture or with endothelium-derived cell lines. Most workers have used monolayers adherent to glass coverslips, others have used cells in suspension. Techniques that permit the study of signal transduction in endothelial cells in situ may soon be available.

GENERAL PROPERTIES OF CALCIUM SIGNALLING IN ENDOTHELIAL CELLS

Perhaps the first evidence for Ca^{2+} mobilisation following stimulation of endothelial cells came from measurements of ^{45}Ca uptake in response to thrombin and bradykinin (1). This was followed by the discovery that Ca^{2+} ionophores could stimulate the release of prostaglandin I_2 (PGI_2) (2) and the production of endothelium-derived relaxing factor (EDRF) (3), indicating that elevated $[Ca^{2+}]_i$ is an effective cell stimulus. Removal of extracellular Ca^{2+} often attenuates endothelial cell responsiveness (4), although this is not conclusive evidence for a role of $[Ca^{2+}]_i$ elevation because Ca^{2+} removal can influence processes at the external surface of the cell membrane. A range of pharmacological agents supposed to interfere with the entry, release, or action of Ca^{2+}, such as the Ca antagonists TMB-8 and W7, have also been found to reduce PGI_2 release but, as pointed out by Hallam et al. (5), these agents are often not selective, particularly at the concentrations employed in these experiments.

Convincing results have come from experiments with intracellular fluorescent Ca^{2+} indicator dyes, including indo-1 and fura-2. Several groups have shown in human, porcine, and bovine endothelial cells in monolayer culture that several ligands, including thrombin, ATP, bradykinin, and histamine, can elevate $[Ca^{2+}]_i$ from a basal level near 100 nM to many hundred nM within a few seconds [see Hallam et al. (5), and refs. cited therein]. The pattern of response in these multicellular preparations is typical of that in many nonexcitable cells. The initial peak is very similar in extent and timing in the presence or absence of external Ca^{2+} and thus reflects receptor-mediated discharge of Ca^{2+} from an internal store. In the absence of external Ca^{2+}, $[Ca^{2+}]_i$ then declines to the basal level over 10s of seconds, and the application of a second agonist typically elicits little response, indicating depletion of the dischargeable internal store. Measurement of $^{45}Ca^{2+}$ efflux supports the view that most of the discharged Ca^{2+} is pumped out of the cell under these conditions (6). In the presence of external Ca^{2+}, the initial transient is typically followed by a maintained plateau phase, which depends on the continued presence of both the external Ca^{2+} and the agonist. This phase of the response is attributable to some form of receptor-mediated Ca^{2+} entry (RMCE) from outside the cell into the cytosol. As in most cells, it seems likely that the internal release is triggered by inositol (1,4,5)-trisphosphate (IP_3) acting at the IP_3 receptor–channel complex and formed by receptor-mediated phosphodiesterase cleavage of phosphatidylinositol bisphosphate. Several agonists are known to promote IP_3 production in endothelium, and IP_3 can release $^{45}Ca^{2+}$ taken up by internal organelles in saponin-permeabilised endothelial cells (6).

RECEPTOR-MEDIATED CALCIUM ENTRY

The route and mechanism of RMCE thought to underly the plateau phase of the $[Ca^{2+}]_i$ response are less clear. The available evidence argues against a significant role for voltage-operated Ca^{2+} channels. Potassium depolarisation does not elevate $[Ca^{2+}]_i$ (7) and, in most cases, calcium antagonists, at concentrations that block genuine Ca^{2+} entry via voltage-operated Ca^{2+} channels, have little effect on $[Ca^{2+}]_i$ signals or PGI_2 and EDRF production. Furthermore, no voltage-operated calcium currents or channels have been demonstrated electrophysiologically (see below).

The nature of RMCE has been recently investigated in human umbilical vein endothelial cells (8–10) using Mn^{2+} as a surrogate for Ca^{2+}. This technique, first used with platelets (11), relies on the detection of Mn^{2+} entry by its ability to quench fura-2 fluorescence. Using Mn^{2+}, it can be shown that not only does an agonist such as histamine or thrombin stimulate Mn^{2+} entry in a similar way to Ca^{2+} entry, but this stimulated entry of Mn^{2+} can be observed after the removal of the agonist, provided that the internal Ca^{2+} stores are still empty (9,10). This is effected by applying agonist in Ca^{2+}-free solution to discharge the internal store, removing the agonist action either by washing off or by addition of an antagonist, and then exposing the cells to Mn^{2+}. This crucial observation, also reported for some other cell types, suggests that RMCE entry is not a direct consequence of receptor binding, i.e., the Ca^{2+} channel is not linked directly to the receptor or operated by a second messenger generated by receptor agonist binding. Instead, it appears that the influx of Ca^{2+} is controlled by the fullness of the internal Ca^{2+} stores and is stimulated when these stores are depleted. A further correlation between Ca^{2+} and Mn^{2+} entry is the ability of a divalent cation such as Ni^{2+} to block both the plateau phase of elevated $[Ca^{2+}]_i$ and the stimulated Mn^{2+} entry that follow agonist stimulation (8,10).

The presence of RMCE does not define the pathways through which it occurs. One possibility is direct entry into the cytosol via a channel in the plasma membrane. Other more complex pathways have been proposed, such as a direct route from the external medium into the $InsP_3$-dischargeable store, bypassing the cytosol, as originally proposed for exocrine gland cells and smooth muscle (12,13). The ability of some individual endothelial cells to "reload" their Ca^{2+} stores, following discharge in Ca^{2+}-free medium, during a brief exposure to external Ca^{2+} without a significant rise in $[Ca^{2+}]_i$ would be explained by the existance of such an indirect pathway (10).

CYTOSOLIC CALCIUM AS A TRIGGER FOR PGI$_2$ RELEASE

The evidence, briefly alluded to above, suggests that elevated [Ca^{2+}]$_i$ is a signal for EDRF production and for PGI$_2$ production and release. The relationship between [Ca^{2+}]$_i$ and PGI$_2$ production has been studied in some detail in human umbilical vein cells using varying concentrations of the Ca^{2+} ionophore, ionomycin, or thrombin to elevate [Ca^{2+}]$_i$ over a range of values (5). [Ca^{2+}]$_i$ was monitored in fura-2-loaded cells adherent to a coverslip wedged across the corners of a cuvette. PGI$_2$ production was followed by sampling the medium in the cuvette at intervals and measuring the stable hydrolysis product 6-oxo-PGF$_{1\alpha}$. There was little increase in PGI$_2$ production until [Ca^{2+}]$_i$ approached a 1-μM threshold, with a steeply increasing production as peak [Ca^{2+}]$_i$ increased to 3 μM. The similarity in the [Ca^{2+}]$_i$–response relationship determined using ionomycin or thrombin suggested that cytosolic Ca^{2+} was the major stimulus and that other pathways used by thrombin such as diacylglycerol and C-kinase were not important. Subsequent work showed similar results comparing ATP and ionomycin as stimuli (14). This result is quite different from that found for secretion from platelet amine storage granules, where higher levels of [Ca^{2+}]$_i$ are required when ionophore translocates Ca^{2+} into the cytosol than when thrombin is the stimulus (15). This seems to reflect synergy between the C-kinase and Ca^{2+} pathways in stimulating exocytosis in platelets. Interestingly, a further analysis (16) has shown that persistent stimulation of C-kinase by the phorbol ester, phorbol myristate acetate (PMA), for many minutes can promote adenosine triphosphate (ATP)-induced PGI$_2$ formation, even though the rise in [Ca^{2+}]$_i$ produced by ATP is at the same time depressed. PMA appears to increase the [Ca^{2+}]$_i$ sensitivity of PGI$_2$ production, perhaps by an action on phospholipase A$_2$.

CALCIUM SPIKING

When measuring the [Ca^{2+}]$_i$ response in a population of human umbilical vein cells, reducing the agonist concentration reduces the magnitude of the response without a change in the basic shape of the response (17), except for the disappearance of the initial peak at the lowest dose (0.1 μM). However, when the same measurement is carried out on single endothelial cells, a strikingly different type of behaviour is seen. The response to a maximal dose of an agonist (in this case histamine) is much the same as seen in a population of cells, but when the histamine concentration is reduced, repetitive spikes of [Ca^{2+}]$_i$, peaking at $\sim$500 nM are generated (18). The frequency of spiking is related to the dose of histamine with the frequency typically increasing from 0.005 to 0.03 Hz as the histamine dose increases from 0.1 to 3 μM. At higher concentrations of histamine, the spikes merge to generate the maintained elevated [Ca^{2+}]$_i$ plateau mentioned above. Although the frequency of spiking depends on the dose of histamine, the shape of the individual spikes, e.g., their height and width, are virtually independent of the dose (18). We have also examined the response of endothelial cells to different agonists. Although we have seen oscillations in response to ATP (19) and thrombin (20), the oscillations are less easy to investigate than are those induced by histamine; this is because of the desensitization of the ATP response and the inability to wash off thrombin completely.

If extracellular Ca^{2+} is removed while the cell is spiking in response to a low dose of histamine, or if a low dose of histamine is applied in Ca^{2+}-free solution, some spiking activity is seen, although the activity eventually decays away (18). This finding indicates that the spikes are generated by a cyclic release of Ca^{2+} from an internal store, although prolonged repetitive spiking requires extracellular Ca^{2+} to maintain a steady state. Presumably, in the absence of extracellular Ca^{2+}, some Ca^{2+} is lost during each spike, and this must be replenished from outside the cell if long-term activity is to be maintained.

The spiking activity is virtually unaffected by putting the cells into a high K^+ depolarizing medium (18), suggesting that, in contrast to the spiking of $[Ca^{2+}]_i$ seen in excitable cells such as cardiac myocytes, voltage-operated Ca^{2+} channels are not involved in the generation of the $[Ca^{2+}]_i$ spikes in endothelial cells. This is consistent with the apparent absence of any voltage-operated calcium channels in endothelial cells (see below).

If the spiking activity is monitored in a confluent layer of human umbilical vein endothelial cells, using digital image processing, it is clear that the $[Ca^{2+}]_i$ in neighbouring cells is uncoupled because the spikes in neighbouring cells occur asynchronously (18,21). Also noticeable is a lag time before the first Ca^{2+} spike following the application of histamine; the lag time is most pronounced at the lowest doses of histamine (0.1–0.3 μM) and is variable from cell to cell. The asynchronous nature of the response can account for the absence of the observation of oscillations in population measurements on human umbilical vein endothelial cells (17). At the lowest doses of histamine, the variable pronounced lag time presumably accounts for the loss of the initial transient peak in the response of a population of human umbilical vein endothelial cells (17).

The asynchronous $[Ca^{2+}]_i$ spiking could have important consequences for the functioning of a monolayer of endothelial cells. Presumably, an increase in permeability of the endothelial cell monolayer, which requires the opening of intercellular pathways as a consequence of cellular contraction (22), may not occur if cells are contracting asynchronously, since a contracting cell might merely pull its relaxed neighbours towards itself. This may explain why an increase in endothelial cell permeability requires relatively high doses (10–100 μM) of histamine (23), since this is the range within which histamine causes the coordinated contraction of neighbouring cells. By contrast, the stimulation by histamine of the secretion of various compounds such as platelet activating factor (PAF) (24) and von Willebrand factor (vWf) (25) is achieved by lower doses of histamine (0.1–10 μM), and this could be because the asynchronicity of the spiking of $[Ca^{2+}]_i$ that occurs in this dose range has no effect on the secretory function of the individual cells. A spiking $[Ca^{2+}]_i$ response has other advantages: (i) It avoids prolonged levels of elevated $[Ca^{2+}]_i$, which activate both Ca^{2+} ATPases, thereby increasing energy consumption, and phospholipases, which can degrade the membranes; (ii) it permits a more accurate signal transduction; and (iii) it offers the possibility of conveying more information because instead of one variable, the level of the $[Ca^{2+}]_i$ plateau, there are three potential variables, i.e., the height of the spikes, the duration of the spikes, and the frequency of spiking.

Although the oscillatory activity in neighboring human umbilical vein endothelial cells in confluent culture appears to be uncoordinated, this is not necessarily the case with other endothelial cell types. Measurements of $[Ca^{2+}]_i$ in a population of confluent bovine pulmonary artery endothelial cells in monolayer culture showed substantial oscillations superimposed on the plateau phase following stimulation by 10 μM bradykinin (26). The occurrence of these oscillations depended on the cultures being initially thinly seeded; the oscillations were not observed in monolayers formed after dense seeding. The presence of these oscillations in a measurement made over many thousands of cells clearly implies the presence of synchronised $[Ca^{2+}]_i$ oscillations. The results also indicate that the nature of the implied intercellular communication may depend on the culture conditions.

ELECTROPHYSIOLOGICAL STUDIES

A number of electrophysiological studies of single endothelial cells have been reported in recent years, despite the technical difficulties of applying the patch-clamp technique to such thin cells. These studies have characterised the resting membrane and also measured the response evoked by agonists and mechanical stimuli.

The Resting Cell

Whole-cell patch-clamp studies of aortic and arterial endothelial cells indicate resting potentials in the order of -60 to -70 mV (27–31). These values lie close to the K^+ equilibrium potential, indicating that the resting membrane is dominated by a K^+ conductance. Whole-cell current-voltage studies indicate the presence of an inwardly rectifying K^+ current, with a marked increase in inward current when the cell is hyperpolarised from the resting potential (27–30,32). A calcium-activated K^+ current may underline the small outward current observed in whole cells at strongly depolarised potentials. Ca^{2+}-activated K^+ currents are readily demonstrated in cells in which $[Ca^{2+}]_i$ is elevated by the application of an agonist or calcium ionophore (27,32,33). In guinea pig coronary endothelial cells, the substantial hyperpolarization that follows stimulation by bradykinin appears to be due to a Ca^{2+}-activated K^+ current (34). Failure of some investigators to observe a Ca^{2+}-activated K^+ current (28) can be ascribed to the inclusion of EGTA in their pipette filling solutions. Both the inwardly rectifying (28,29) and Ca^{2+}-activated (30,32) K^+ currents have been studied at the single-channel level in cell-attached and excised membrane patches.

Human umbilical vein endothelial cells show some differences from the arterial cells described above; resting potentials are lower, around -30 mV, and the inwardly rectifying K^+ channel is absent (35). Possible differences between arterial and venous endothelia require further investigation.

Studies of cells in confluent coronary artery monolayers indicate that the input resistance is about 200 times lower than that of single cells (36). This can be attributed to electrical coupling of cells by gap junctions. Electrical coupling has also been demonstrated in human umbilical vein endothelial cells (37). The significance of this coupling is uncertain. For example, the possibility that it contributes to the synchrony of agonist-evoked oscillations in $[Ca^{2+}]_i$ observed in bovine pulmonary artery endothelial cells (26) remains to be tested.

Lack of Evidence for Voltage-Operated Calcium Channels

No evidence for voltage-gated inward Ca^{2+} (or Na^+) currents has been forthcoming from single-cell electrophysiological studies. Such conclusions have been reached on the basis of the absence of inward currents at depolarised potentials (27–29,35,38). However, it cannot be excluded that small Ca^{2+} currents might be undetectable in whole-cell current-voltage relationships. For example, Johns et al. (28) calculated that a whole-cell Ca^{2+} current of only 1.5 pA could account for the thrombin-evoked Ca^{2+} entry measured in isotopic studies. A current of this magnitude would be below the resolution of whole-cell voltage-clamp experiments.

Recently, however, we have investigated the potential dependence of $[Ca^{2+}]_i$ in single endothelial cells, loaded with the fluorescent Ca^{2+} indicator indo-1 and held under whole-cell voltage clamp (38). $[Ca^{2+}]_i$ decreased continuously with depolarisation from -70 to $+60$ mV, a result offering strong evidence for the absence of voltage-operated Ca^{2+} channels in the endothelial cell membrane.

Agonist-Evoked Conductance Changes

The absence of voltage-operated Ca^{2+} channels in endothelial cells suggests that some form of receptor-mediated Ca^{2+} entry accounts for the ability of agonists to evoke Ca^{2+} influx in these cells. Johns et al. (28) reported that thrombin or bradykinin rapidly activated a large inward current in bovine pulmonary artery endothelial cells. These currents, which showed no latency, were abolished in Na^+- and Ca^{2+}-free solutions. On the basis of this evidence, it was suggested that this current was conducted by nonselective receptor-operated cation channels in the plasma membrane. By contrast, we have been unable to demonstrate any bradykinin-evoked inward currents during the early stages of activation in the same cell type (38). Our result cannot be attributed to a failure of the cells to respond to the agonist, since the indo-1 in the cells clearly indicated an increase in $[Ca^{2+}]_i$. In our experiments, there was a latency of 3 s between agonist application and the commencement of the rise in $[Ca^{2+}]_i$. Colden-Stanfield et al. (27) reported a similar lack of increased inward current in bradykinin-stimulated bovine aortic endothelial cells. Although these investigators had no direct measure of $[Ca^{2+}]_i$ it seems likely that their cells did respond, since they described an increase in outward current that was attributed to the opening of Ca^{2+}-activated K^+ channels in the endothelial cell membrane (see below). Stretch-activated channels might open in response to shear stresses generated by the pressure-injected flow of agonist solution over the cell. If the current described by Johns et al. (28) was mechanically activated, this could explain the lack of latency in the response.

Whereas we were unable to detect any increase in inward currents during the early stages of bradykinin activation, we did find an increase in inward current that developed about 30 s after agonist application (38). This late-developing current was not involved in mediating the initial rise in $[Ca^{2+}]_i$, since it commenced after the rise in $[Ca^{2+}]_i$ had peaked. However, this current, which appeared to be conducted by a nonselective cation channel, might contribute Ca^{2+} to the plateau phase of the agonist-evoked response. The latency of this bradykinin-evoked inward current may be compatible with evidence from fluorescence studies indicating that divalent cation entry lags behind the discharge of the intracellular Ca^{2+} stores (8).

Bregestovski et al. (35) reported an inward, nonselective cation current evoked by histamine in human umbilical vein endothelial cells. This current, which showed a latency of >60 s, was mimicked by application of the Ca^{2+} ionophore, A23187. Hence, it was suggested that the histamine-evoked current was conducted by Ca^{2+}-activated nonselective cation channels. This histamine-evoked current resembles that evoked by bradykinin in bovine pulmonary artery endothelial cells (38) and may likewise be involved in the plateau phase of the agonist-evoked response. Histamine has also been shown to evoke single-channel activity in cell-attached membrane patches (37). Responses were elicited by application of histamine outside the patch pipette, favouring the idea that the response is mediated by a second-messenger operated, rather than a receptor-operated channel.

Thus, to date, electrophysiological studies of endothelial cells have produced conflicting evidence as to the mechanism of agonist-evoked Ca^{2+} entry. Some of these discrepancies may arise from differences between species or between endothelium from different vessels within the same species, or different experimental procedures and design. Further studies are clearly needed.

Mechanically Evoked $[Ca^{2+}]_i$ and Conductance Changes

Vascular endothelium is subjected to a range of haemodynamically generated shear-stress forces that evoke changes in morphology (39) and biochemistry (40). These changes may, at least in part, be mediated by a shear-stress-induced rise in $[Ca^{2+}]_i$; Ando et al. (41) reported that the $[Ca^{2+}]_i$ in bovine aortic endothelial cells responded to a shear stress with a biphasic response of an initial transient peak followed by a small elevated plateau. We have seen shear-stress-induced $[Ca^{2+}]_i$ transients as a result of turning on the superfusion over human umbilical vein endothelial cells, although there is no sustained plateau phase. These transient shear responses are quite variable; not only does their magnitude vary between cells from one culture, but they are also completely absent from some cultures. We have yet to make a systematic study of these transients, but an example is shown in Figure 1, compared with the response to a maximal dose of histamine.

Lansman et al. (42) reported single, stretch-activated channels in porcine aortic endothelial cells. These channels were activated in cell-attached patches by suction on the patch-pipette and were shown to be cation selective and Ca^{2+} permeable. Stretch-activated cation channels might contribute to elevations in $[Ca^{2+}]_i$ evoked by haemodynamic stresses.

A different type of shear-stress-activated current has been described in bovine aortic endothelial cells (31). In ingenious experiments, whole-cell recordings were made from cells grown in glass capillary tubes through which the flow of medium could be controlled. The flow-induced current was K^+ selective and resulted in hyperpolarisation of the cell under physiological conditions. Since basal $[Ca^{2+}]_i$ in endothelial cells has been shown to be potential sensitive (38), shear-stress-evoked hyperolarisation might result in elevated $[Ca^{2+}]_i$. Consistent with this idea is that the plateau phase of the shear stress response of bovine aortic endothelial cells appears to depend on the presence of extracellular Ca^{2+}.

CONCLUSION

Recent developments in the measurement of $[Ca^{2+}]_i$ coupled with the application of modern electrophysiological techniques are beginning to provide us with an understanding of how $[Ca^{2+}]_i$ is regulated in endothelial cells. However, we still need to know, for example, how Ca^{2+} entry is controlled, how complex patterns of $[Ca^{2+}]$ response (e.g., spiking and

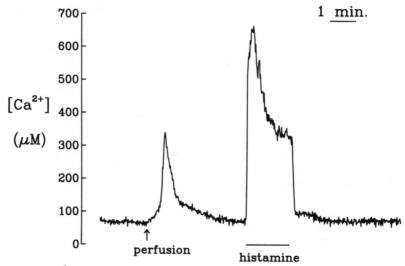

Fig. 1. $[Ca^{2+}]_i$ recorded from a single human umbilical vein endothelial cell loaded with fura-2; see Jacob et al. (18) for a description of the methods. *(arrow)* The time when the superfusion was turned on. Bar shows the period of application of 100 µM histamine.

oscillations) are generated, how mechanical stimulation can affect $[Ca^{2+}]_i$ regulation, and how Ca^{2+} entry and membrane potential might interact. Knowledge of such aspects of $[Ca^{2+}]_i$ regulation will be necessary for a fuller understanding of Ca^{2+} in signal transduction.

REFERENCES

1. D'Amore P, Shepro D. Stimulation of growth and calcium influx in cultured bovine endothelial cells by platelets and vasoactive substances. J Cell Physiol 1977;92:177–184.
2. Weksler BB, Ley CW, Jaffe EA. Stimulation of endothelial cell prostacyclin production by thrombin, trypsin, and the ionophore A23186. J Clin Invest 1978;62:923–930.
3. Furchgott RF. Role of the endothelium in response of vascular smooth muscle. Circ Res 1983;53:557–573.
4. Vanhoutte PM. Vascular endothelium and Ca^{2+} antagonists. J Cardiovasc Pharmacol 1988;12:521–528.
5. Hallam TJ, Pearson JD, Needham LA. Thrombin-stimulated elevation of human endothelial cell cytoplasmic free calcium concentration causes prostacyclin production. Biochem J 1988;251:243–249.
6. Johns A, Freaz AD, Adams DJ, Lategan TW, Ryan US, van Breeman C. Role of calcium in the activation of endothelial cells. J Cardiovasc Pharmacol 1988; 12:5119–5123.
7. Hallam TJ, Pearson JD. Exogenous ATP raises cytoplasmic free calcium in fura-2 loaded piglet aortic endothelial cells. FEBS Lett 1986;207:95–96.

8. Hallam TJ, Jacob R, Merritt JE. Evidence that agonists stimulate bivalent-cation influx into human endothelial cells. Biochem J 1988;255:170–184.

9. Hallam TJ, Jacob R, Merritt JE. Influx of bivalent cations can be independent of receptor stimulation in human endothelial cells. Biochem J 1989;259:125–129.

10. Jacob R. Agonist stimulated divalent cation entry into single cultured human umbilical vein endothelial cells. J Physiol (Lond) 1990;421:55–77.

11. Hallam TJ, Rink TJ. Agonists stimulate divalent cation channels in the plasma membrane of human platelets. FEBS Lett 1985;186:175–179.

12. Putney JW Jr. A model for receptor-regulated calcium entry. Cell Calcium 1986;7:1–12.

13. Merritt JE, Rink TJ. Regulation of cytosolic free calcium in fura-2-loaded rat parotid acinar cells. J Biol Chem 1987;262:17362–17369.

14. Carter TD, Hallam TJ, Cusack NJ, Pearson JD. Regulation of P_{2y}-purinoceptor-mediated prostacyclin release from human endothelial cells by cytoplasmic calcium concentration. Br J Pharmacol 1988;95:1181–1190.

15. Rink TJ, Sanchez A, Hallam TJ. Diacylglycerol and phorbol ester stimulate secretion without raising cytoplasmic free calcium in human platelets. Nature (Lond) 1983;305:317–319.

16. Carter TD, Hallam TJ, Pearson JD. Protein kinase C activation alters the sensitivity of agonist-stimulated endothelial cell prostacyclin production to intracellular Ca^{2+}. Biochem J 1989;262:431–437.

17. Rotrosen D, Gallin JI. Histamine type I receptor occupancy increases endothelial cytosolic calcium, reduces F-actin, and promotes albumin diffusion across cultured endothelial cell monolayers. J Cell Biol 1986;103:2379–2387.

18. Jacob R, Hallam TJ, Merritt JE, Rink TJ. Repetitive spikes in cytoplasmic calcium evoked by histamine in human endothelial cells. Nature (Lond) 1988;335:40–45.

19. Jacob R, Newton J. Response of single cultured human umbilical vein endothelial cells to ATP. J Physiol (Lond) 1989;417:76P.

20. Rink TJ, Hallam TJ. Calcium signalling in non-excitable cells: Notes on oscillations and store refilling. Cell Calcium 1989;10:385–395.

21. Jacob R. Imaging cytoplasmic free calcium in histamine stimulated endothelial cells and in fMet-Leu-Phe stimulated neutrophils. Cell Calcium 1990;11:241–249.

22. Crone C. When capillary permeability increases. News Physiol Sci 1987;2:16–18.

23. Killackey JF, Johnston MG, Movat HZ. Increased permeability of micro carrier-cultured endothelial monolayers in response to histamine and thrombin. Am J Pathol 1986;122:50–61.

24. McIntyre TM, Zimmerman GA, Satoh K, Prescott SM. Cultured endothelial cells synthesize both platelet-activating factor and prostacyclin in response to histamine, bradykinin and adenosine triphosphate. J Clin Invest 1985;76:271–280.

25. Hamilton KK, Sims PJ. Changes in cytosolic Ca^{2+} associated with von Willebrand factor release in human endothelial cells exposed to histamine. J Clin Invest 1987;79:600–608.

26. Sage SO, Adams DJ, van Breeman C. Synchronised oscillations in cytoplasmic free calcium concentration in confluent bradykinin-stimulated bovine pulmonary artery endothelial monolayers. J Biol Chem 1989;264:6–9.

27. Colden-Stanfield M, Schilling WP, Ritchie AK, Eskin SG, Navarro LT, Kunze D L. Bradykinin-induced increases in cytosolic calcium and ionic currents in bovine aortic endothelial cells. Circ Res 1987;61:632–640.

28. Johns A, Lategan TW, Lodge NJ, Ryan US, van Breeman C, Adams DJ. Calcium entry through receptor-operated channels in bovine pulmonary artery endothelial cells. Tissue Cell 1987;19:733–745.

29. Takeda K, Schini V, Stoeckel H. Voltage-activated potassium, but not calcium currents, in cultured bovine aortic endothelial cells. Pflügers Arch 1987;410: 385–393.

30. Fichtner H, Frobe U, Busse R, Kohlhardt M. Single non-selective cation channels and Ca^{2+}-activated channels in aortic endothelial cells. J Membr Biol 1987;98:125–133.

31. Olesen SP, Clapham DE, Davies P. Haemodynamic shear stress activates a K^+ current in vascular endothelial cells. Nature (Lond) 1988;331:168–170.

32. Sauve R, Simoneau C, Roy G. External ATP triggers a biphasic activation process of a calcium-dependent K^+ channel in cultured bovine aortic endothelial cells. Pflügers Arch 1988;412:469–481.

33. Busse R, Fichtner H, Luckhoff A, Kohlhardt M. Hyperolarisation and increased free calcium in acetylcholine-stimulated endothelial cells. Am J Physiol 1988;255:H965–H969.

34. Daut J, Dischner A, Mehrke G. Bradykinin induces a transient hyperpolarization of cultured guinea-pig coronary endothelial cells. J Physiol (Lond) 1989;410:48P.

35. Bregestovski P, Bakhramov A, Davilov S, Moldobaeva A, Takeda K. Histamine-induced inward currents in cultured endothelial cells from human umbilical vein. Br J Pharmacol 1988;95:429–436.

36. Daut J, Merke G, Nees S, Newman WH. Passive electrical properties and electrogenic sodium transport of cultured guinea-pig coronary endothelial cells. J Physiol (Lond) 1987;402:237–254.

37. Bakhramov A, Bregestovski P, Takeda, K. Histamine-dependent currents in endothelial cells isolated from human umbilical vein. J Physiol (Lond) 1988;406:90P.

38. Cannell MB, Sage SO. Bradykinin-evoked changes in cytosolic calcium and membrane currents cultured bovine pulmonary artery endothelial cells. J Physiol (Lond) 1989;419:555–568.

39. Flaherty JT, Pierce JE, Ferrans VJ, Patel DJ, Tucker WK, Fry DL. Endothelial nuclear patterns in the canine arterial tree with particular reference to haemodynamic events. Circ Res 1972;30:23–34.

40. Davies PF, Dewey CF, Bussolari SR, Gordon EJ, Gimbrone MA. Influence of haemodynamic forces on vascular endothelial function. J Clin Invest 1984;73:-1121–1129.

41. Ando J, Komatsuda T, Kamiya A. Cytoplasmic calcium response to fluid shear stress in cultured vascular endothelial cells. In Vitro Cell Dev Biol 1988;24:871–877.

42. Lansman JB, Hallam TJ, Rink TJ. Single stretch-activated ion channels in endothelial cells: A vascular mechanotransducer?. Nature (Lond) 1987;325: 811–813.

The Endothelium: An Introduction to Current Research, pages 45–51
© 1990 Wiley-Liss, Inc.

5

Receptors Linked to Adenylate Cyclase on Endothelial Cells

J.R. McEWAN, H. PARSAEE, D.C. LEFROY, AND J. MacDERMOT

Department of Clinical Pharmacology, Royal Postgraduate Medical School, London W12 ONN, England

INTRODUCTION

Endothelial cells cover the luminal surface of blood vessels and provide a mechanical barrier between the solutes and cellular components of blood within the vascular lumen and the pro-aggregatory collagen-containing surface of the subendothelial matrix. However, in addition to this structural role, endothelial cells are also intimately involved in the control of vascular tone; stimulation of endothelial cells by adenine nucleotides, thrombin, histamine, or bradykinin is followed by a transient synthesis and release of prostacyclin and endothelium-derived relaxing factor (EDRF).

THE RELEASE OF PROSTACYCLIN AND EDRF

There is now compelling evidence that the release of prostacyclin (and probably EDRF as well) is triggered by a rise in intracellular calcium (1–6). The rapid rise in calcium is largely due to the release of calcium from intracellular stores under the control of inositol 1,4,5-trisphosphate (7), but there is an accompanying slower and more sustained rise in calcium that is derived from calcium which enters from the exterior of the cell (8).

The pathway of receptor-mediated hydrolysis of phosphatidylinositol 4,5-bisphosphate, the release of inositol 1,4,5-trisphosphate (IP3), and the subsequent calcium transient and activation of phospholipase A2 may be modified in two separate ways by the activity of protein kinase C (9). First, phorbol ester has been shown to decrease the rapid rise in calcium which is due to release from intracellular stores. This could possibly be due to a phosphorylation site on the IP3 receptor, but the authors have argued in favour of a phosphorylation site on the G-protein (Gp) that couples the receptor (in this case, the P2y receptor for adenine nucleotides) to phospholipase C. The second effect of phorbol ester is to increase the sensitivity of phospholipase A2 to rises in intracellular calcium. To date, there is no clear indication of whether this latter effect is due directly to phosphorylation of phospholipase A2. An alternative possibility (which, once again, is preferred by the authors of this work) might be the phosphorylation of a regulatory protein such as lipocortin or a G-protein with subsequent changes in the calcium sensitivity of phospholipase A2. A mechanism of this sort has been reported in other cell types (10,11).

RECEPTORS LINKED TO ADENYLATE CYCLASE
β-Adrenoceptors

The first receptor in this group was identified on rabbit endothelial cells and was the β-adrenoceptor (12). Since that time, this observation has been confirmed (13); similar receptors have been reported in endothelium from cow (13,14), dog (13,15), and rat (13). In bovine aortic endothelial cells, radioligand binding suggests a single class of receptors (14) and inhibition by selected agonists, and the antagonists available at that time (propranolol, which is nonselective; practolol, which is β_1-selective; butoxamine, which is β_2-selective) indicated β_2-selectivity in these cells. Recent results from this laboratory (Parsaee and Lefroy, unpublished observations) confirm the capacity of isoprenaline to activate adenylate cyclase in human and bovine aortic endothelial cells. However, the availability of more selective β_1-adrenoceptor antagonists (CGP 20712A) and β_2-adrenoceptor antagonists (ICI 118,551) suggest that both receptor subtypes are present in bovine aortic endothelium, and that the response mediated by isoprenaline is dependent on each class for about half the response. Binding data are not yet available to quantify the numbers of each β-adrenoceptor subtype.

The expression of β-adrenoceptors on bovine aortic endothelial cells is controlled, at least in part, by agonist occupation, and prolonged exposure of AG4762 bovine aortic endothelial cells to isoprenaline reduced the maximum isoprenaline-dependent activation of adenylate cyclase (Parsaee H: unpublished results). Preliminary results suggest that this is purely homologous desensitisation, with no modification of responses mediated by other adenylate cyclase-linked receptors.

A2-Purinoceptors

Recently, we identified adenosine A2 purinoceptors on bovine aortic endothelial cells (16). Analysis of the capacity of 5'-(N-ethylcarboxamido)adenosine (NECA, a stable adenosine analogue) to activate adenylate cyclase suggested a single class of receptors. This result was confirmed by measurement of the inhibition of the response by selected antagonists, and the A2-purinoceptor was identified by the rank order of potency of the compounds.

Prolonged exposure of bovine aortic endothelial cells to NECA results in very substantial (about 70%) desensitisation. Further examination revealed that the effect of NECA on the endothelial cells in culture was to reduce the maximum NECA-dependent increase in adenylate cyclase activity, without altering the concentration of NECA required for half-maximum enzyme activation (Kact). Experimental results are not available to confirm the presumed reduction in adenosine A2 receptors, as no suitable radioligand is available. The problems associated with the interpretation of NECA binding have been described fully recently (17).

Bovine aortic endothelial cells can be shown to resensitise after removal of the desensitising agent. The experiments were performed with cells that had been treated for 24 h with cytosine arabinofuranoside to arrest cell division, and minimise the contribution in "resensitised" cells of daughter cells from recent mitoses. Sensitivity to NECA was restored slowly over many hours (16), and the process was inhibited in the presence of cycloheximide (Luty and MacDermot, unpublished results). This suggests that restoration of adenosine A2 responsiveness in bovine aortic endothelial cells is dependent on de novo protein synthesis.

CGRP Receptors

We have recently identified receptors for CGRP in endothelium from human umbilical vein (18) and bovine aorta (19). CGRP appears to activate the adenylate cyclase by interaction with a single class of receptors in endothelial cell homogenates from either species. In common with other examples of receptor-linked activation of adenylate cyclase, the effects of CGRP are dependent on the presence of GTP, which suggests that coupling of the receptor to the enzyme is mediated by Gs (the stimulatory guanine nucleotide-binding regulatory protein). The interpretation that these effects are mediated by a single class of CGRP receptors was based solely on agonist concentration curves. More recently however at least two antagonists (20,21) and a partial agonist (19) have been identified, and it should be possible now to address this question more rigorously.

The partial agonist at CGRP receptors (19) on bovine aortic endothelial cells incorporates a [°TYR]-substitution on CGRP. The maximum stimulation of adenylate cyclase mediated by [°TYR]-CGRP is about half that mediated by authentic CGRP, and it inhibits enzyme activity in the presence of CGRP at saturating concentrations.

THE FUNCTION OF ADENYLATE CYCLASE-LINKED RECEPTORS IN ENDOTHELIUM

The function of this class of receptors on endothelial cells remains unknown, although a number of points in this respect can be made. A striking finding has been the similarity in the magnitude of the responses in endothelial cells to either β-adrenoceptor, adenosine A2, or CGRP receptor agonists. While the actual response in vivo clearly depends also on the concentration of these agonists and their affinities for their respective receptors, it seems probable (at least in the case of adrenaline and adenosine) that the cells could respond to concentrations of these compounds that are found at the luminal surface of blood vessels.

In preliminary experiments performed in this laboratory (McEwan, unpublished observations), we have observed an inhibitory affect of both isoprenaline and forskolin (a compound that activates directly the adenylate cyclase molecule) on the release of prostacyclin when bovine endothelial cells are stimulated with bradykinin. It seems probable that this effect would be mediated by protein kinase A, with phosphorylation of a protein involved in the complex cascade of bradykinin-dependent release of prostacyclin. In many diverse tissues, activation of protein kinase A by cAMP reduces the amplitude of the calcium transient. This process may involve one of several mechanisms, including (i) sequestration of calcium into the sarcoplasmic reticulum of heart muscle by phosphorylation of a regulatory protein, phospholamban (22); (ii) decreased activity of phospholipase C in airway smooth muscle, most probably by phosphorylation of the enzyme or related G-protein (23); and (iii) diminished release of calcium from endoplasmic reticulum by phosphorylation of the IP3 receptor in brain (24). A purely hypothetical scheme is shown in Figure 1 to illustrate some of the possible sites for protein kinase A-dependent phosphorylation in the cascade of bradykinin-dependent release of prostacyclin. These phosphorylation sites have been identified in other tissues (see above), but their presence has still to be confirmed in endothelium.

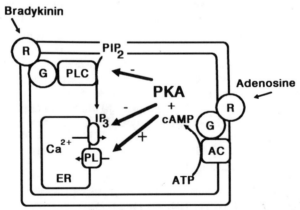

Fig. 1.   Hypothetical scheme for the functional role of adenylate cyclase-linked receptors in endothelial cells. The figure shows receptors for bradykinin or adenosine (R) that link through their particular G-proteins (G) to either phospholipase C (PLC) or adenylate cyclase (AC); other abbreviations: phophatidylinositol 4,5-bisphosphate (PIP2), inositol 1,4,5-trisphosphate (IP3), endoplasmic reticulum (ER), and phospholamban (PL).

There is already good evidence for a protein kinase C phosphorylation site on phospholipase A2 (or one of its regulatory proteins), and the G-protein that links bradykinin receptors to phospholipase C (9). It seems likely therefore that there is a complex pattern of inhibitory feedback on the molecular components of the pathway(s) involved in the stimulation of endothelial cells by bradykinin, thrombin, adenine nucleotides, etc. One element of the inhibitory process appears to involved activation of protein kinase C by diacylglycerol (a product of phospholipase C activation), and another may well be the activation of protein kinase A by cAMP.

It is interesting to speculate further in this context. An inhibitory feedback pathway within the cell has been described for ATP or ADP which trigger release of both prostacyclin and EDRF from the cell. The release mechanism involves activation of phospholipase C, release of IP3 into the cytoplasm, and release of calcium from the endoplasmic reticulum. The inhibitory pathway (as described above) is mediated by diacylglycerol, the other product of phospholipase C. However, there is also another pathway that could serve to inhibit the ATP-dependent release of prostacyclin. There are abundant hydrolases on the surface of endothelial cells that are competent to hydrolyse ATP and ADP to adenosine (22), which would then be available to bind to surface adenosine A2 receptors and activate adenylate cyclase. This would then initiate the second inhibitory pathway involving protein kinase A (Fig. 2).

Lastly, the question of the effect(s) of protein kinase A or C on the release of EDRF requires to be elaborated. It seems likely that the pathway for the

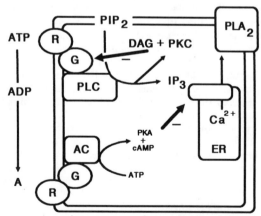

Fig. 2. Hypothetical scheme for the dual inhibitory effects of protein kinases A (PKA) and C (PKC) on the capacity of receptors for ATP (P2y purinoceptors) to activate a cascade that results in activation of phospholipase A2. Protein kinase C (PKC) is activated by diacylglycerol (DAG); other abbreviations as in Figure 1.

synthesis and release of EDRF will be published within the next year, and since the process appears to be intimately linked with the development of a calcium transient, the expectation must be that it will be regulated by a complex pattern of phosphorylation similar to that involved with the release of prostacyclin.

REFERENCES

1. Hallam TJ, Pearson JD. Exogenous ATP raises cytoplasmic free calcium in fura-2 loaded pig aortic endothelial cells. FEBS Lett 1986;207:95–99.
2. Luckhoff A, Busse R. Increased free calcium in endothelial cells under stimulation with adenine nucleotides. J Cell Physiol 1986;126:414–420.
3. Jaffe EA, Grulich J, Weksler BB, Hampel G, Watanabe K. Correlation between thrombin-induced prostacyclin production and inositol trisphosphate and cytosolic free calcium levels in cultured human endothelial cells. J Biol Chem 1987;262:8557–8565.
4. Rotrosen D, Gallin JI. Histamine type I receptor occupancy increases endothelial cytosolic calcium, reduces F-actin, and promotes albumin diffusion across cultured endothelial monolayers. J Cell Biol 1986;103:2379–2380.
5. Morgan-Boyd R, Stewart JM, Vavrek RJ, Hassid A. Effects of bradykinin and angiotensin 11 on intracellular calcium ion dynamics in endothelial cells. Am J Physiol 1987;253:C588–C598.
6. Moncada S, Palmer RMJ, Higgs EA. Biosynthesis of nitric oxide from L-arginine. A pathway for the regulation of cell function and communication. Biochem Pharmacol. 1989;38:1709–1715.
7. Bartha K, Muller-Peddinghaus R, Van Rooijen LAA. Bradykinin and thrombin effects on polyphosphoinositide hydrolysis and prostacyclin production in endothelial cells. Biochem J 1989;263:149–155.
8. Carter TD, Hallam TJ, Cusack NJ, Pearson JD. Regulation of P2y-purinoceptor-mediated prostacyclin release from human endothelial cells by cytoplasmic calcium concentration. Br J Pharmacol 1988;95:1181–1190.
9. Carter TD, Hallam TJ, Pearson JD. Protein kinase C activation alters the sensitivity of agonist-stimulated endothelial cell prostacyclin production to intracellular calcium. Biochem J 1989;262:431–437.
10. Wallner BP, Mattaliano RJ, Hession C, Cate RL, Tizard R, Sinclair LK, Foeller C, Chow EP, Browning JL, Ramachandran KL, Pepinsky RB. Cloning and expression of human lipocortin, a phospholipase A2 inhibitor with potential anti-inflammatory activity. Nature (Lond) 1986;320:77–81.
11. Axelrod J, Burch RM, Jelsema CL. Receptor-mediated activation of phospholipase-A2 via GTP-binding proteins—arachidonic acid and its metabolites as 2nd messengers. Trends Neurosci. 1988;11:117–123.
12. Buonassisi V, Venter JC. Hormone and neurotransmitter receptors in an established vascular endothelial cell line. Proc Natl Acad Sci USA 1976;73:1612–1616.
13. Stephenson JA, Summers RJ. Autoradiographic analysis of receptors on vascular endothelium. Eur J Pharmacol 1987;134:35–43.
14. Steinberg SF, Jaffe EA, Bilezikian JP. Endothelial cells contain beta adrenoceptors. Naunyn-Schmiedebergs Arch Pharmacol 1984;325:310–313.

15. Macdonald PS, Dubbin PN, Dusting GJ. β-Adrenoceptors on endothelial cells do not influence release of relaxing factor in dog coronary arteries. Clin Exp Pharmacol Physiol 1987;14:525–534.
16. Luty J, Hunt JA, Nobbs PK, Kelly E, Keen M, MacDermot J. Expression and desensitisation of A2 purinoceptors on cultured bovine aortic endothelial cells. Cardiovasc Res 1989;23:303–307.
17. Keen M, Kelly E, Nobbs P, MacDermot J. A selective binding site for ^{3}H-NECA that is not an adenosine A2 receptor. Biochem Pharmacol 1989;38:3827–3833.
18. Crossman D, McEwan J, MacDermot J, MacIntyre I, Dollery CT. Human calcitonin gene-related peptide activates adenylate cyclase and releases prostacyclin from human umbilical vein endothelial cells. Br J Pharmacol 1987;92:695–701.
19. McEwan JR, Ritter JM, MacDermot J. Calcitonin gene related peptide (CGRP) activates adenyate cyclase of bovine aortic endothelial cells: Guanosine 5'-triphosphate dependence and partial agonist activity of a tyrosinated analogue. Cardiovasc Res 1989;23:921–927.
20. Maton PN, Webber P, Sutliff VE, Zhou Z-C, Gardner JD, Jensen RT. Spectrum of activities of calcitonin gene-related peptide (CGRP) and related peptides at the CGRP receptor. Biomed Res 1988;65:(suppl1) (abst).
21. Chiba T, Yamaguchi A, Yamatani T, Nakamura A, Morishita T, Inui T, Fukase M, Noda T, Fujita T. Calcitonin gene-related peptide receptor antagonist human CGRP-(8-37). Am J Physiol 1989;256:E331–E335.
22. Exton JH. Calcium signalling in cells, molecular mechanisms. Kidney Int 1987;32(suppl 23):S68–S76.
23. Hall IP, Donaldson J, Hill SJ. Inhibition of histamine-stimulated inositol phospholipid hydrolysis by agents which increase cyclic AMP level in bovine tracheal smooth muscle. Br J Pharmacol 1989;97:603–613.
24. Suppattapone S, Danoff SK, Thiebert A, Joseph SK, Steiner J, Snyder SH. Cyclic AMP-dependent phosphorylation of a brain inositol trisphosphate receptor decreases its release of calcium. Proc Natl Acad Sci USA 1988;85:8747–8750.
25. Pearson JD, Gordon JL. Nucleotide metabolism by endothelium. Annu Rev Physiol 1985;47:617–627.

The Endothelium: An Introduction to Current Research, pages 53–63
© 1990 Wiley-Liss, Inc.

6

Adenine Nucleotides and the Endothelium

J.M. BOEYNAEMS, S. PIROTTON, D. DEMOLLE, AND
A. VAN COEVORDEN
*Institute of Interdisciplinary Research, School of Medicine, Free
University of Brussels, B-1070 Brussels, Belgium*

INTRODUCTION

Adenosine triphosphate (ATP) plays an essential role as energy source in the cytoplasm of cells, where it is present at millimolar concentrations. In addition, extracellular ATP and other nucleotides, at concentrations ranging from nanomolar to millimolar, produce a large variety of pharmacological actions (1). ATP released into the extracellular space from cell lysis, selective permeabilization of the plasma membrane (as in endothelial cells), or exocytosis of secretory granules (in platelets and neurons), can therefore play a physiological role as intercellular mediator. The various effects of extracellular nucleotides exhibit distinct characteristics, in terms of effective concentrations (from nM to mM), agonist specificity (ATP effect mimicked or not by adenosine diphosphate (ADP)) and mechanism of action (phosphorylation reaction or noncovalent interaction with a receptor site). Examples include the following:

1. In snail neurons, nanomolar concentrations of ATP activate Ca^{2+} channels, an effect mimicked by the nonhydrolysable analogue adenylylimidodiphosphate (APPNP) and partially by ADP.
2. In Ehrlich ascites tumour cells, ATP at micromolar concentrations induces a rapid mobilization of intracellular Ca^{2+} and a slow influx of extracellular Ca^{2+}; these effects are mimicked neither by ADP nor by nonhydrolysable analogues of ATP.
3. ATP at millimolar concentrations induces the depolarization of mouse macrophages, promotes Na^+ influx and K^+ efflux and inhibits phagocytosis.
4. ATP (> 100 μM) produces a general increase in the membrane permeability of transformed fibroblasts, associated with the phosphorylation of a 44-kD membrane protein.

5. Whereas ADP triggers platelet aggregation in the 0.1 to 10-μM range, ATP behaves as a competitive antagonist (K_i = 20 μM).
6. Histamine secretion from mast cells is induced selectively by a minor component of total ATP, the tetrabasic acid ATP^{4-}.

Some responses to ATP contraction of the bladder such as contraction and relaxation of several blood vessels, relaxation of the trachea, secretion of surfactant by alveolar pneumocytes, secretion of fluid and amylase by the parotid gland, insulin secretion, and activation of liver glycogenolysis share several features (1). They are elicited by ATP and ADP (whereas AMP and adenosine are inactive), they are not inhibited by methylxanthines, and they are not associated with changes in cyclic adenosine monophosphate (cAMP) level. In 1978, Burnstock proposed that these responses were mediated by a particular subtype of receptor that he called P_2, as opposed to P_1-receptors, which interact preferentially with adenosine and of which methylxanthines are competitive antagonists (2).

The availability of several chemical analogues of ATP has led recently to a further subdivision of P_2-purinergic receptors into P_{2x} and P_{2y} (3). P_{2x} responses are characterized by the following order of potency: α, β-methylene ATP (APCPP) $\sim \beta, \gamma$-methylene ATP > ATP = 2-methylthio-ATP. The P_{2y} subtype displays a different rank order of potency: 2-methythio ATP > ATP > α, β-methylene ATP $\sim \beta, \gamma$-methylene ATP. However, the lack of a truly potent and selective antagonist has precluded a biochemical characterization of P_2-receptors by the classical methods of radioligand binding.

The physiological significance of P_2-purinoceptors has also remained elusive. Evidence has accumulated to support the role of ATP as a neurotransmitter in the central nervous system, and as a co-transmitter of noradrenaline in sympathetic nerves (4); in the guinea pig vas deferens, the phasic and tonic components of contraction are mediated respectively by ATP and noradrenaline (4). Large quantities of ATP are stored in the dense granules of platelets, from which they are released in response to aggregating agents. Studies during the past 7 years have indicated that ATP is likely to be an important mediator in the interactions between platelets and the vascular endothelium. By contrast, cultured aortic endothelial cells have proved a useful model to investigate the biochemical mechanisms coupled to P_2-purinoceptors.

ACUTE EFFECTS OF ATP ON ENDOTHELIAL CELLS

In several blood vessels, ATP produces an endothelium-dependent relaxation (3,5,6); this observation was the first indication that P_2-receptors might be present on endothelial cells. It was shown in 1983 that ATP releases prostacyclin (PGI_2), the most potent inhibitor of platelet aggregation identified so far from the endothelium of the rabbit aorta, the rabbit pulmonary artery, and the rat aorta (7). This finding was confirmed later using cultured endothelial cells from bovine (8), porcine (9), and human (10) aorta. This ATP-induced release of PGI_2 is typically a P_2-purinergic response: ADP and ATP are equiactive and equipotent, whereas AMP and adenosine are completely inactive. Further studies by Needham et al. (11) showed that the rank order of potency for various ATP analogs is consistent with the involvement of P_{2y}-receptors. The same receptors are involved in endothelium-dependent relaxation by ATP, which is mediated by the generation of nitric oxide (NO:12,13). In general, the productions of PGI_2 and NO are tightly coupled. The release of PGI_2 in response to ATP is rapid in onset (within 2 min), transient (< 10 min) and followed by a period of refractoriness to a new challenge, mainly due to a process of homologous desensitization (14). The ATP-induced release of PGI_2 results from an increased synthesis that can be explained entirely by the enhanced mobilization of free arachidonic acid.

ATP and ADP stimulate the production of PGI_2 by cultured aortic endothelial cells in the 1- to 100-μM range. Although these concentrations are high, they may still be physiological. Indeed, in the platelet-dense granules, the concentrations of ATP and ADP reach values as high as 430 mM and 650 mM, respectively. Following platelet activation by thrombin, the serum concentration of ATP rises to 12 μM, and the sum of ADP and ATP concentrations is approximately 20 μM (1). Even higher concentrations would be available locally at sites of active platelet–vessel wall interactions. Sources other than platelets such as hemolysed erythrocytes (15) and damaged endothelial cells themselves (16) could release ADP and ATP in the vicinity of the endothelium. It is therefore likely that ATP and ADP could be the physiological mediators of a negative feedback loop, which limits the extent of platelet aggregation thus helping to localize thrombus formation to areas of endothelium damage (Fig. 1).

These in vitro findings are consistent with observations that several disease states characterized by an intravascular activation of platelets are associated with an increased biosynthesis of PGI_2, which might represent a compensatory response. These pathological states include severe atherosclerosis of lower limbs (17), unstable angina, and acute myocardial infarction (18). ATP and ADP are not the only factors, generated or released during the haemostatic response, that increase vascular PGI_2. Endothelial cells convert platelet prostaglandin endoperoxides into PGI_2 (19). Thrombin increases the release of PGI_2 from human umbilical vein endothelial cells (20). Serotonin and platelet-derived growth factor produce a synergistic stimulation of PGI_2 synthesis in cultured aortic smooth muscle cells (21).

It has also been shown that ATP, and mostly its stable analogue ATPγS, stimulate the synthesis of PGI_2 in bovine aortic smooth muscle cells (22). The actions of ATP on endothelial and smooth muscle cells from the bovine

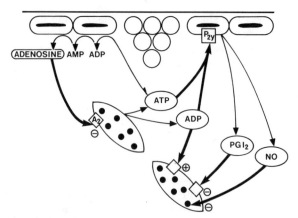

Fig. 1. Role of endothelial P_2-purinergic receptors in the interaction between platelets and a lesion of the arterial wall. During their aggregation on the site of an endothelial lesion, platelets release the content of their dense granules, including ADP and ATP. This triggers the operation of several regulatory loops: ADP recruits additional platelets; ADP is sequentially degraded by endothelial ectonucleotidases (44) into adenosine, which inhibits platelets via A_2 receptors; and ADP and ATP, co-released from platelets, activate P_{2y}-receptors on the surface of endothelial cells, resulting in the release of prostacyclin (PGI_2) and NO, which synergize to inhibit platelet aggregation.

aorta are very different. In smooth muscle cells, ADP and ADPβS have no effect and the action of ATPγS is sustained for several hours. This stimulation of PGI_2 production by ATP seems to be mediated by receptors distinct from the P_{2y}-purinoceptors involved in the release of PGI_2 from endothelial cells, as well as from the P_{2x}-purinoceptors responsible for the contraction of vascular smooth muscle. These discrepancies underscore the heterogeneity of P_2-purinergic receptors.

MITOGENIC ACTION OF ATP ON AORTIC ENDOTHELIAL CELLS

It was recently shown that, in addition to their acute effects on PGI_2 and NO release, adenine nucleotides exert a long-term mitogenic action on aortic endothelial cells (23). Bovine aortic endothelial cells were cultured for 18 h in a serum-free medium containing the various agents tested; then they were incubated in presence of ^{3}H-thymidine and the number of labelled nuclei was counted. At 10 μM, ATP, ADP, ATPγS, and ADPβS produced a significant increase in the percentage of labelled nuclei; this effect had however a smaller magnitude than that of fetal calf serum (10%). The action of ATP was mimicked by the nonhydrolysable analogue APPNP (100 μM), whereas APCPP had no effect at 10 μM and a slight effect at 100 μM. This pattern of agonist specificity is consistent with a role of P_{2y}-purinoceptors. However, adenosine (10–100 μM) also induced a mitogenic response of a magnitude comparable to that of ATP. Apparently, this response does not involve P_1-receptors, belonging to either A1 or A2 subclass. Indeed, it was not inhibited by the P_1-antagonist 8-phenyltheophylline and was reproduced neither by 5'-N-ethylcarboxamidoadenosine (NECA), an A_2 agonist, nor by L-phenylisopropyladenosine (L-PIA), an A_1 agonist, but it was mimicked by inosine and hypoxanthine.

As shown later, ATP induces several biochemical events in aortic endothelial cells, classically associated with a mitogenic action; activation of the Na^+/H^+ antiport (24), phosphorylation of 28-kD proteins (25), and release of choline from phosphatidylcholine via activation of phospholipase D (26). None of these effects is reproduced by adenosine, and the mechanism of the mitogenic action of adenosine on endothelial cells remains unclear. The mitogenic action of adenine nucleotides that we have observed in vitro suggests that in vivo, ATP, released from platelets deposited on an endothelial lesion, might promote the repair of that lesion.

BIOCHEMICAL MECHANISMS COUPLED TO THE P_2-RECEPTORS OF ENDOTHELIAL CELLS
Inositol Trisphosphate and Calcium

ADP and ATP, in the 1- to 100-μM range of concentrations, increase the formation of inositol phosphates in bovine aortic endothelial cells (27). The accumulation of inositol trisphosphate in response to adenine nucleotides is rapid (maximum at 15 sec) and transient. This material was identified as the biologically active isomer inositol 1,4,5-trisphosphate on the basis of its retention time in high-performance liquid chromatography (HPLC) on an anion-exchange resin. AMP and adenosine have no effect on inositol phosphates. The action of ATP and ADP was mimicked with an equal potency and activity by their phosphorothioate analogues, ATPγS and ADPβS, and with a lower potency by APPNP, whereas APCPP was inactive. This agonist specificity is consistent with the involvement of P_{2y}-receptors. It can be concluded that, in aortic endothelial cells, P_2-purinergic receptors of the P_{2y}-subtype are coupled to the hydrolysis of phosphatidylinositol bisphosphate by a phospholipase C. Activation of P_{2y}-receptors also increased the level of inositol phosphates in rat hepatocytes (28), capillary endothelial cells from the adrenal medulla (29), and turkey erythrocytes (30).

The use of the fluorescent Ca^{2+}-sensitive dyes, quin-2 or fura-2, has permitted the demonstration that ATP increases the cytoplasmic concentration of free Ca^{2+} in bovine and porcine aortic endothelial cells (31,32). This Ca^{2+} transient was maintained in a calcium-free medium, which is consistent with the release by inositol 1,4,5-trisphosphate of Ca^{2+} sequestered in the endoplasmic reticulum. It is likely that the release of PGI_2 (33) and NO in response to ATP is a direct consequence of this rise in cytosolic Ca^{2+}.

It was recently shown that the P_{2x}-receptor of vascular smooth muscle cells is coupled to a Ca^{2+} channel (34). Ca^{2+} is thus a second messenger of adenine nucleotides in both endothelial cells, where P_{2y}-receptors are present, and smooth muscle cells that express P_{2x}-receptors. However, the mechanism of the increase in cytosolic Ca^{2+} is different for the two receptors: an influx of extracellular Ca^{2+} through Ca^{2+} channels for the P_{2x}-subtype, a mobilization of intracellular Ca^{2+} by inositol 1,4,5-trisphosphate for the P_{2y}-subtype.

GTP-Binding Proteins

The coupling of many receptors to the hydrolysis of phosphatidylinositol bisphosphate by phospholipase C has been shown to involve GTP-binding regulatory proteins. These G-proteins seem to be heterogeneous, in particular as concerns their sensitivity to bacterial toxins. We have observed that pretreatment of bovine aortic endothelial cells with pertussis toxin produces a partial inhibition of inositol phosphate accumulation in response to ATP, whereas cholera toxin has no effect (35). This result was confirmed recently in the HL-60 human promyelocytic leukemia cell line (36). There are two explanations for the incomplete action of pertussis toxin: either the G-protein ADP-ribosylated by the toxin remains partially active or the activation of phospholipase C by P_2-receptors is mediated by both pertussis toxin-sensitive and -insensitive mechanisms. At any rate, these data strongly suggest that a G-protein is involved in the coupling of P_{2y}-receptors to phospholipase C.

Phosphorylation of Endothelial Cell Proteins

In many systems, the effects of second messengers, such as Ca^{2+}, appear to be mediated by the activation of specific proteins kinases that phosphorylate a variety of substrate proteins. Protein kinases that have been detected in extracts of bovine aortic endothelial cells include cyclic adenosine monophosphate (cAMP)-dependent kinase, calmodulin-dependent kinases II and III, and protein kinase C (37). Using mono- and bidimensional gel electrophoresis, it was demonstrated that ATP, via P_{2y}-receptors, induces or stimulates the phosphorylation of a dozen proteins in bovine aortic endothelial cells (25). These various events were mimicked by the Ca^{2+} ionophore A23187, whereas phorbol 12-myristate, 13-acetate (PMA), an activator of protein kinase C, reproduced only some of them with a slighter intensity. This suggests that the action of ATP is mostly mediated by Ca^{2+}-dependent kinases distinct from kinase C, essentially calmodulin-dependent kinases II and III.

Three major substrates are of particular interest. ATP induces the phosphorylation of a 95-kD protein, with a rapid and transient time course closely agreeing with that of the cytosolic Ca^{2+} increase. According to its molecular weight and isoelectric point, this protein appears identical to an ubiquitous substrate of calmodulin-dependent kinase III, recently identified as elongation factor-2 (38). Since phosphorylation reduces the activity of this factor, it is possible that ATP produces a transient inhibition of protein synthesis in aortic endothelial cells, although the physiological significance of such an action is unclear. ATP also stimulates the phosphorylation of a doublet of 18-kD proteins, which are probably identical to myosin light chain. This action is rapid in onset, sustained with time and emphasizes that the transient rise of cytosolic Ca^{2+} can be translated into a long-lived signal. This is probably via the autophosphorylation of calmodulin-dependent kinase II, which converts this enzyme into a permanently activated state. Finally, ATP produces a delayed and sustained stimulation of 28-kD proteins phosphorylation. The same substrates are phosphorylated in response to tumor necrosis factor-α (TNF), which does not increase cytosolic Ca^{2+} in endothelial cells; this phosphorylation actually represents the earliest biochemical event detected in response to TNF (39). These 28-kD proteins have been identified as stress proteins (39). Their phosphorylation is thus a common feature of distinct signalling pathways and might play a key role in the regulation of endothelial cell functions.

Metabolism of Choline

Hydrolysis of phosphatidylinositol bisphosphate by a phospholipase C generates two second messengers: inositol 1,4,5-trisphosphate, which releases Ca^{2+}; and diacylglycerol, which activates protein kinase C. Phosphatidylcholine represents an alternative source of intracellular mediators whereby the hydrolysis by phospholipase C releases diacylglycerol (and phosphorylcholine), while phospholipase D generates phosphatidic acid (and choline). Phosphatidic acid may be a mitogenic signal; indeed, several mitogens activate the hydrolysis of phosphatidylcholine by either phospholipase C or D. It was recently shown that ATP increases the level of choline inside bovine aortic endothelial cells and stimulates its release into the extracellular space, presumably as a result of the activation of a phospholipase D hydrolyzing phosphatidylcholine (26). This effect was abolished in endothelial cells depleted of protein kinase C by prolonged exposure to PMA. These data suggest that the following sequence of events is induced by ATP in aortic endothelial cells; the initial hydrolysis of phosphatidylinositol bisphosphate by a phospholipase C generates diacylglycerol, which stimulates protein kinase C; kinase C then activates a phospholipase D, which cleaves phosphatidylcholine into choline and phosphatidic acid. Phosphatidic acid might play a role in the mitogenic action of ATP.

K^+ Channels

ATP induces a transient increase in the efflux of ^{86}Rb from aortic endothelial cells (40). Recent electrophysiological studies have demonstrated the opening of Ca^{2+}-activated K^+ channels in ATP-stimulated endothelial cells (41). The resulting hyperpolarization might represent an important

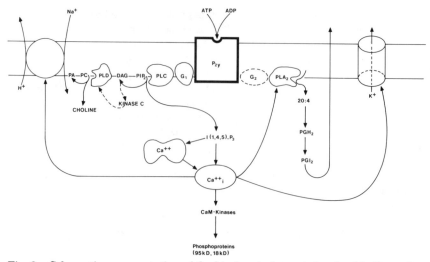

Fig. 2. Schematic representation of the biochemical events involved in the action of adenine nucleotides on aortic endothelial cells. P_{2y}-receptors are coupled, via a GTP-binding protein (G_1), to a phospholipase C (PLC), which hydrolyzes phosphatidylinositol bisphosphate (PIP_2) into inositol trisphosphate [$I(1,4,5)-P_3$] and diacylglycerol (DAG). $I(1,4,5)-P_3$ releases Ca^{2+} from the endoplasmic reticulum, while DAG activates protein kinase C. The increase in cytosolic Ca^{2+} activates several processes: phosphorylation of specific proteins by calmodulin-dependent kinases (Ca M-kinases), mobilization of free arachidonic acid (20:4) by a phospholipase A_2 (PLA_2), resulting in an enhanced synthesis and release of prostacyclin (PGI_2), efflux of K^+ through Ca^{2+}-activated K^+ channels, cytoplasmic alkalinization mediated by a Na^+/H^+ antiport. The increased activity of a phospholipase D (PLD), hydrolyzing phosphatidylcholine (PC) into phosphatidic acid (PA) and choline, is likely to result from the stimulation of kinase C. A direct coupling between the P_{2y}-receptors and phospholipase A_2, via a specific GTP-binding protein (G_2), remains hypothetical.

signal. Indeed, the earliest event induced by haemodynamic shear stress in endothelial cells is the activation of a specific K^+ current (42). It has been speculated that the hyperpolarization caused either by ATP and other agonists, or by shear stress, might play a role in endothelium-dependent relaxation, either by direct junctional conductance to smooth muscle cells or by stimulating the endothelial cells themselves to release NO or PGI_2. However, the insensitivity of PGI_2 release to changes in endothelial membrane potential argues against this last hypothesis (43).

CONCLUSION

ATP and ADP stimulate the release of prostacyclin from aortic endothelial cells and increase their rate of proliferation. These two actions might have a physiological importance in the interaction between platelets, a rich source of adenine nucleotides, and the vascular endothelium (see Fig. 1). The release of PGI_2 will limit the extent of platelet aggregation following a lesion of the endothelium, while the mitogenic effect will accelerate the repair of that lesion.

It is now established that P_{2y}-receptors of ATP and ADP in aortic endothelial cells are coupled to a phospholipase C by a GTP-binding protein (Fig. 2). The rise of cytoplasmic Ca^{2+} that results from this initial event mediates several effects of ATP and ADP. The direct activation of a Ca^{2+}-sensitive phospholipase A_2 can explain the increased synthesis of PGI_2, while the phosphorylation of several proteins by calmodulin-dependent kinases will modulate other endothelial cell functions.

REFERENCES

1. Gordon JL. Extracellular ATP: Effects, sources and fate. Biochem J 1986;233: 309–319.
2. Burnstock G. A basis for distinguishing two types of purinergic receptor. In: Straub RW, Bolis L, eds. Cell Membrane Receptors for Drugs and Hormones. A Multi-disciplinary Approach. New York: Raven Press, 1978;107–118.
3. Burnstock G, Kennedy C. A dual function for ATP in the regulation of vascular tone. Circ Res 1986;58:319–330.
4. Sneddon P, Westfall DP, Fedan JD. Cotransmitters in the motor nerves of the guinea pig vas deferens: Electrophysiological evidence. Science 1982;218:693–695.
5. De Mey JG, Vanhoutte PM. Role of the intima in cholinergic and purinergic relaxation of isolated canine femoral arteries. J Physiol (Lond) 1981;316:347–355.
6. Furchgott RF. The requirement of endothelial cells in the relaxation of arteries by acetylcholine and some other vasodilators. Trends Pharmacol Sci 1981;2: 173–176.
7. Boeynaems JM, Galand N. Stimulation of vascular prostacyclin synthesis by extracellular ADP and ATP. Biochem Biophys Res Commun 1983;112:290–296.
8. Van Coevorden A, Boeynaems JM. Physiological concentrations of ADP stimulate the release of prostacyclin from bovine aortic endothelial cells. Prostaglandins 1984;27:615–626.
9. Pearson JD, Slakey LL, Gordon JL. Stimulation of prostaglandin production through purinoceptors on cultured porcine endothelial cells. Biochem J 1983; 214:273–276.
10. Boeynaems JM, Pirotton S, Van Coevorden A, Raspe E, Demolle D, Erneux C. P_2-purinergic receptors in vascular endothelial cells: From concept to reality. J Receptor Res 1988;8:121–132.
11. Needham L, Cusack NJ, Pearson JD, Gordon JL. Characteristics of the P2 purinoceptor that mediates prostacyclin production by pig aortic endothelial cells. Eur J Pharmacol 1987;134:199–209.
12. Palmer RMJ, Ashton DS, Moncada S. Vascular endothelial cells synthesize nitric oxide from L-arginine. Nature (Lond) 1988;333:664–666.
13. Kelm M, Feelisch M, Spahr R, Piper HM, Noak E, Schrader J. Quantitative and kinetic characterization of nitric oxide and EDRF released from cultured endothelial cells. Biochem Biophys Res Commun 1988;154:236–244.

14. Toothill, VJ, Needham L, Gordon JL, Pearson JD. Desensitization of agonist-stimulated prostacyclin release in human umbilical vein endothelial cells. Eur J Pharmacol 1988;157:189–196.

15. Born GVR, Wehmeier A. Inhibition of platelet thrombus formation by chlorpromazine acting to diminish haemolysis. Nature (Lond) 1979;282:212–213.

16. Pearson JD, Gordon JL. Vascular endothelial and smooth muscle cells in culture selectively release adenine nucleotides. Nature (Lond) 1979;281:384–386.

17. FitzGerald GA, Smith B, Pedersen AK, Brash AR. Increased prostacyclin biosynthesis in patients with severe atherosclerosis and platelet activation. N Engl J Med 1984;310:1065–1068.

18. Fitzgerald DJ, Roy L, Catella F, FitzGerald GA. Platelet activation in unstable coronary disease. N Engl J Med 1986;315:983–989.

19. Marcus AJ, Weksler BB, Jaffe EA, Broekman MJ. Synthesis of prostacyclin from platelet-derived endoperoxides by cultured human endothelial cells. J Clin Invest 1980;66:979–986.

20. Weksler BN, Ley CW, Jaffe EA. Stimulation of endothelial cell PGI_2 production by thrombin, trypsin and the ionophore A23187. J Clin Invest 1976;62:923–930.

21. Coughlin SR, Moskowitz MA, Antoniades HN, Levin L. Serotonin receptor-mediated stimulation of bovine smooth muscle cell prostacyclin synthesis and its modulation by platelet-derived growth factor. Proc Natl Acad Sci USA 1981;78:7134–7138.

22. Demolle D, Lagneau C, Boeynaems JM. Stimulation of prostacyclin release from aortic smooth muscle cells by purine and pyrimidine nucleotides. Eur J Pharmacol 1988;155:339–343.

23. Van Coevorden A, Roger P, Boeynaems JM. Mitogenic action of adenine nucleotides and nucleosides on aortic endothelial cells. Thromb Haemost 1989;62:190.

24. Kitazono T, Takeshige K, Cragoe EJ, Minakami S. Intracellular pH changes of cultured bovine aortic endothelial cells in response to ATP addition. Biochem Biophys Res Commun 1988;152:1304–1309.

25. Demolle D, Lecomte M, Boeynaems JM. Pattern of protein phosphorylation in aortic endothelial cells: Modulation by adenine nucleotides and bradykinin. J Biol Chem 1988;263:18459–18465.

26. Pirotton S, Robaye B, Lagneau C, Boeynaems JM. Adenine nucleotides modulate phosphatidylcholine metabolism in aortic endothelial cells. J Cell Physiol 1990;142:449–457.

27. Pirotton S, Raspe E, Demolle D, Erneux C, Boeynaems JM. Involvement of inositol (1,4,5) trisphosphate and calcium in the action of adenine nucleotides on aortic endothelial cells. J Biol Chem 1987;262:17461–17469.

28. Charest R, Blackmore PF, Exton JM. Characterization of responses of isolated rat hepatocytes to ATP and ADP. J Biol Chem 1985;260:15789–15794.

29. Forsberg EJ, Feuerstein G, Shohami E, Pollard HB. Adenosine triphosphate stimulates inositol phospholipid metabolism and prostacyclin formation in adrenal medullary endothelial cells by means of P_2-purinergic receptors. Proc Natl Acad Sci USA 1987;84:5630–5634.

30. Berrie CP, Hawkins PT, Stephens LR, Harden TK, Downes CP. Phosphatidylinositol 4,5-bisphosphate hydrolysis in turkey erythrocytes is regulated by P_{2y} receptors. J Pharmacol Exp Ther 1989;35:526–532.

31. Luckoff A, Busse R. Increased free calcium in endothelial cells under stimulation with adenine nucleotides. J Cell Physiol 1986;126:414–420.
32. Hallam TJ, Pearson JD. Exogenous ATP raises cytoplasmic free calcium in fura-2 loaded piglet aortic endothelial cells. FEBS Lett 1986;207:95–99.
33. Carter TD, Hallam TJ, Cusack NJ, Pearson JD. Regulation of P_{2y}-purinoceptor-mediated prostacyclin release from human endothelial cells by cytoplasmic calcium concentration. Br J Pharmacol 1988;95:1181–1190.
34. Benham CD, Tsien RW. A novel receptor operated Ca^{2+}-permeable channel activated by ATP in smooth muscle. Nature (Lond) 1987;328:275–278.
35. Pirotton S, Erneux C, Boeynaems JM. Dual role of GTP-binding proteins in the control of endothelial prostacyclin. Biochem Biophys Res Commun 1987;147: 1113–1120.
36. Dubyak GR, Cowen DS, Meuller LM. Activation of inositol phospholipid breakdown in HL60 cells by P_2-purinergic receptors for extracellular ATP. J Biol Chem 1988;263:18108–18117.
37. Mackie K, Lay Y, Nairn AC, Greengard P, Pitt B, Lazo JS. Protein phosphorylation in cultured endothelial cells. J Cell Physiol 1986;128:367–374.
38. Mackie KP, Nairn AC, Hampel G, Lam G, Jaffe EA. Thrombin and histamine stimulate the phosphorylation of elongation factor 2 in human umbilical vein endothelial cells. J Biol Chem 1989;264:1748–1753.
39. Robaye B, Hepburn A, Lecocq R, Fiers W, Boeynaems JM, Dumont JE. Tumor Necrosis Factor-α induces the phosphorylation of 28 kDa stress proteins in endothelial cells: Possible role in protection against cytotoxicity. Biochem Biophys Res Commun 1989;163:301–308.
40. Gordon JL, Martin W. Endothelium-dependent relaxation of the pig aorta: Relationship to stimulation of ^{86}Rb efflux from isolated endothelial cells. Br J Pharmacol 1983;79:531–541.
41. Sauve R, Parent L, Simoneau C, Roy G. External ATP triggers a biphasic activation process of a calcium-dependent K^+ channel in cultured bovine aortic endothelial cells. Pflugers Arch. 1988;412:469–481.
42. Olesen SP, Clapham DE, Davies FF. Haemodynamic shear stress activates a K^+ current in vascular endothelial cells. Nature (Lond):1988;331:168–171.
43. Boeynaems JM, Ramboer I. Effects of changes in extra- and intracellular K^+ on the endothelial production of prostacyclin. Br J Pharmacol 1989;98:966–972.
44. Pearson, JD, Gordon, JL. Nucleotide metabolism by endothelium. Annu Rev Physiol 1985;47:617–627.

The Endothelium: An Introduction to Current Research, pages 65–80
© 1990 Wiley-Liss, Inc.

7

Circulating and Tissue Renin-Angiotensin Systems: The Role of the Endothelium

DAVID J. WEBB AND JOHN R. COCKCROFT

Department of Pharmacology and Clinical Pharmacology, St George's Hospital Medical School, London SW17 0RE, England (D.J.W.); Department of Clinical Pharmacology, RPMS, Hammersmith Hospital, London W12 0NN, England (J.R.C.)

INTRODUCTION

In 1898, Tigerstedt and Bergman (1) established a role for the kidney in blood pressure regulation. They showed that intravenous injection of an extract of rabbit kidney produced hypertension in dogs and named the pressor component of this extract renin. Elegant experiments by Goldblatt and colleagues (2) confirmed the contribution of the kidney to blood pressure control, demonstrating renal renin release, and the development of hypertension, in response to renal ischaemia in dogs. Subsequently, autonomic and humoral mechanisms have also been shown to contribute to the regulation of renal renin release (3). Although Goldblatt's experiments demonstrated a relationship between renin and hypertension, it soon became clear that the presence of plasma was necessary for the pressor activity of renin (4). This was subsequently explained, in 1940, when it was shown (5,6) that renin is not directly pressor but, through its action as a proteolytic enzyme, raises blood pressure indirectly, via generation of a pressor peptide, from a plasma substrate, angiotensinogen.

Two potent and short-acting pressor peptides, a decapeptide and an octapeptide (7), subsequently identified as angiotensin I and angiotensin II, were isolated following the incubation of renin with plasma. The later discovery of an enzyme (converting enzyme), which converts angiotensin I to angiotensin II (8), led to the widely held belief that this conversion occurred mainly in circulating blood. This belief was strengthened by the observation, in isolated vascular strips, that angiotensin I was incapable of producing contraction while angiotensin II remained active (9). However, at this time, the importance of the preservation of endothelium for the action of converting enzyme was not fully appreciated. Indeed, contraction to angiotensin I in rabbit aortic rings has since been shown to be endothelium dependent (10), and vasoconstriction to angiotensin I is present in experiments with the saline-perfused, blood-free dog hindquarters, where the endothelium is likely to be intact (11). Such early experiments stimulated further research, leading to the demonstration, by Ng and Vane (12), of conversion of angiotensin I to angiotensin II across the pulmonary vascular bed. As angiotensin II is generated only slowly in blood, they concluded that the lung is the principal site of angiotensin II production.

These experiments led to the classical view of the circulating renin-angiotensin system (13,14), with renal release of renin, in response to a variety of stimuli, leading to generation of angiotensin I from its circulating plasma substrate, angiotensinogen. Subsequent generation of the pressor peptide angiotensin II was thought to occur across the pulmonary circulation. The role of renally released renin, acting on plasma angiotensinogen, in the maintenance of plasma angiotensin II, is supported by the hypotensive action of angiotensinogen antibodies (15), and by the marked fall in circulating renin and angiotensin II levels following nephrectomy (16).

However, during the 1960s, renin-like activity was detected in blood vessel walls (17), and in cross-circulation studies the prolonged pressor response of a nephrectomised rat to exogenous renin was not associated with a prolonged persistence of renin in the blood (18). Furthermore, large amounts of the angiotensin receptor antagonist, saralasin, are needed to block the effects of endogenous angiotensin II in the rat, although to antagonise the effect of exogenous, infused peptide only relatively small amounts are sufficient (19). These findings suggest that there is a site of endogenous generation of angiotensin II, which is inaccessible to a plasma-borne inhibitor. Taken together, these findings led to speculation that renin might play a role in regulation of vascular tone through mechanisms other than plasma generation of angiotensin II and drew attention to a wider role for renin in extrarenal tissues.

TISSUE RENIN-ANGIOTENSIN SYSTEMS
Evidence for a Vascular Renin-Angiotensin System

Renin-like enzymes have now been detected in a number of tissues, including the walls of arteries (20,21) and veins (22), the brain (23), and the adrenal gland (24). This review focuses primarily on vessel wall renin. Although renin-like enzymes have been detected in blood vessel walls, it is not clear whether these enzymes are indeed true renin, as other tissue-located enzymes have the capacity to generate angiotensin II from substrate (25–27). This has since been resolved using renin-specific monoclonal antibodies which show that blood vessels do, indeed, contain true renin (28,29). In the aorta and large vessels, renin is found in the entire thickness of the vessel wall, though particularly in the intima, the outer part of the medial muscular layer, and in the peri-adventitial region. The peri-adventitial staining for renin is pronounced around noradrenergic nerve endings and the vaso vasorae. Smaller blood vessels show uniform staining, and staining is found in the smooth muscle layer of veins.

If, as appears the case, true renin exists in extra-renal tissues, it may be generated locally, or may be taken up from plasma at extra-renal sites (19). Here, we provide evidence that true renin is generated locally within the walls of peripheral blood vessels, as well as in other tissues, rather than derived from plasma (Fig. 1).

Tissue Culture

Evidence in support of local generation of renin is provided by demonstration of renin synthesis in studies with cultured cells. Specific renin immunoreactivity has been detected in cultures of both vascular smooth

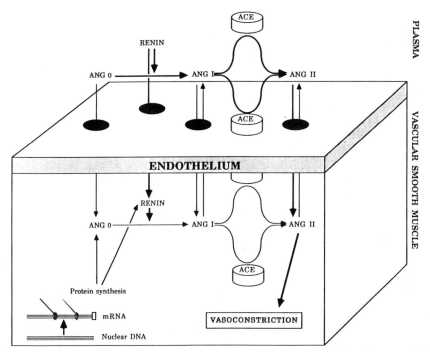

Fig. 1. Proven *(wide lines; large arrows)* and putative pathways *(fine lines; small arrows)* for generation of angiotensin II within peripheral blood vessels. Pathways for conversion of angiotensinogen (ANG 0) to angiotensin I (ANG I) and for subsequent generation of angiotensin II (ANG II) by the action of plasma and tissue-located angiotensin converting enzyme (ACE) are shown.

muscle (30) and vascular endothelium (31). Evidence also exists for the synthesis of both angiotensinogen (32) and converting enzyme (33) by human vascular endothelial and smooth muscle cells.

Molecular Biology

Advances in molecular biology have provided the most convincing evidence for the existence of functional renin-angiotensin systems in extrarenal tissue. Renin-like mRNA has been demonstrated in extrarenal tissue in animals (34–36) and in human subjects (28). However, the most important advance has been the sequencing of the renin gene itself (37–39), which has provided convincing evidence for functional renin-angiotensin systems in the peripheral vasculature (40). The renin gene has three major promotor elements on which the action of RNA polymerase yields as many as 4 different renin precursors. The major promotor is found predominantly in the human kidney (41) and produces a renin precursor with a hydrophobic N-terminal leader sequence, thus facilitating its entry to the endoplasmic reticulum of the cell prior to secretion to the exterior. However, a second promotor region yields a renin precursor with a hydrophilic N-terminal leader sequence (42), thus preventing its entry to the endoplasmic reticulum. Renin produced from this promotor region would not be secreted and might have an intracellular role. The third promotor region can yield renin precursors with either hydrophobic or hydrophilic leader sequences (43). The ability to secrete renin appears to be limited to the juxtaglomerular cells, so the renin generated by extrarenal tissues may well remain at an intracellular level generating angiotensin I, which is then converted to angiotensin II by the action of endothelially located converting enzyme (44). It is, however, possible that angiotensin II may be generated intracellularly, as it has been found in secretory granules from juxtaglomerular cells (45). It has, however, been suggested that this intragranular angiotensin II may have an extracellular origin (46) (Fig. 1).

In addition to the evidence for local renin generation, there is also evidence for the presence of angiotensinogen within blood vessel walls (47). Furthermore, there are data showing that the angiotensinogen gene is expressed in a number of tissues other than liver, including brain (48), kidney (49), and blood vessels (50). The co-localisation of renin, and its substrate, within the blood vessel wall allows for the possibility that angiotensin II may be generated locally.

Physiological Role of the Vascular Renin-Angiotensin System

In the case of the tissue renin-angiotensin systems of brain and adrenal, there is evidence to suggest that regulation may be independent of changes in circulating renin (51) and may thus play an independent role in regulation of cardiovascular physiology. This may also be the case with vascular renin, though in many experimental models vascular renin appears to correlate relatively closely with plasma renin, except in non-steady-state situations (52), for example, immediately following nephrectomy. However, the techniques for measuring vascular renin are relatively insensitive and, using techniques involving measurement of mRNA, it appears that renin expression in some tissues, such as brain and liver, is not regulated by changes in salt intake in the same manner as kidney mRNA. There is no equivalent evidence for vascular renin.

Experiments using both animal (53) and human resistance vessels (54) show that these vessels have the capacity to generate angiotensin II from tetradecapeptide renin substrate, and that this effect can be blocked by specific renin inhibitors (55). These findings suggest that vascular renin, regardless of source, may play a role in the regulation of peripheral vascular tone. Further indirect evidence of a role for vascular renin in maintenance of vascular tone comes from experiments in animals and human subjects, in which hypotensive responses to the inhibition of converting enzyme (56) or renin (57,58) do not parallel the changes in plasma renin. It is also widely recognised that converting enzyme inhibitors may produce major reduction of blood pressure in hypertensive patients, even when plasma renin activity is normal or suppressed (59). However, under these circumstances, other extrarenal sources of renin may also be involved.

Vascular renin could influence local vascular tone in a variety of ways. Locally generated angiotensin II may contribute directly to tone within vascular smooth muscle. It might also be ideally situated for modulation of peripheral sympathetic neurotransmission. Indeed, it has been suggested that isoprenaline-induced β-mediated facilitation of noradrenergic neurotransmission may act by local release of angiotensin II, which in turn increases noradrenaline release from sympathetic nerve terminals (44). Locally released angiotensin II may also play an important role as a local vascular growth factor (60).

ENDOTHELIALLY LOCATED ACE
Studies in Animals and In Vitro Preparations

In their experiments, Ng and Vane (12) showed that the rate of conversion of angiotensin I to angiotensin II in blood proceeds at too slow a rate to account for the rapid onset of the pressor effect associated with systemic infusion of the decapeptide. Using organ superfusion bioassay techniques to estimate generation of angiotensin II, they concluded that approximately 80% of an intravenous dose of angiotensin I was converted in a single passage through the pulmonary vascular bed of the dog.

Following this work, studies in a number of species, both in intact animals and in isolated lung preparations have confirmed that the pulmonary vascular bed is a major site of angiotensin I conversion (61–63); indeed, isolated pulmonary arteries appear to convert angiotensin I more readily than arteries from other sites (64). However, bioassay methods may underestimate the contribution of peripheral tissues to angiotensin conversion, as the lung appears to be the only tissue that does not possess angiotensinases (62). The strong evidence for pulmonary conversion drew attention away from other possibly important sites of angiotensin conversion, although an early study using the systemic pressor response as a measure of angiotensin I conversion, suggested that peripheral vascular conversion might be of greater importance (65). A number of studies have demonstrated conversion of angiotensin I to angiotensin II in vascular beds other than the lung; these include the peripheral vascular (11,65), renal (11,66), splanchnic (67), and coronary circulations (68).

Angiotensin converting enzyme is a ubiquitous enzyme, found in plasma, and occurring as a membrane-bound ectoenzyme predominantly on endothelial and epithelial cells (69–72). Confirmation of these sites of localisation has been provided by both immunohistochemical and in vitro autoradiographic techniques, with the latter using converting enzyme inhibitors as the radioligand (73). Although this enzyme is found predominantly on the luminal surface of the vascular endothelium (74) and is not found in endothelial cell cytoplasm (75), some converting enzyme activity has been demonstrated within the tunica media and adventitia of blood vessels (76). This indirect evidence for the presence of converting enzyme in vascular smooth muscle is supported by studies with [^{3}H]captopril, in which specific binding is found in the intima and adventitia of vascular smooth muscle, with little binding in the media. However, different lines of evidence are conflicting, and a report that the enzyme located in the adventitial layer in vascular smooth muscle (76) is insensitive to inhibition with the converting enzyme inhibitors captopril and ramipril, suggests that this enzyme may not be identical with the classical converting enzyme of the intimal endothelium.

The role of the endothelium in regulating responses to angiotensin I has been investigated directly. Saye and colleagues (10) studied the conversion of angiotensin I to II in rabbit aortic rings, and showed that both contractions to angiotensin I, and generation of angiotensin II, were initially attenuated by disruption of the endothelium. Responses to angiotensin I, either with or without endothelium, were inhibited by pretreatment with the converting enzyme inhibitor teprotide. Generation of angiotensin II, albeit slow, did, however, occur after de-endothelialisation, suggesting that the aortic smooth muscle does contain some converting enzyme activity. These experiments are open to the criticism that residual converting enzyme activity, present after de-endothelialisation, may be located on the endothelial surface of the vasa vasorae rather than within vascular smooth muscle. In order to overcome this problem, Pipili and colleagues (77) repeated these experiments, denuding the vessels using either infusion of deoxycholate or gentle endothelial scraping, and found that de-endothelialisation produced a 30% reduction in enzyme activity, with the remaining activity captopril sensitive. They suggest that residual activity is within vascular smooth muscle, and in these circumstances the enzyme cannot be the converting enzyme inhibitor-insensitive enzyme detected in the adventitia (76). In these experiments, the evidence for complete removal of the endothelium is presumed from the absence of relaxation to infused acetylcholine (78). It is possible, however, that the methods used here to disrupt endothelial cells interfere with the functional pathway for endothelium-dependent vasodilatation, but do not entirely remove endothelial plasma membrane-bound converting enzyme. The evidence that converting enzyme exists in the vascular smooth muscle, and that it has sufficient activity to have a physiological role in angiotensin II generation, remains inconclusive.

Relatively little is known about the regulation of vascular converting enzyme activity. A marked reduction in aortic converting enzyme activity has been reported (79) following a 4-week period of sodium loading in spontaneously hypertensive rats (SHR), suggesting that vascular converting enzyme activity may play a role in the regulation of vascular tone. Interestingly, this manoeuvre increased converting enzyme activity in the rat midbrain, suggesting independent regulation of vascular and midbrain converting enzyme activity. By contrast, other workers were unable to demonstrate consistent changes in rat aortic converting enzyme activity across a wide range of sodium intakes (80). Vascular converting enzyme has, however, been shown to increase after experimental induction of hypertension in dogs (81) and rats (82) and to be increased in SHR compared with Wistar Kyoto rats (83,84). Interestingly, this increase correlates with blood pressure throughout the development of hypertension in SHR. Glucocorticoids (85) and vascular growth factors (86) have been shown to stimulate converting enzyme activity in cultured endothelial cells from the bovine aorta, raising the possibility that peripheral vascular angiotensin II generation may be controlled by humoral factors, through regulation of tissue converting enzyme activity. Finally, in rat aortic tissue the ratio of angiotensin I to II is much higher than in plasma (22), from which it has been concluded that angiotensin I is generated locally within vascular tissue. Moreover, the relatively high ratio of angiotensin I to angiotensin II in this vascular tissue suggests that the activity of vascular converting enzyme may be a rate-limiting step in local vascular angiotensin II generation. Proven and putative pathways for generation of angiotensin II within plasma and vascular tissue are shown in Figure 1.

Studies in Man

Studies using the systemic pressor response to angiotensin I as a measure of pulmonary conversion, suggest a lesser degree of pulmonary conversion (0–40%) (87,88) in humans than in most of the animal studies, although this method only demonstrates pulmonary conversion in situations where peripheral conversion is less than complete. Further evidence for a lesser degree of conversion across the lung, in man, is provided by studies measuring plasma angiotensin I and angiotensin II concentrations in the main pulmonary artery and left ventricle of subjects undergoing diagnostic cardiac catheterisation (89,90). In both studies, angiotensin I conversion was rather less substantial than in earlier animal studies, with pulmonary conversion being in the order of 30%. Furthermore, in subjects on cardiopulmonary bypass, circulating levels of angiotensin II are appropriate for the prevailing plasma renin activity (91), suggesting that there is substantial capacity for peripheral angiotensin I conversion when the lung is temporarily disconnected from the systemic vascular circuit.

Measurements of angiotensin I have been made in plasma drawn from arterial and venous blood, from both animals (92) and human subjects (93). On the basis of rates for conversion and inactivation of angiotensin I by the peripheral blood vessels, it has been concluded that there must be substantial production of angiotensin I by peripheral tissues (94). Using estimates for angiotensin I conversion in peripheral tissues, and known rates for inactivation of infused angiotensin I, a model for angiotensin production has been developed (94). This model suggests that the vast majority of angiotensin I in venous blood (80–90%) is derived from local production in peripheral tissues. A similar model for angiotensin II suggests that most of the active peptide is also generated in peripheral vessels. More direct evidence in support of this hypothesis has recently been obtained from studies in man, where measurements of arteriovenous differences for angiotensin I in a variety of vascular beds have been made during systemic infusion of radiolabelled (^{125}I) angiotensin I (95). There is marked clearance of the radio-labelled peptide in peripheral vessels, though measured arteriovenous differences for angiotensin I are small. These studies suggest that substantial amounts of the angiotensin I in venous blood draining peripheral vascular beds are generated locally.

Further confirmation of substantial converting enzyme activity in peripheral blood vessels in man has been obtained in studies with local infusion of angiotensin I into dorsal hand veins. Here, it has been shown that local angiotensin I, but not angiotensin II, induced venoconstriction is markedly attenuated by local infusion of the nonapeptide converting enzyme inhibitor, teprotide. This strongly suggests the presence of converting enzyme activity in limb veins in man (96). Whether this converting enzyme activity is also present in peripheral arterial vessels in man was not resolved at this time, although it was inferred from the local vasoconstriction associated with intra-arterial infusion of angiotensin I into the forearm circulation (96).

In studies in man, in whom peptides have been infused into the brachial artery, both angiotensin I and II have been shown to produce dose-dependent reductions in forearm blood flow (96–98). Recent studies show that co-infusion of a converting enzyme inhibitor markedly reduces responses to angiotensin I, such that 100-fold greater doses are required to produce an equivalent reduction in local blood flow to that achieved in the absence of converting enzyme inhibition (97,98); however, responses to angiotensin II are unchanged (Fig. 2). These findings confirm the conclusion of Ng and Vane (12) that vasoconstriction to angiotensin I is mediated through generation of angiotensin II.

Conversion of angiotensin I to angiotensin II occurs only slowly in blood in vitro (12) compared with the transit time of the forearm arterial circulation in vivo. Thus the conversion of angiotensin I to II following local intra-arterial infusion is likely to be an effect of the endothelially located enzyme (see Fig. 1). Furthermore, in experiments in which infusion of the converting enzyme inhibitor was stopped, but infusion of angiotensin I continued, redevelopment of angiotensin I induced vasoconstriction was markedly delayed as compared with the development of the maximal response to infusion of angiotensin I alone (20 mm compared with 2 min). Inhibition of plasma converting enzyme cannot account for this response, as plasma-bound inhibitor is rapidly cleared from the forearm, and it is presumably mediated by inhibition of the endothelially located enzyme. Other enzymes may generate angiotensin II from angiotensin I in vitro (22). However, these experiments show that substantial generation of angiotensin II from angiotensin I by other enzymes is unlikely to occur in vivo, as the response to angiotensin I is so markedly attenuated by inhibition of converting enzyme.

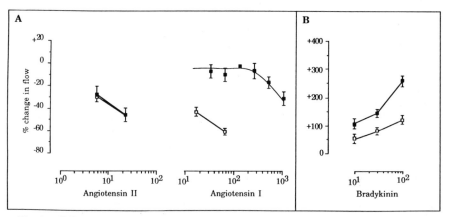

Fig. 2. Effect of intra-arterial infusion of angiotensin II and angiotensin I (**A**) and bradykinin (**B**) on forearm blood flow in the absence (open symbols) and presence (closed symbols) of local infusion of the converting enzyme inhibitor enalaprilat. Reproduced from Benjamin et al. (98), with permission of the Physiological Society.

In the absence of local converting enzyme inhibition the potency of angiotensin I, on a molar basis, is only slightly less than that of angiotensin II. This implies substantial conversion of angiotensin I to angiotensin II within a single passage through the arterial side of the forearm circulation. Indeed, the degree of conversion across the forearm (40%) is at least as great as that across the pulmonary circulation in man (30%) (89,90). Thus peripheral vascular beds in man are capable of substantial generation of circulating angiotensin II.

The action of converting enzyme is nonspecific, catalysing the release of carboxy-terminal dipeptides from a variety of peptide substrates. Converting enzyme degrades the vasodilator peptide bradykinin to inactive fragments (99). When bradykinin is infused into the forearm of man, via the brachial artery, it produces a dose dependent increase in local blood flow. If accompanied by co-infusion of a converting enzyme inhibitor, there is a substantial increase in the vasodilatation to bradykinin (98), suggesting a role for endothelially located converting enzyme in its degradation in the human forearm (Fig. 2). Kininase I and other proteolytic enzymes (100) provide an important alternative route for bradykinin metabolism in vitro. By contrast, this does not appear to be the case for arterially administered bradykinin in the human peripheral circulation. This difference may reflect the endothelial location of the enzyme (74), which is presumably particularly favourable for the metabolism of intravascular peptides. It is possible that one function of endothelially located converting enzyme is to prevent kinins, formed in the blood, from diffusing into tissues. This could have pathophysiological importance in disorders in which intravascular kinin concentrations may be increased, such as diffuse intravascular coagulation, septicaemia and hereditary angio-oedema.

In healthy sodium replete subjects, intra-arterial infusion of the converting enzyme inhibitor enalaprilat into the forearm circulation had no effect on local blood flow (98), whereas in the same subjects, when sodium depleted, there was a small but significant increase in local blood flow (101). In a further group of normotensive and hypertensive subjects, using another converting enzyme inhibitor, ramiprilat, intra-arterial infusion of the inhibitor did not affect local blood flow, but individual changes in blood flow correlated significantly with the prevailing plasma renin concentration (97). Overall, local converting enzyme inhibition appears to have a relatively small effect in the forearm resistance vessels in man.

In view of the evidence suggesting that there is substantial angiotensin generation across a number of vascular beds in man (94,95), a lack of any major effect of local converting enzyme inhibition on forearm blood flow is, perhaps, unexpected. It appears to suggest that angiotensin II is not generated to any significant degree within this particular vascular bed, unless produced at a site distal to the resistance vessels. Alternatively, angiotensin II may be generated by an enzyme other than the converting enzyme

(22), or at a site that is inaccessible to the converting enzyme inhibitors employed in these experiments (102). In the future, evidence of a role for local tissue generation of angiotensin within blood vessels in man may be obtained with the development of tissue-specific converting enzyme inhibitors (102) or by the use of specific renin inhibitors, the action of which may depend, in part, on inhibition of tissue renin (58,103). Until these issues are resolved, the role of vascular angiotensin generation in hypertension and other vascular diseases remains unclear.

REFERENCES

1. Tigerstedt R, Bergman PG. Niere und Kreislauf. Skand Ark Physiol 1898;8: 223–272.
2. Goldblatt H, Lynch J, Hanzal RF, Summerville WW. Studies on experimental hypertension I. The production of persistent elevation of systolic blood pressure by means of renal ischemia. J Exp Med 1934;59:347–379.
3. Vander AJ. Control of renin release. Physiol Rev 1967;47:359–382.
4. Kohlstaedt KG, Helmer OM, Page IH. Activation of renin by blood colloids. Proc Soc Exp Biol 1938;39:214–215.
5. Braun-Menendez E, Fasciolo JC, Leloir LF, Munoz JM. The substance causing renal hypertension. J Physiol (Lond) 1940;98:283–298.
6. Page IH, Helmer OM. A crystalline pressor substance (angiotonin) resulting from the reaction between renin and renin activator. J Exp Med 1940;71:29–42.
7. Skeggs LT, Marsh WH, Kahn JR, Shumway WP. The existence of two forms of hypertensin. J Exp Med 1954;99:275–282.
8. Skeggs LT, Kahn JR, Shumway NP. The preparation and function of the hypertensin converting enzyme. J Exp Med 1956;103:295–299.
9. Helmer OM. Differentiation between two forms of angiotonin by means of spirally cut strips of rabbit aorta. Am J Physiol 1957;188:571–577.
10. Saye JA, Singer HA, Peach MJ. Role of endothelium in conversion of angiotensin I to angiotensin II in rabbit aorta. Hypertension 1984;6:216–221.
11. Aiken JW, Vane JR. Inhibition by converting enzyme of the renin angiotensin system in kidneys and hind legs of dogs. Circ Res 1972;30:263–273.
12. Ng KKF, Vane JR. Fate of angiotensin I in the circulation. Nature (Lond) 1968;218:144–150.
13. Peart WS. The renin-angiotensin system. Pharmacol Rev 1965;17:140–182.
14. Peach MJ. Renin-angiotensin system: Biochemistry and mechanisms of action. Physiol Rev 1977;57:313–370.
15. Gardes J, Bouhnick J, Clauser E, Corvol P, Ménard J. Role of angiotensinogen in blood pressure homeostasis. Hypertension 1982;4:185–189.
16. Medina A, Bell PRF, Briggs JD, Brown JJ, Fine A, Lever AF, Morton JJ, Paton AM, Robertson JIS, Tree M, Waite MA, Weir R, Winchester J. Changes of blood pressure, renin, and angiotensin after bilateral nephrectomy in patients with chronic renal failure. Brit Med J 1972;4:694–696.
17. Gould AB, Skeggs LT, Kahn JR. The presence of renin activity in blood vessel walls. J Exp Med 1964;119:389–399.
18. Schaechtelin G, Regoli D, Gross F. Quantitative assay and disappearance rate of circulating renin. Am J Physiol 1964;206:1361–1364.

19. Swales JD. Arterial wall or plasma renin in hypertension? Clin Sci 1979;56:293–298.
20. Ganten D, Hermann K, Unger T, Lang RE. The tissue renin-angiotensin systems: Focus on brain angiotensin, adrenal gland and arterial wall. Clin Exp Hypertension 1983;5:1099–1118.
21. Swales JD, Loudon M, Bing RF, Thurston H. Renin in the arterial wall. Clin Exp Hypertension 1983;5:1127–1136.
22. Rosenthal JH, Pfiefle B, Michailov ML, Pschorr J, Jacob ICM, Dahlheim H. Investigations of components of the renin-angiotensin system in rat vascular tissue. Hypertension 1984;6:383–390.
23. Inagami T, Clemens T, Hirose S, Okamura T, Naruse K, Takii Y, Yokasawa H. Brain renin. Clin Exp Hypertension 1982;4:607–622.
24. Naruse M, Sussman CR, Naruse K, Jackson RV, Inagami T. Renin exists in human adrenal tissue. J Clin Endocrinol Metab 1983;57:483–487.
25. Dorer FE, Lentz KE, Kahn JR, Levine M, Skeggs LT. A comparison of the substrate specificities of cathepsin D and pseudo-renin. J Biol Chem 1978;187:647–653.
26. Dzau VJ, Bremner A, Emmet N, Haber E. Identification of renin and renin-like enzymes in rat brain by a renin-specific antibody. Clin Sci 1980;59:455–475.
27. Maruta H, Arakawa K. Confirmation of direct angiotensin formation by kallikrein. Biochem J 1983;213:193–200.
28. Dzau VJ. Circulating versus local renin-angiotensin systems in cardiovascular homeostasis. Circulation 1988;77(suppl 1):1–4.
29. Dzau VJ. Vascular renin-angiotensin system in hypertension: New insights into the mechanism of angiotensin converting enzyme inhibitors. Am J Med 1988;84(suppl 4A):4–8.
30. Re R, Fallon JT, Dzau V, Quay SC, Haber E. Renin synthesis by canine aortic smooth muscle cells in culture. Life Sci 1982;30:99–106.
31. Lilley LS, Pratt RE, Alexander RW. Renin expression by vascular endothelial cells in culture. Circ Res 1985;57:312–318.
32. Eggena P, Chu CL, Barrett JD, Sambhi M. Purification and partial characterisation of human angiotensinogen. Biochim Biophysi Acta 1976;427:208–217.
33. Hial V, Gimbrone MA, Peyton MP, Wilcox GM, Pilano JJ. Angiotensin metabolism by cultured human vascular endothelial and smooth muscle cells. Microvasc Res 1979;17:314–329.
34. Field LJ, McGowan RA, Dickinson DP, Gross KW. Tissue and gene specificity of mouse renin expression. Hypertension 1984;6:597–603.
35. Samani NJ, Morgan K, Brammar WJ, Swales JD. Detection of renin messenger RNA in rat tissues: Increased sensitivity using an RNAase protection technique. J Hypertension 1987;5(suppl 2):S19–S21.
36. Samani NJ, Swales JD, Brammar WJ. Expression of the renin gene in extrarenal tissues of the rat. Biochem J 1988;253:907–910.
37. Morris BJ, Catanzaro DF, Hardman J, Mesterovic N, Tellam J, Hort Y, Bennetts BH, Shine J. Structure of human renin and expression of the renin gene. Clin Exp Pharmacol Physiol 1984;11:369–374.
38. Hardman JA, Hort YJ, Catanzaro DF, Tellam JT, Baxter JD, Morris BJ, Shine J. Primary structure of the human renin gene. DNA 1984;3:457–468.

39. Miyazaki H, Fukamizu A, Hirose S, Hayashi T, Hori H, Ohkubo H, Nakanishi S, Murakami K. Structure of the human renin gene. Proc Natl Acad Sci USA 1984;81:5999–6003.

40. Morris BJ. New possibilities for intracellular renin and inactive renin now that the structure of the human renin gene has been elucidated. Clin Sci 1986;71: 345–355.

41. Imai T, Miyazaki H, Hirose S, Hori H, Hayashi T, Kageyama R, Ohkubo H, Nakanishi S, Murakami K. Cloning and sequence analysis of cDNA for human renin precursor. Proc Nat Acad Sci USA 1983;80:7405–7409.

42. Panthier J-J, Dreyfus M, Tronik-Le Roux D, Rougeon F. Mouse kidney and submaxillary gland renin genes differ in their 5' putative regulatory sequences. Proc Nat Acad Sci USA 1984;81:5489–5493.

43. Hobart PM, Fogliano M, O'Connor BA, Schaefer IM, Chirgwin JM. Human renin gene: Structure and sequence analysis. Proc Nat Acad Sci USA 1984;81: 5026–5030.

44. Nakamura M, Jackson EK, Inagami T. Beta-adrenoceptor mediated release of angiotensin II from mesenteric arteries. Am J Physiol 1986;250:H144–H148.

45. Cantin M, Gutkowska J, Lacasse J, Ballac M, Ledoux S, Inagami T, Beuzeron J, Genest J. Ultrastructural and immunocytochemical localisation of renin and angiotensin II in the juxtaglomerular cells of the ischaemic kidney in experimental hypertension. Am J Pathol 1984;115:212–224.

46. Taugner R, Manneck E, Nobling R, Buhrle CP, Hackenthal E, Ganten D, Inagami T, Schroder H. Co-existence of renin and angiotensin II in epithelioid cell secretory granules of rat kidney. Histochemistry 1984;81:39–45.

47. Desjardins-Giasson S, Gutkowska J, Garcia R, Genest J. Renin substrate in rat mesenteric artery. Can J Physiol Pharmacol 1981;59:528–532.

48. Campbell DJ, Bouhnick J, Menard J, Corvol P. Identity of angiotensinogen precursors in rat brain and liver. Nature (Lond) 1984;308:206–208.

49. Gomez RA, Lynch KR, Chevalier RL, Everett AD, Johns DW, Wilfong N, Peach MJ, Carey RM. Renin and angiotensinogen gene expression and intrarenal renin distribution during ACE inhibition. Am J Physiol 1988;254:F900–F906.

50. Campbell DJ, Habener JF. Angiotensinogen gene is expressed and differentially regulated in multiple tissues of the rat. J Clin Invest 1986;78:31–39.

51. Dzau VJ. Implications of local angiotensin production in cardiovascular physiology and pharmacology. Am J Cardiol 1985;59:59A–65A.

52. Swales JD, Heagerty AM. Vascular renin-angiotensin system: The unanswered questions. J Hypertension 1987;5(suppl 2):S1–S5.

53. Juul B, Aalkjaer C, Mulvany MJ. Contractile effects of tetradecapeptide renin substrate on rat femoral resistance vessels. J Hypertension 1987;5(suppl 2):S7–S10.

54. Juul B, Aalkjaer C, Heagerty AM, Leckie B, Lever AF. The generation of angiotensin II from tetradecapeptide substrate in human skin resistance vessels. J Hypertension 1990; in press.

55. Oliver JA, Sciacca RR. Local generation of angiotensin II as a mechanism of regulation of peripheral vascular tone in the rat. J Clin Invest 1984;74:1247–1256.

56. Bing RF, Russell GI, Swales JD, Thurston H. Effect of 12-hour infusions of saralasin or captopril on blood pressure in hypertensive conscious rats. J Lab Clin Med 1981;98:302–310.
57. Blaine EH, Schorn TW, Boger T. Statine-containing renin inhibitor: Dissociation of blood pressure lowering and renin inhibition in sodium-deficient dogs. Hypertension 1984;6:I111–I118.
58. Webb DJ, Manhem PJO, Leckie BJ, Lever AF, Morton JJ, Robertson JIS, Semple PF, Szelke M. Severe hypotension with bradycardia during renin inhibition with H142 in sodium deplete man. J Hum Hypertension 1989;3:227–232.
59. Brunner HR, Gavras H, Waeber B. Oral angiotensin-converting enzyme inhibitor in long-term treatment of hypertensive patients. Ann Intern Med 1979;2:1317–1323.
60. Jackson TR, Blair LAC, Marshall J, Goedert M, Hanley MR. The mas oncogene encodes an angiotensin receptor. Nature (Lond) 1988;335:437–440.
61. Bakhle YS, Reynard AM, Vane JR. Metabolism of the angiotensins in isolated perfused tissues. Nature (Lond) 1969;222:956–959.
62. Vane JR. Sites of conversion of angiotensin I. In: Genest J, Koiw E, eds. Hypertension. 1972. New York: Springer-Verlag, 1972;523–532.
63. Erdös EG. The angiotensin I converting enzyme. Fed Proc 1977;36:1760–1765.
64. Aiken JW, Vane JR. The renin-angiotensin system: Inhibition of converting enzyme in isolated tissues. Nature (Lond) 1970;228:30–34.
65. Kreye VAW, Gross F. Conversion of angiotensin I to angiotensin II in peripheral vascular beds of the rat. Am J Physiol 1971;220:1294–1296.
66. Di Salvo J, Peterson A, Montefusco C, Menta M. Intrarenal conversion of angiotensin I to angiotensin II in the dog. Circ Res 1971;29:398–406.
67. Di Salvo J, Britton S, Galvas P, Sanders TW. Effects of angiotensin I and angiotensin II on canine hepatic vascular resistance. Circ Res 1973;32:85–92.
68. Britton S, Di Salvo J. Effects of angiotensin I and angiotensin II on hindlimb and coronary vascular resistance. Am J Physiol 1973;225:1226–1231.
69. Caldwell PRB, Seegal BC, Hsu KC, Das M, Soffer RL. Angiotensin-converting enzyme: Vascular endothelial localisation. Science 1976;191:1050–1051.
70. Cushman DW, Cheung HS. Concentrations of angiotensin-converting enzyme in tissues of the rat. Biochim Biophys Acta 1971;250:261–265.
71. Erdös EG, Skidgel RA. The angiotensin I converting enzyme. Lab Invest 1987;56:345–348.
72. Johnston CI, Kohzuki M. Angiotensin converting enzyme: Localisation, regulation and inhibition. In: MacGregor GA, Sever PS, eds. Current Advances in ACE Inhibition. Edinburgh: Churchill Livingstone, 1989;3–7.
73. Strittmatter SM, Kapiloff MK, Snyder SH. [^{3}H] Captopril binding to membrane associated angiotensin converting enzyme. Biochem Biophys Res Commun 1983;112:1027–1033.
74. Ryan US, Ryan JW, Whitaker C, Chiu A. Localisation of angiotensin-converting enzyme (kininase II). Immunocytochemistry and immunofluorescence. Tissue Cell 1976;8:125–145.
75. Catravas JD, Watkins CA. Plasmalemmal activities in cultured calf pulmonary artery endothelial cells. Res Commun Chem Pathol Pharmacol 1985;50:163–179.

76. Okunishi H, Miyazaki M, Okamura T, Toda N. Different distribution of two types of angiotensin II-generating enzymes in the aortic wall. Biochem Biophys Res Commun 1987;149:1186–1192.
77. Pipili E, Manolopoulos VG, Catravas JD, Maragoudakis ME. Angiotensin converting enzyme activity is present in the endothelium-denuded aorta. Br J Pharmacol 1989;98:333–335.
78. Furchgott RF, Zawadzki JV. The obligatory role of endothelial cells in the relaxation of arterial smooth muscle by acetylcholine. Nature (Lond) 1980;288: 373–376.
79. Mizuno K, Hata S, Fukuchi S. Effect of sodium intake on angiotensin-converting enzyme activity of aorta in rats. Clin Sci 1981;61:249–251.
80. Jackson B, Cubela R, Johnston CI. Angiotensin converting enzyme (ACE): Characterisation by 125I MK351A binding studies of plasma and tissue ACE during variation of salt status in the rat. J Hypertension 1986;4:759–765.
81. Miyazaki M, Okunishi H, Okamura T, Toda N. Elevated vascular angiotensin converting enzyme in chronic two-kidney, one clip hypertension in the dog. J Hypertension 1987;6:105–110.
82. Wilson SK, Lynch DR, Snyder SH. Angiotensin-converting enzyme labelled with ^{3}H-captopril: Tissue localization and changes in different models of hypertension in the rat. J Clin Invest 1987;80:841–851.
83. Nakata K, Nishimura K, Takada T, Ikuse T, Yamauchi H, Iso T. Effects of an angiotensin-converting enzyme (ACE) inhibitor, SA446, on tissue ACE activity in normotensive, spontaneously hypertensive, and renal hypertensive rats. J Cardiovasc Pharmacol 1987;9:305–310.
84. Nakamura Y, Nakamura K, Matsukura T. Vascular angiotensin converting enzyme activity in spontaneously hypertensive rats and its inhibition with cilazapril. J Hypertension 1988;6:105–110.
85. Mendelsohn FAO, Lloyd CJ, Kachel C, Funder JW. Induction by glucocorticoids of angiotensin converting enzyme production from bovine endothelial cells in culture and rat lung in vivo. J Clin Invest 1981;70:684–693.
86. Okabe T, Yamagata K, Fujisawa M, Takaku F, Hidaka H, Umezawa Y. Induction by fibroblast growth factor of angiotensin converting enzyme in vascular endothelial cells in vitro. Biochem Biophys Res Commun 1987;145:1211–1216.
87. Biron P, Campeau L, David P. Fate of angiotensin I and II in the human circulation. Am J Cardiol 1969;24:544–547.
88. Freidli B, Biron P, Fouron J-C, Davignon A. Conversion of angiotensin I in pulmonary and systemic vascular beds of children. Acta Paediatri Scand 1974; 63:17–22.
89. Walker WG, Horvath JS, Moore MA, Russell RP, Conti CR, Mitch WE. Pulmonary generation and peripheral uptake of endogenous angiotensin II in man. Trans Assoc Am Physicians 1973;86:226–236.
90. Semple PF. The concentration of angiotensins I and II in blood from the pulmonary artery and left ventricle of man. J Clin Endocrinol Metab 1977;44: 915–920.
91. Favré L, Valloton MB, Muller AF. Relationship between plasma concentrations of angiotensin I, angiotensin II and plasma renin activity during cardiopulmonary bypass in man. Eur J Clin Inves 1974;4:135–140.

92. Fei DTW, Scoggins BA, Tregear GW, Coghlan JP. Angiotensin I, II and III in sheep: A model of angiotensin production and metabolism. Hypertension 1981;3:730–737.

93. Semple PF, Boyd AS, Dawes PM, Morton JJ. Angiotensin II and its heptapeptide (2–8), hexapeptide (3–8) and pentapeptide (4–8) metabolites in arterial and venous blood of man. Circ Res 1976;39:671–678.

94. Campbell DJ. The site of angiotensin production. J Hypertension 1985;3:199–207.

95. Schalekamp MADH, Admiraal PJJ, Derkx FHM. Estimation of regional metabolism and production of angiotensins in hypertensive subjects. Brit J Clin Pharmacol 1989;28:105S–113S.

96. Collier JG, Robinson BF. Comparison of effects of locally infused angiotensin I and II on hand veins and forearm arteries in man; evidence for converting-enzyme activity in limb vessels. Clin Sci Mol Med 1974;47:189–192.

97. Webb DJ, Collier JG. Influence of ramipril diacid on the peripheral vascular effects of angiotensin I. Am J Cardiol 1987;59:45D–49D.

98. Benjamin N, Cockcroft JR, Collier JG, Dollery CT, Ritter JM, Webb DJ. Local inhibition of converting enzyme and vascular responses to angiotensin and bradykinin in the human forearm. J Physiol (Lond) 1989;412:543–555.

99. Dorer FE, Kahn JR, Lentz KE, Levine M, Skeggs LT. Hydrolysis of bradykinin by angiotensin-converting enzyme. Circ Res 1974;34:824–827.

100. Regoli D, Barabé, J. Pharmacology of bradykinin and related kinins. Pharmacol Rev 1980;32:1–46.

101. Webb DJ, Collier JG, Seidelin P, Struthers AD. Regulation of regional vascular tone: The role of angiotensin conversion in human forearm resistance vessels. J Hypertension 1988;6(suppl 3):S57–S59.

102. Cushman DW, Wang FL, Fung WC, Harvey CM, DeForrest JM. Differentiation of angiotensin-converting enzyme (ACE) inhibitors by their selective inhibition of ACE in physiologically important target organs. Am J Hypertension 1989;2:294–306.

103. Kleinert HD, Martin D, Chekal MA, Kadam J, Luly JR, Plattner JJ, Perun TJ, Luther RR. Effects of the renin inhibitor A-64662 in monkeys and rats with varying baseline plasma renin activity. Hypertension 1988;11:613–619.

The Endothelium: An Introduction to Current Research, pages 81–93
© 1990 Wiley-Liss, Inc.

8
Endothelial Function in Vascular Remodeling

GARY H. GIBBONS AND VICTOR J. DZAU

Division of Vascular Medicine, Department of Medicine, Molecular and Cellular Vascular Research Laboratory, Brigham & Women's Hospital, Harvard Medical School, Boston, Massachusetts 02115

INTRODUCTION

It has become increasingly clear that the role of the endothelium in the circulation extends far beyond its function as a nonthrombogenic surface lining the blood vessel wall. Indeed, the entire vessel wall can no longer be conceptualized as a passive conduit responding to circulating hormones from distant endocrine organs. A growing body of evidence supports the concept that the vasculature is an organ capable of (i) sensing changes within its milieu; (ii) integrating and modulating these signals by intercellular communication; and (iii) responding and adapting by the local production of various mediators that influence function as well as structure. The vasculature as an integrated unit is not only capable of short-term responses to acute stimuli, such as the autoregulatory change in tone in response to changes in perfusion pressure, but is also capable of responding to chronic stimuli by long-term structural changes that modify function. This review examines the role of the endothelium in this process of vascular remodeling.

ENDOTHELIUM AS A SIGNAL SENSOR AND TRANSDUCER

Because of its unique localization, the endothelium is ideally situated to sense changes within the circulation. Thus, alterations in hemodynamic forces, such as blood flow and pressure, should first affect the endothelium. Similarly, as the major interface with the bloodstream, the endothelium senses changes in humoral factors (e.g., hormones, vasoactive substances, serum electrolytes), which may influence vessel tone or structure. This role as sensor and transducer also extends to the inflammatory response via its interaction with endotoxins, cytokines, and inflammatory cells. Endothelial cells contain receptors, ion channels, and other membrane-bound structures that may function as sensors detecting specific changes in the milieu and thereby triggering adaptive responses.

The endothelium responds to a variety of ligands by specific receptor-coupled events. Bradykinin, histamine, acetylcholine (ACh), adenosine triphosphate (ATP), platelet-activating factor (PAF), and thrombin all trigger an increase in intracellular calcium within the endothelial cell (1–4). Indeed, many of the endothelial cell responses evoked by these ligands can also be elicited by calcium ionophores. The receptor-mediated calcium signal appears to be mediated by an activation of phospholipase C-induced hydrolysis of inositol phospholipids resulting in the generation of inositol 1,4,5-trisphosphate (IP3) and 1,2-diacylglycerol (DAG). IP3 binds to intracellular sites and causes a release of calcium into the cytoplasm whereas DAG activates protein kinase C. Thus, the calcium ion appears to play an important role in the signal transduction function of the endothelium.

There is also evidence to suggest that endothelial cells respond to humoral stimuli via activation of ion channels. Both bradykinin and acetylcholine have been reported to activate potassium channels in endothelial cells (2,5). Similarly, platelet activating factor, histamine, and thrombin appear to activate endothelial cell ion channels (4,6). Although there are some conflicting data, voltage-sensitive calcium channels do not appear to play a significant signal transduction role. The precise role of these signals in stimulus–secretion coupling or other functional responses is still not well defined.

Endothelial cells also respond to hemodynamic stimuli. Studies in vivo and in vitro suggest that endothelial cells increase synthesis of prostacyclin, endothelial-derived relaxing factor (EDRF), histamine, and endothelin in response to increased flow (7–11). Harder and co-workers (12) have also reported that the autoregulatory increase in vascular tone induced by increased perfusion pressure is an endothelium-dependent response in the cerebral vasculature. These data suggest that the endothelial cell can sense changes in flow or pressure and thereby modulate the vascular response by releasing vasoactive substances.

The precise signal-transduction pathway mediating these responses remains to be clarified. The capacity to sense pressure could be transduced by the recently described stretch-activated ion channel on endothelial cells (13). Flowing blood exerts a tractive force on endothelial cells defined as shear stress. Endothelial cells may sense shear stress via an inwardly rectifying potassium channel recently described by Olesen et al. (14). Moreover, shear stress can also induce an increase in intracellular calcium (15). The stimulus–secretion coupling events linking shear stress, potassium channels, intracellular calcium, and mediator release (e.g., EDRF, endothelin) have not been fully characterized. However, such a linkage can be inferred from recent studies in our laboratory in which flow-mediated release of EDRF was inhibited by pharmacologic blockade of calcium-activated potassium channels (Cooke JP, et al: personal communication). These data support the postulate that hemodynamic stimuli may activate endothelial cells by signal transduction pathways similar to those employed by vasoactive agents and other agonists. Indeed, it is noteworthy that the calcium ion appears to play a central role in mediating endothelial cell activation in a variety of biologic settings such as hemostasis, inflammation, or blood flow control. It is therefore less surprising that rather diverse types of stimuli result in similar secretory responses such as eicosanoid or EDRF release (1,16,17).

ENDOTHELIUM AS A PRODUCER OF BIOLOGICAL MEDIATORS FOR VASCULAR REMODELING

In addition to sensing and transducing the signals, the endothelium can mediate or trigger the blood vessel to undergo structural and geometric changes by the transfer of these signals to underlying vascular smooth muscle cells (VSMC) via tight junctions or by the synthesis and release of effector molecules. The effector substances may be growth promoting, growth inhibitory, vasoactive or extracellular matrix modulators.

Vasoactive Substances in Vascular Remodeling

Peptide growth factors such as platelet-derived growth factor (PDGF) and epidermal growth factor (EGF) have been shown to possess vasoconstrictor properties (18,19). These data suggest that growth factors and vasoactive agents may share similar signal transduction pathways. Indeed, both vasoactive agents and several VSMC mitogens activate phospholipase C and generate IP3 and DAG in association with increased intracellular calcium and cellular alkalinization (20). On the basis of these findings, it is not surprising that there is a substantial body of in vitro evidence that vasoactive substances influence VSMC growth.

Studies in our laboratory and others have shown that the vessel wall (including the endothelium) contains not only angiotensin-converting enzymatic activity but also renin and angiotensinogen as well (21,22). Thus, there is a paracrine renin-angiotensin system in addition to the circulating hormonal system that may influence vascular structure. This paracrine system may modify vascular reactivity as well as modulate vascular remodeling.

In confluent quiescent vascular smooth muscle cells in culture, angiotensin II induces cellular hypertrophy (23,24). We have shown that this hypertrophic response is in association with increased mRNA levels of proto-oncogenes c-fos, c-myc, and the autocrine growth factors PDGF-A chain and transforming growth factor-β (24) (Gibbons GH: personal communication). These autocrine growth factors may mediate angiotensin-induced hypertrophy. Angiotensin may also potentiate serum or fibroblast growth factor-induced DNA synthesis (25,26). These data suggest that angiotensin may modulate the proliferative response to autocrine/paracrine growth factors. Similarly, other endothelium-derived vasoactive substances also possess growth regulatory properties. We have shown that endothelin induces increased expression of c-myc in association with VSMC proliferation (27). Growth promoting effects of vasoconstrictors on VSMC have also been described for thromboxane, leukotrienes, substance P, and serotonin (28–31). By contrast, vasodilators such as prostaglandins and nitrosovasodilators appear to inhibit VSMC proliferation (32,32b).

These data suggest that circulating or locally produced vasoactive substances may influence VSMC growth and thereby modulate vascular remodeling. Given that endothelial cells produce prostacyclin and nitrosovasodilators and generate angiotensin and endothelin locally, it is tempting to speculate that the endothelium may contribute to vascular remodeling by the synthesis of these potentially growth-modulating substances.

Endothelium-Derived Growth Factors

The endothelium produces several VSMC growth promoting factors such as PDGF, basic fibroblast growth factor (FGF), insulin-like growth factor I (IGF-1), and interleukin 1 (IL-1) (33–37). Both the A and B chains of PDGF are synthesized by the endothelium such that theoretically all three isoforms of PDGF may be produced. This may be of significance, since there are two PDGF receptors, α and β, which have different binding affinities for each isoform (38). Differences in receptor isoform activation could influence the response response (19,39). Indeed, studies in our laboratory suggest that the PDGF AA homodimer is a weaker VSMC as compared with the BB homodimer (39). Production of either the AB or BB isoforms promotes VSMC migration and proliferation and may play a role in some forms of vascular remodeling.

Both the PDGF A and B chain messenger RNA (mRNA) levels are increased in microvascular endothelium in response to phorbol esters, thrombin, and transforming growth factor-β (TGF-β) (33). This response appears to be primarily due to an effect on transcription rate (40). Increased cAMP appears to block the increased transcription of PDGF B chain induced by these agents (33). Tissue necrosis factor, interleukin-1 and endotoxin (possibly mediated by IL-1) also promote secretion of PDGF by endothelial cells (34,35).

The regulation of IL-1, IGF-1, and FGF expression, and the role of these agents in vascular remodeling is poorly defined. IL-1 expression is increased by substances such as endotoxin. Administration of the peptide induces VSMC proliferation only during prostaglandin synthesis blockade (41). The IL-1 proliferative response appears to be mediated by inducing autocrine production of PDGF-AA (42). The role of IGF-1 in endothelial cells is poorly defined, but data suggest that it plays a growth promoting role in microvascular endothelial cells (43). Regenerating endothelium appears to express IGF-1 after balloon injury (36) and may play a role in endothelial cell migration. In the presence of growth factors such as PDGF or FGF, IGF-1 potentiates VSMC hyperplasia (44), whereas in the absence of these competence factors it promotes hypertrophy (45).

FGF is a potent autocrine growth factor for endothelial cells as well as a potent VSMC mitogen (26,46). In vitro studies with neutralizing antibodies suggest that FGF plays a critical role in endothelial cell proliferation, cell migration, cell invasion, matrix alterations, and angiogenesis (46,47). FGF-induced production of endothelial plasminogen activators appears to be important in vascular cell invasion into tissues (47).

The endothelium also modulates vascular structure via the production of growth inhibitory substances. Campbell and others have observed that confluent endothelial cells secrete growth inhibitory substances that appear to maintain VSMC in the most quiescent, differentiated-appearing phenotype (48). Studies by Karnovsky and colleagues have suggested that heparan sulfate produced by endothelial cells has a growth inhibitory effect on VSMC (49,50). Recent studies also suggest that the endothelium produces transforming growth factor beta (TGF) (51). This multifunctional growth factor has the autocrine effects of inhibiting endothelial cell proliferation and migration in some conditions but promoting angiogenesis in other circumstances (52–54). TGF-β has a bifunctional effect on VSMC in that it either inhibits mitogen-induced proliferation of VSMC or promotes hypertrophy and matrix production of quiescent VSMC (55,56). On the basis of the available data, we would speculate that TGF-β and heparan sulfate produced by the endothelium may also contribute to vascular remodeling. Factors such as TGF-β may be particularly important in structural changes in which lumen size decreases or vessels undergo rarefaction or regression, i.e., settings in which cell involution and matrix production are important.

Vascular Remodeling: Role of the Matrix

Alterations of vascular structure not only involve cellular hypertrophy, hyperplasia, or regression but must also involve the structural elements and binding elements present within the extracellular compartment of the vessel wall. The endothelium may also participate in vascular remodeling by the production of extracellular matrix and proteolytic enzymes. It has become increasingly clear that these matrix proteins play an important role in modulating cell phenotype and function as well as provide structural support (57,58). For example, the amount of fibronectin or laminin within the extracellular matrix can influence whether VSMCs in culture express a more proliferative "synthetic" phenotype versus the more quiescent "differentiated" phenotype (48,59). Conversely, the extracellular matrix synthesized by cells in culture is modulated by the cell phenotype (59,60). Matrix proteins such as thrombospondin are not growth factors per se, but they appear to be necessary agents for mitogen-induced proliferation of VSMCs (61). This growth-promoting role of the matrix protein thrombospondin is in contrast to the growth inhibiting role of heparin sulfate described above (49,50). The finding that PDGF activates gene expression of thromobospondin suggests that the regulation of cell growth involves an interaction between autocrine/paracrine growth factors and matrix proteins (61). Thus, matrix components produced by vascular cells can influence vascular structure by modulating cell phenotype and growth response to mitogens.

Vascular remodeling also entails changes in the mass and cell composition of the vessel wall. This process must involve a reconstruction of the matrix scaffolding and therefore a process of active proteolysis and resynthesis of these proteins. Similarly, the migration of VSMC from the media to the subintimal space must involve a complex process of ligand-receptor binding, coupling and proteolysis. The cytoskeletal scaffolding (e.g., actin) must change with cell movement, the points of contact with the extracellular matrix mediated by integrins and other membrane receptor proteins must change with movement, and the barrier created by the scaffolding and ground substance of the extracellular matrix must be destroyed by proteolytic action (62–64).

As discussed above, vascular cells have the capacity to synthesize the collagens, glycoproteins, and proteoglycans that compose the extracellular matrix (57,58,60). It is also apparent that these cells have the capacity to produce the proteases necessary for vascular remodeling. Endothelial cells synthesize the plasminogen activators urokinase and tissue plasminogen activator (16,64). The inactive proenzyme plasminogen binds to the matrix and is abundant in the vasculature (64). The plasmin produced by plasminogen activation is not only the critical protease in thrombolysis but is also capable of activating procollagenases and participating in the proteolysis of other matrix proteins. In addition to its effect on matrix proteins, plasmin also converts the latent TGF-β precursor into its active form (54). Hence, the production of plasmin not only modifies the matrix as a result of its own proteolytic activity but also through its effect on other protease enzymes and matrix-modulating growth factors.

It is noteworthy that other agents such as FGF, thrombin and phorbol esters also induce increased plasminogen activator synthesis by endothelial cells (16,46,65). Indeed, it has recently been reported that shear stress stimulates the secretion of tissue plasminogen activator by endothelial cells (66). These data suggest that hemodynamic or humoral factors may modulate vascular remodeling by activating factors that regulate the proteolytic activity within the vessel wall.

The regulation of vessel wall proteolytic activity not only involves the plasminogen activator/plasmin system, but also interstitial and type IV collagenases, stromelysin, tissue inhibitor of metalloproteinases, as well as plasminogen activator inhibitor (63,64,67). Vascular smooth muscle cells may modulate this proteolytic activity by secreting plasminogen activator inhibitor into the matrix (69).

Thus, matrix proteins, cell-derived proteases, and cell-derived protease inhibitors provide a critically important element of the endothelial cell effector system modulating vascular structure. The interaction between vasoactive substances, hemodynamic stimuli, autocrine/paracrine growth factors, matrix proteins, and matrix-modulating proteases will be an area of fruitful research.

MODELS OF VASCULAR REMODELING

Given the pivotal role of the endothelium in regulating vascular structure, it should not be surprising that endothelium dysfunction may result in pathological structural changes of the blood vessel. To discuss this possibility, we will examine several animal models in which vascular remodeling is a prominent feature.

For many years, pathologists have described structural alterations in the veins of patients with long-standing elevation in venous pressure or in the portal veins of patients with cirrhosis of the liver. Studies of animal models of venous hypertension such as partial portal vein ligation have described VSMC hypertrophy without hyperplasia (70). Similarly, animal models of arterial hypertension demonstrate VSMC hypertrophy and increased matrix production within the conduit vessel walls (71). These in vivo observations have been confirmed by in vitro models of mechanical stretch that demonstrate that VSMC adapt to mechanical stretch by hypertrophy and increased matrix production (72). Tozzi et al. recently observed that in the pulmonary vasculature, the induction of increased matrix production in response to mechanical stretch is an endothelium-dependent process (73). These studies suggest that the vasculature remodels itself in response to increased intraluminal pressure transduced by the endothelium.

The vasculature also responds to changes in flow or shear stress. Changes in shear stress not only involve acute adaptive changes in vascular tone but also appear to modulate vascular structure. An artery exposed to chronically high shear stress dilates over time and thereby normalizes the shear stress (74). Recently, Langille et al. provided confirmatory data by demonstrating that an artery exposed to a chronic decrease in shear stress undergoes an adaptive decrease in caliber. This response appears to be endothelium dependent and involves alterations in the matrix and cell involution but not cell proliferation (75). Thus, shear stress appears to be an important determinant of vascular remodeling mediated by the endothelium.

Another model of vascular remodeling of particular clinical relevance is the adaptation of vein grafts to the arterial circulation. Vein grafts in the arterial circulation are characterized by a process of myointimal hyperplasia that is most prominent at the site of anastomosis. The vein grafts with prominent myointimal hyperplasia also exhibit endothelial dysfunction as demonstrated by impaired EDRF release in response to ACh, ADP, and thrombin (76). Clinicians have observed that vein grafts exposed to high flow rates in the renal circulation have higher patency rates than do those in other circulatory beds. In animal models, grafts established with a distal fistula and increased shear stress have minimal myointimal hyperplasia compared with grafts with distal stenosis and decreased flow (77). These data suggest that the vascular remodeling of vein grafts is influenced by hemodynamic stimuli. The role of the endothelium in this process remains to be further elucidated.

Finally, the myointimal hyperplasia observed after balloon injury of an artery is another example of vascular remodeling secondary to endothelium denudation/dysfunction. In the absence of endothelium, platelets aggregate and release VSMC growth factors, such as PDGF and serotonin. In addition, the subintimal smooth muscle cells migrate, proliferate and express PDGF even in the presence of a regenerated endothelium several weeks later (68). Moreover the regenerated endothelium is dysfunctional as documented by impaired EDRF release (Cooke JP, et al: personal communication). We would speculate that the dysfunctional endothelium may produce less growth inhibitory mediators such as nitric oxide, prostaglandins, heparan sulfate, and TGF-β and/or increased growth promoting factors such as FGF, PDGF, and IGF-1. The regenerated endothelium may also participate in the proteolysis and resynthesis of the matrix to promote VSMC invasion into the subintimal space. It is intriguing to note that three factors appear to inhibit myointimal hyperplasia in vivo: shear stress, heparin, and angiotensin converting enzyme inhibitors (50,77,78). The importance of the endothelium in the remodeling process can be inferred from the fact that these three factors are either transduced or synthesized by the endothelium. These observations are consistent with the hypothesis that endothelial denudation/dysfunction results in an imbalance of inhibitory and stimulatory forces that promote VSMC proliferation and migration. We speculate that future developments in effective therapy of myointimal hyperplasia may involve the enhancement of growth inhibitory mediators (e.g., heparin) or the blockade of growth promoting mediators (e.g., angiotensin II).

SUMMARY

The endothelium appears to play an important role in vascular remodeling by detecting changes in humoral or hemodynamic conditions within the circulation, by transducing the signals to the underlying blood vessel wall, and by producing mediators that modify vascular structure. An alteration in endothelial function may promote adaptive changes in vascular structure that may assume pathophysiologic significance such as myointimal hyperplasia.

ACKNOWLEDGMENTS
This work is supported by NIH grants HL35610, HL35792, HL19259, HL35252, HL40210, HL42663, NIH Specialized Center of Research in Hypertension HL36568. Dr. Gary Gibbons is a recipient of a Robert Wood Johnson Foundation Minority Faculty Development Fellowship. We wish to thank Ms. Donna MacDonald for her expert secretarial assistance.

REFERENCES

1. Brock TA, Capasso EA. Thrombin and histamine activate phospholipase C in human endothelial cells via a phorbol ester-sensitive pathway. J Cell Physiol 1988;136:54–62.
2. Colden-Stanfield M, Schilling WP, Ritchie AK, Eskin SG, Navarro LT, Kunze DL. Bradykinin-induced increases in cytosolic calcium and ionic currents in cultured bovine aortic endothelial cells. Circ Res 1987;61:632–640.
3. Danthuluri NR, Cybulsky MI, Brock TA. Ach-induced calcium transients in primary cultures of rabbit aortic endothelial cells. Am J Physiol 1988; 255:H1549–H1553.
4. Ryan US. Endothelium as a transducing surface. J Mol Cell Cardiol 1989;21(suppl 1):85–90.
5. Olesan S-P, Davies PF, Clapham DE. Muscarinic-activated K^+ current in bovine aortic endothelial cells. Circ Res 1988;62:1059–1064.
6. Johns A, Lategan TW, Lodge NJ, Ryan US, Van Breeman C, Adams DJ. Calcium entry through receptor-operated channels in bovine pulmonary artery endothelial cells. Tissue Cell 1987;19:733–745.
7. DeForrest JM, Hollis TM. Shear stress and aortic histamine synthesis. AM J Physiol 1978;234:H701–H705.
8. Frangos VA, Eskin SG, McIntire LV, Ives CL. Flow effects on prostacyclin production by cultured human endothelial cells. Science 1985;227:1477–1479.
9. Kaiser L, Hull SS, Sparks HV. Methylene blue and ETYA block flow-dependent dilation in canine femoral artery. Am J Physiol 1986;250:H974–H987.
10. Pohl U, Holtz J, Busse R, Bassenge E. Crucial role of endothelium in the vasodilator response to increased flow in vivo. Hypertension 1986;8:37–44.
11. Yoshizumi M, Korihara H, Sugiyama T, Takaku F, Yanagisawa M, Masaki T, Yazaki Y. Hemodynamic shear stress stimulates endothelin production by cultured endothelial cells. Biochem Biophys Res Commun 1989;161:859–864.
12. Harder DR. Pressure-induced myogenic activation of cat cerebral arteries is dependent on intact endothelium. Circ Res 1987;60:102–107.
13. Lansman JB, Hallam TJ, Rink TJ. Single stretch-activated ion channels in vascular endothelial cells as mechanotransducers? Nature (Lond) 1987;325: 811–813.
14. Olesen S-P, Clapham DE, Davies PF. Hemodynamic shear stress activates a K^+ current in vascular endothelial cells. Nature (Lond) 1988;331:168–170.
15. Ando J, Komatsuda T, Kamiya A. Cytoplasmic calcium response to fluid shear stress in cultured vascular endothelial cells. In Vitro 1988;24:871–877.
16. Gross JL, Moscatelli D, Jaffe EA, Rifkin DB. Plasminogen activator and collagenase production by cultured capillary endothelial cells. J Cell Biol 1982;95:974–981.

17. Jaffe EA, Grulich J, Weksler BB, Hampel G, Watanabe K. Correlation between thrombin-induced prostacyclin production and inositol triphosphate and cytosolic free calcium level in cultured human endothelial cells. J Biol Chem 1987; 262:8557–8565.
18. Berk BC, Brock TA, Webb RC, Taubman MB, Atkinson WJ, Gimbrone MA, Alexander RW. Epidermal growth factor, a vascular smooth muscle mitogen, induces rat aortic contraction. J Clin Invest 1985;75:1083–1086.
19. Block LH, Emmans LR, Vogt E, Sachinidis A, Vetter W, Hoppe J. Ca^{2+}-channel blockers inhibit the action of recombinant platelet-derived growth factor in vascular smooth muscle cells. Proc Natl Acad Sci USA 1989;86:2388–2392.
20. Berk BC, Brock TA, Gimbrone MA, Alexander RW. Early agonist-mediated ionic events in cultured vascular smooth muscle cells: Calcium mobilization is associated with intracellular acidification. J Biol Chem 1987;262:5065–5072.
21. Kifor I, Dzau VJ. Endothelial renin-angiotensin pathway: Evidence for intracellular synthesis and secretion of angiotensins. Circ Res 1987;60:422–428.
22. Lilly LS, Pratt RE, Alexander RW, Larson DM, Ellison KE, Gimbrone MA, Dzau VJ. Renin expression by vascular endothelial cells in culture. Circ Res 1985;57:312–218.
23. Geisterfer AAT, Peach MJ, Owens GK. Angiotensin II induces hypertrophy, not hyperplasia, of cultured rat aortic smooth muscle cells. Circ Res 1988;62:749–756.
24. Naftilan AJ, Pratt RE, Dzau VJ. Induction of platelet-derived growth factor A-chain and c-myc gene expressions by angiotensin II in cultured rat vascular smooth muscle cells. J Clin Invest 1989;83:1419–1424.
25. Campbell-Boswell M, Robertson AL. Effects of angiotensin II and vasopressin on human smooth muscle cells in vitro. Exp Mol Pathol 1981;35:265–276.
26. Gibbons GH, Pratt RE, Stevenson LF, Dzau VJ. Angiotensin: A bifunctional modulator of vascular smooth muscle cell growth. (submitted).
27. Dubin D, Pratt RE, Cooke JP, Dzau VJ. Endothelin, a potent vasoconstrictor is a vascular smooth muscle mitogen. J Vasc Med Biol 1989;1:150–154.
28. Ishimitsu T, Uehara Y, Ishii M, Ikeda T, Matsuoka H, Sugimoto T. Thromboxane and vascular smooth muscle cell growth in genetically hypertensive rates. Hypertension 1988;12:46–51.
29. Nemecek GM, Coughlin SR, Handley DA, Moskowitz MA. Stimulation of aortic smooth muscle cell mitogenesis by serotonin. Proc Natl Acad Sci USA 1986;83:674–678.
30. Nilsson J, von Euler AM, Dalsgaard C-J. Stimulation of connective tissue cell growth by substance P and substance K. Nature (Lond) 1985;315:61–63.
31. Palmberg L, Claesson H-E, Thyberg J. Leukotrienes stimulate initiation of DNA synthesis in cultured arterial smooth muscle cells. J Cell Sci 1987;88:151–159.
32. Loesberg C, Wijk RV, Zandbergen J, Van Aken WG, Van Mourik JA, DeGroot PhG. Cell cycle-dependent inhibition of human vascular smooth muscle cell proliferation by prostaglandin El. Exp Cell Res 1985;160:117–125.
32b. Garg UC, Hassid A. Nitric oxide-generating vasodilators and 8-bromo-cyclic guanosine monophosphate inhibit mitogenesis and proliferation of cultured rat vascular smooth muscle cells. J Clin Invest 1989;83:1774–1777.

33. Daniel TO, Gibbs VC, Milfay DF, Williams LT. Agents that increase cAMP accumulation block endothelial c-sis induction by thrombin and transforming growth factor-B. J Biol Chem 1987;262:11893–11896.

34. Fox PL, DiCorleto PE. Regulation of production of a platelet-derived growth factor-like protein by cultured bovine aortic endothelial cells. J Cell Physiol 1984;121:298–308.

35. Hajjar KA, Hajjar DP, Silverstein RL, Nachman RL. Tumor necrosis factor-mediated release of platelet-derived growth factor from cultured endothelial cells. J Exp Med 1987;166:235–245.

36. Hansson H-A, Jennische E, Skottner A. Regenerating endothelial cells express insulin like growth factor-1 immunoreactivity after arterial injury. Cell Tissue Res 1987;250:499–505.

37. Vlodavsky I, Folkman J, Sullivan R, Fridman R, Ishai-Michaeli R, Sasse J, Klagsbrun M. Endothelial cell-derived basic fibroblast growth factor: Synthesis and deposition into subendothelial extracellular matrix. Proc Natl Acad Sci USA 1987;84:2292–2296.

38. Hart CE, Forstrom JW, Kelly JD, Seifert RA, Smith RA, Ross R, Murray MJ, Bowen-Pope DF. Two classes of PDGF receptor recognize different isoforms of PDGF. Science 1988;240:1529–1531.

39. Gibbons GH, Pratt RE, Dzau VJ. Platelet-derived growth factor isoforms differ in mitogenic effect on adult vascular smooth muscle cells. Circulation 1989 (abst).

40. Starksen NF, Harsh GR, Gibbs VC, Williams LT. Regulated expression of the platelet-derived growth factor A chain gene in microvascular endothelial cells. J Biol Chem 1987;262:14381–14384.

41. Libby P, Warner SJC, Friedman GB. Interleukin 1: A mitogen for human vascular smooth muscle cells that induces the release of growth inhibitory prostanoids. J Clin Invest 1988;81:487–498.

42. Raines EW, Dower SK, Ross R. Interleukin-1 mitogenic activity for fibroblasts and smooth muscle cells is due to PDGF-AA. Science 1989;243:393–395.

43. King GL, Goodman AD, Buzney S, Moses A, Kahn CR. Receptors and growth promoting effects of insulin and insulinlike growth factors on cells from bovine retinal capillaries and aorta. J Clin Invest 1985;75:1028–1036.

44. Clemmons DR. Interaction of circulating cell-derived and plasma growth factors in stimulating cultured smooth muscle cell replication. J Cell Physiol 1984;121:425–430.

45. Libby P, O'Brien KV. Culture of quiescent arterial smooth muscle cells in a defined serum-free medium. J Cell Physiol 1983;115:217–223.

46. Sato Y, Rifkin DB. Autocrine activities of basic fibroblast growth factor: Regulation of endothelial cell movement, plasminogen activator synthesis, and DNA synthesis. J Cell Biol 1988;107:1199–1205.

47. Mignatti P, Tsuboi R, Robbins E, Rifkin DB. In vitro angiogenesis on the human amniotic membrane: requirement for basic fibroblast growth factor-induced proteinases. J Cell Biol 1989;108:671–682.

48. Campbell JH, Campbell GR. Endothelial cell influences on vascular smooth muscle phenotype. Annu Rev Physiol 1986;48:295–306.

49. Castellot JJ, Farreau LV, Karnovsky MJ, Rosenberg RD. Inhibition of vascular smooth muscle cell growth by endothelial cell-derived heparin: Possible role of a platelet endoglycosidase. J Biol Chem 1982;257:11256–11260.

50. Hoover RL, Rosenberg R, Haering W, Karnovsky MJ. Inhibition of rat arterial smooth muscle cell proliferation by heparin. II. In vitro studies. Circ Res 1980; 47:578–583.
51. Antonelli-Orlidge A, Saunders KB, Smith S, D'Amore PA. An activated form of transforming growth factor-beta is produced by cocultures of endothelial cells and pericytes. Proc Natl Acad Sci USA 1989;86:4544–4548.
52. Heimark RL, Twardzik DR, Schwartz SM. Inhibition of endothelial regeneration by type-beta transforming growth factor from platelets. Science 1986;233: 1078–1080.
53. Roberts AB, Sporn MB, Assoian RK, Smith JM, Roche NS, Wakefield LM, Heine UI, Liotta LA, Falanga V, Kehrl JH, Fauci AS. Transforming growth factor type beta: rapid induction of fibrosis and angiogenesis in vivo and stimulation of collagen formation in vitro. Proc Natl Acad Sci USA 1986;83:4167–4171.
54. Sato Y, Rifkin DB. Inhibition of endothelial cell movement by pericytes and smooth muscle cells: Activation of a latent transforming growth factor-beta 1-like molecule by plasmin during co-culture. J Cell Biol 1989;109:309–315.
55. Majack RA. Beta type transforming growth factor specifies organizational behavior in vascular smooth muscle cultures. J Cell Biol 1987;105:465–471.
56. Owens GK, Geisterfer AAT, Yang YW-H Komoriya A. Transforming growth factor B-induced growth inhibition and cellular hypertrophy in cultured vascular smooth muscle cells. J Cell Biol 1988;107:771–780.
57. Mayne R. Collagenous proteins of blood vessels. Arteriosclerosis 1986;6:585–593.
58. Wight TN. Proteoglycans in pathological conditions: Atherosclerosis. Fed Proc 1985;44:381–385.
59. Hedin U, Bottger BA, Forsberg E, Johansson S, Thyberg J. Diverse effects of fibronectin and laminin on phenotypic properties of cultured arterial smooth muscle cells. J Cell Biol 1988;107:307–319.
60. Stepp MA, Kindy MS, Franzblau C, Sonenshein GE. Complex regulation of collagen gene expression in cultured bovine aortic smooth muscle cells. J Biol Chem 1986;261:6542–6547.
61. Majack RA, Goodman LV, Dixot VM. Cell surface thrombospondin is functionally essential for vascular smooth muscle cell proliferation. J Cell Biol 1988; 106:415–422.
62. Hynes RO. Integrins: A family of cell surface receptors. Cell 1987;48:549–554.
63. Liotta LA, Rao CN, Wewer UM. Biochemical interactions of tumor cells with the basement membrane. Annu Rev Biochem 1986;55:1037–1057.
64. Saksela O, Rifkin DB. Cell-associated plasminogen activation: Regulation and physiological functions. Annu Rev Cell Biol 1988;4:93–126.
65. Levin EG, Marzec U, Anderson J, Harker LA. Thrombin stimulates tissue plasminogen activation release from cultured human endothelial cells. J Clin Invest 1984;74:1988–1995.
66. Diamond SE, Eskin SG, McIntire LV. Fluid flow stimulates tissue plasminogen activator secretion by cultured human endothelial cells. Science 1989;243:1483–1485.
67. Delvos V, Gajdusek C, Sage H, Harker LA, Schwartz SM. Interactions of vascular wall cells with collagen gels. Lab Invest 1982;46:61–72.

68. Walker LN, Bowen-Pope DF, Reidy MA. Production of platelet-derived growth factor-like molecules by cultured arterial smooth muscle cells accompanies proliferation after arterial injury. Proc Natl Acad Sci USA 1986;83:7311–7315.
69. Knudsen BS, Harpel PC, Nachman RL. Plasminogen activator inhibitor is associated with the extracellular matrix of cultured bovine smooth muscle cells. J Clin Invest 1987;80:1082–1089.
70. Uvelius B, Arner A, Johansson B. Structural and mechanical alterations in hypertrophic venous smooth muscle. Acta Physiol Scand 1981;112:463–471.
71. Iwatsuki K, Cardinale GJ, Spector S, Udenfriend S. Hypertension: Increase of collagen biosynthesis in arteries but not in veins. Science 1977;198:403–405.
72. Leung DYM, Glagov S, Mathews MB. Cyclic stretching stimulates synthesis of matrix components by arterial smooth muscle cells in vitro. Science 1976;191: 475–477.
73. Tozzi CA, Poiani GJ, Harangozo AM, Boyd CD, Riley DJ. Pressure-induced connective tissue synthesis in pulmonary artery segments is dependent on intact endothelium. J Clin Invest 1989;84:1005–1012.
74. Kamiya A, Togawa T. Adaptive regulation of wall shear stress to flow change in the canine carotid artery. Am J Physiol 1980;239:H14–H21.
75. Langille BL, Bendeck MP, Keeley FW. Adaptations of carotid arteries of young and mature rabbits to reduced carotid blood flow. Am J Physiol 1989;256:H931–H939.
76. Miller VM, Reigel MM, Hollier LH, Vanhoutte PM. Endothelium-dependent responses in autogenous femoral veins grafted into the arterial circulation of the dog. J Clin Invest 1987;80:1350–1357.
77. Faulkner SL, Fisher RD, Conkle DM, Page DL, Bender HW. Effect of blood flow rate on subendothelial proliferation in venous autografts used as arterial substitutes. Circulation 1975;51/52(suppl I):I-163–I-172.
78. Powell JS, Clozel J-P, Muller RKM, Kuhn H, Hefti F, Hosang M, Baumgartner HR. Inhibitors of angiotensin-converting enzyme prevent myointimal proliferation after vascular injury. Science 1989;245:186–188.

The Endothelium: An Introduction to Current Research, pages 95–105
© 1990 Wiley-Liss, Inc.

9
The Endothelium and Atherosclerosis

J.F. MARTIN AND D.G. HASSALL
*Wellcome Research Laboratories, Beckenham, Kent BR3 3BS, England
(J.F.M., D.G.H.); King's College School of Medicine and Dentistry,
London, England (J.F.M)*

ATHEROSCLEROSIS

The commonest causes of death in industrialised society are myocardial infarction and stroke. Invariably, the underlying condition that leads to arterial occlusion in both these diseases is atherosclerosis. This is a proliferative disease of the vessel wall whose origin is unknown but whose final manifestation is seen at postmortem examination as an amorphous fatty and often calcified lesion. The use of monoclonal antibodies has allowed identification of cellular components within this lesion (1). Both macrophages and lymphocytes are present. Fatty streaks, lesions formed throughout life and even in children, are composed of monocytes under an intact endothelium. Some have claimed that these lesions may progress to adult atherosclerosis (2), but others have argued that they have a different anatomical distribution in the vascular system. There is, however, general agreement that the early human lesion involves proliferation of smooth muscle cells and the formation of foam cells due the accumulation of cholesteryl esters by macrophages derived from circulating monocytes. However, the time of initiation of the lesion and the original cellular events are still debated. There is, however, evidence from animal experiments and human postmortem tissue that several different factors may be involved: release of platelet-derived growth factor from platelets (3), rheological damage to the endothelium, (4), the adhesion of monocytes to endothelium (5), the accumulation of fibrinogen (6), monoclonal proliferation of smooth muscle cells (7), viral initiation of cellular change (8), or abnormal stimulation of the nerve supply to the vessel wall (9).

However, for more than 100 years it has been generally believed that the initiation of atherosclerosis takes place at the interface between the blood and the vessel wall. While Virchow (10), later supported by Ross and Glomset (3), held contrary views to Rokitansky (11) and later Duguid (12), the essential argument was whether the initial lesion in atherosclerosis

was luminal injury or luminal encrustation of thrombus. The commonest animal models of atherosclerosis arise from these theories and are of two types: those involving direct damage to the endothelium (13) and those maintaining elevated levels of blood cholesterol (14). A recently developed model of atherosclerosis questions whether endothelial damage is necessarily involved in the initiation of atherosclerosis (15).

A NEW MODEL OF ATHEROSCLEROSIS

Over the past three decades of atherosclerosis research, many advances have been made in our understanding of the cellular events that lead to the degenerative pathology of lesion formation. Man is unique in the animal kingdom in developing the progressive cellular changes that occur in these lesions (probably because of his environment), making its study in vivo difficult. It is with this in mind that models of atherosclerosis have been studied in other species. However, because of the time course of the development of this disease process, any "model" of atherosclerosis can only approximate the natural history of the cellular elements of early and advanced atherosclerotic plaque in man.

Since the development of the "response to injury" hypothesis supported by Ross and Glomset (3), many models of atherosclerosis have involved direct injury to the vessel wall (13), particularly the endothelium. Current lines of investigation now suggest that atherosclerotic lesions may develop under an endothelium that is at least physically intact.

Recent experimental evidence using a model established in the rabbit that produces a rapid proliferative lesion containing foam cells supports this proposal. A light, biologically inert, flexible Silastic collar is placed around a carotid artery in rabbits. It touches the artery circumferentially at two points; the contralateral artery acts as a control in the same animal. The placing of the "collar" results in a massive proliferation of the intimal region of the vessel wall when left in place 7–14 days. This proliferation consisted of smooth muscle cells (Fig. 1). In groups of animals where, in addition to the collar, the animals were maintained on a high cholesterol diet, the appearance of macrophage-derived foam cells and extracellular lipid were also present within the area defined by the collar over the same time period. There was no evidence of intimal proliferation, foam cell formation or accumulation of extracellular lipid in the control arteries of either dietary groups, indicating that physical manipulation at the time of surgery was not sufficient to generate the lesions. The presence of proliferating smooth muscle cells and foam cells account for two major components of any human atherosclerotic plaque. Analysis of the lipid content of the vessels by measurement of free and esterified cholesterol following extraction demonstrated a significant elevation in the cholesteryl ester content when on a high cholesterol diet consistent with the histological observation of foam cells and extracellular lipid.

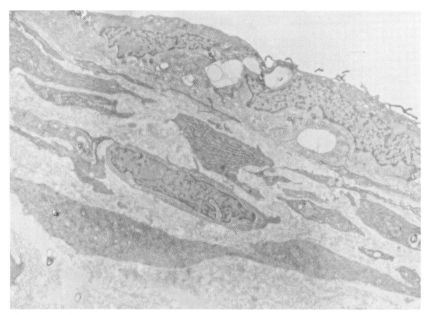

Fig. 1. Endothelial cells overlaying a proliferative lesion in the rabbit model of atherosclerosis described in the text. They appear morphologically intact. There is extensive Golgi apparatus and endoplasmic reticulum, together with many mitochondria, lipid vacuoles, and vesicles. The endothelial cells possess short microvilli and complex cell to cell junctions. ×10,000.

Examination of the lesions under electron microscopy demonstrated that these proliferative changes had occurred under a physically intact endothelium from as early as 24 hr up to 8 weeks in the presence of the collar. Biochemical measurements of prostacyclin production showed similar synthesis rates to control carotids. Also, the demonstration of endothelium-dependent relaxation in response to acetylcholine (ACh) is suggestive of a functionally intact endothelium. The infiltration of circulating mononuclear cells, particularly monocytes, has been demonstrated in man and in models of atherosclerosis (16). These cells marginate on and diapedese through the vascular lining (Fig. 2) by a mechanism that is so far poorly understood.

There is now increasing evidence that these cells require the expression and interaction of specific adherence proteins on the surfaces of both monocytes and endothelial cells. Such molecules on the endothelium include intercellular adhesion molecule-1 (ICAM-1) and endothelial-cell adhesion molecule-1 (ELAM-1) (17). These molecules have been reported to alter their expression following various stimuli suggesting that in response to

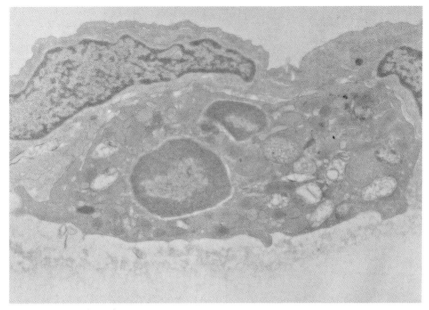

Fig. 2. Leukocytes are associated with early lesion development in the rabbit model of atherosclerosis described in the text. In this instance a leukocyte is observed below the endothelial layer but above the internal elastic lamina. The endothelial cells are morphologically normal. ×20,000.

certain biochemical triggers, the surface of the intact endothelium may express a different pattern of recognition markers for circulating monocytes, lymphocytes, or platelets.

The processes of atherosclerosis are a highly complex sequence of events that are orchestrated by many biochemical and cellular changes. Many of these are, as yet, undefined or poorly understood and warrant further investigation. Of particular importance is the possible functional alteration that may occur in the endothelial cells lining affected arteries. Intrinsic changes, including the expression of receptors, alterations in permeability and biological responses to the many possible stimuli that occur due to the development of atherosclerotic lesions should all be considered. Alternatively, we must begin to consider other possible casual relationships for the development of this disease.

A NEW HYPOTHESIS FOR ATHEROGENESIS

The above model, seen to produce a focal proliferative lesion due to the manipulation of the outer layers of the carotid artery suggests that the development of these lesions may arise due to light pressure on the outside of the vessel, which will almost certainly occlude the vasa vasorum or impair nerves within the adventitial layer. Investigators have interfered with flow through vasa vasorum (18), resulting in medial necrosis, intimal thickening with the proliferation of smooth muscle cells, and production of elastin and collagen. Occlusion of the vasa vasorum would cause hypoxia of medial smooth muscle cells. It has been demonstrated that exposure of cultured endothelial cells or monocytes to hypoxia results in significant increases in their production of mRNA to platelet-derived growth factor (PDGF) (19). PDGF is a potent mitogen for smooth muscle cells. Biochemical enzyme change, including acyl CoA: cholesterol acyl transferase (ACAT) responsible for the esterification of cholesterol has also been reported. ACAT activity has been shown to increase in response to hypoxic conditions in smooth muscle cells (20) and may also increase in macrophages. A similar origin may underlie some forms of human atherosclerosis. Alterations in the function of endothelium lining the vasa vasorum such as changes in surface markers may lead to the deposition of fibrin and result in platelet thrombus formation as has been demonstrated in diabetes (21). Plugging of vessels of the vasa vasorum with platelets and fibrin would again result in medial hypoxia, as well as impair vasomotor tone of the vessels due to nerve damage. The endothelium of the vasa vasorum, which is so far unstudied, might be involved in the pathogenesis of atherosclerosis.

PLATELETS AND ATHEROSCLEROSIS

A pathogenic role has been ascribed to platelets in atherosclerosis (22, 23) and thrombotic disorders (24). Platelets from patients with type IIa hyperlipoproteinaemia are more sensitive to agonists such as adrenaline and adenosine diphosphate than, platelets from normal subjects (25), and this may be significant because the increased concentration of cholesterol-rich low-density lipoproteins (LDL) associated with this disorder has been linked with atherogenesis (26,27). Plasma lipoproteins, particularly LDL, have been shown to enhance the sensitivity of platelet-rich plasma to some agonists (28) and enhance platelet aggregation in isolated systems (29). Platelet sensitivity can also change following the destruction of the circulating platelet pool (30). Platelets so produced in response to thrombocytopenia not only are more reactive but also have a larger mean platelet volume (31).

Myocardial infarction (MI), one of the major consequences of atherosclerosis, is invariably associated with occlusion of the coronary artery by thrombus which, itself, arises because of an altered relationship between platelets and the vessel wall either due to changes in endothelial function or due to rupture of atheromatous plaque (32). In either case, the presence of more reactive platelets in coronary blood is more likely to lead to thrombosis than less reactive platelets. Platelet density and volume have both been shown to increase in acute myocardial infarction (33–35). Shortened bleeding time in MI is also associated with platelet mass (36) which is generally accepted as an indicator of in vivo platelet activity (37). Platelets are produced from the cytoplasm of megakaryocytes; these cells are unique in that they can increase their nuclear DNA content (ploidy) without undergoing mitotic cell division. The regulation of platelet production is poorly understood but an increase in megakaryocyte ploidy and size occurs in response to platelet consumption, as for example in experimental thrombocytopenia (30). The appearance of large megakaryocytes is paralleled by the appearance of large, more reactive platelets (30) associated with a shortened bleeding time (38).

Further evidence that megakaryocyte and platelet heterogeneity might be altered in vascular disease comes from rabbit and guinea pig models (39,40). Increased cholesterol is a major risk factor for death from myocardial infarction (27). Cholesterol feeding of animals can lead to alterations in platelet responses to agonists (41). Platelets themselves do not take up cholesterol from lipoproteins in the circulation, but it is incorporated directly into the megakaryocyte, which in turn will produce cholesterol-enriched platelets (40). Similarly, platelet count and megakaryocyte size and ploidy are found to be increased when rabbits are fed a high cholesterol diet that induces atheromatous lesions (39,40). In more recent experiments, the maintenance of rabbits on a high cholesterol diet, when combined with the induction of thrombocytopenia, resulted in an acceleration of the atherogenic process (Fig. 3), as well as increases in megakaryocyte size and ploidy (42).

Platelet involvement in atherosclerosis may also include the development of foam cell formation by monocytes. Recent evidence suggests that the presence of platelet aggregation products leads to the enhancement of lipid accumulation by monocyte-derived macrophages in vitro (43). Clearly, the cellular events leading to initiation and development of atherosclerosis are complex and have been suggested to include changes in endothelial cells, monocytes, macrophages, lymphocytes, smooth muscle cells, and platelets (5), as well as a variety of extracellular matrix components. The relative importance of these cells is still unknown and appears to depend on the choice of experimental model. Platelets may be crucial in initiating the movement of smooth muscle cells into the intima following endothelial injury but do not appear to initiate their proliferation (44). Enhancement of platelet sensitivity due to a disturbance in the platelet–megakaryocyte axis or due to direct influence of blood-borne components or alteration in endothelial function may also occur singly or as a complex process. This will influence the behaviour of other cell types such as monocytes and resident vessel macrophages. Further study is required for all these elements in order to establish their relevance in the initiation and ultimate progression of atherosclerosis.

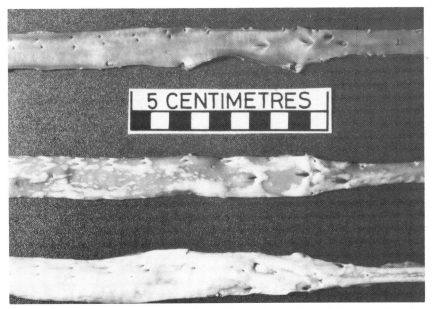

Fig. 3. Macroscopic atheromatous plaque formation in the rabbit aorta following high-cholesterol diet. The three aortae shown are representative from a group of male siblings. The upper aorta is from a rabbit on normal diet sacrificed at the same time as the other two. The aorta in the centre is from a rabbit sacrificed after 12-week high-cholesterol diet; atheromatous plaque occupies 45% of the aorta. The rest of the endothelium is intact as in the control above it. The lower aorta is from a rabbit that underwent platelet destruction 7 days before sacrifice. It was also on a high-cholesterol diet. Platelet and megakaryocyte changes occurred during the 7 days of accelerated atherogenesis, leading to the 97% coverage of the aorta with atheroma as shown.

MONOCYTES, THE ENDOTHELIUM, AND SECOND MESSENGERS

The endothelial cell is a complex cell that fulfills many specific functions. These include the maintenance of a semipermeable barrier between the blood and the cells that comprise the vessel wall. Also the endothelium is responsible for the synthesis and secretion of many vasoactive substances including prostacyclin (PGI_2), nitric oxide (NO), endothelin, tissue plasminogen activator and factor VIII, possessing both pro- and anticoagulant properties. Studies on the relationship between blood-borne cells and endothelium have been mainly based on ex vivo experiments or in vitro tissue culture studies. The discovery of PGI_2 and NO and their involvement in the inhibition of platelet function are well documented and have been discussed fully elsewhere in this book. From these results, it is suggested that the inhibition of platelet function may account for the antithrombotic nature of the endothelial cell surface and may therefore act as a defence mechanism against blood-borne cell invasion.

Experimental results obtained in vitro lend some support for this. The potent effect of PGI_2 and NO have already been described for platelets. Other cellular responses to these agents have been observed in monocytes. The adherence of blood monocytes to the arterial endothelium and subsequent migration into the arterial intima are early events in the development of atherosclerotic lesions (16). The factors that initiate these responses in vivo are unknown. Similarly, factors that may oppose monocyte adherence and chemotaxis are also unknown. Monocytes have been studied for their ability to adhere to layers of endothelial cells in culture and in response to chemotactic signals in Boyden chambers. Using both PGI_2 and NO as probes to study their effects in cellular behaviour, it has been demonstrated that PGI_2 can inhibit monocyte chemotaxis in a dose-dependent manner when moncytes are exposed to a chemotactic gradient of N-formyl-methionyl-leucyl-phenylalanine (fMLP). This effect can be enhanced by the presence of a cyclic adenosine monophosphate (cAMP) phosphodiesterase inhibitor (HL725) (45). NO, when added to unstimulated monocytes, results in a reduction in the basal adherence of these cell types (46). These difficult experiments provide some support for the existence of a regulatory role for endothelium in modulating blood-borne cells (Fig. 4). Monocyte cAMP is raised after stimulation by PGI_2, and cyclic guanine monophosphate (cGMP) is raised after NO stimulation. The interplay between these second messenger systems may therefore serve to prevent the margination and chemotaxis of resting cells. These processes may then be overridden when strong pro-adherent/pro-chemotactic signals are re-

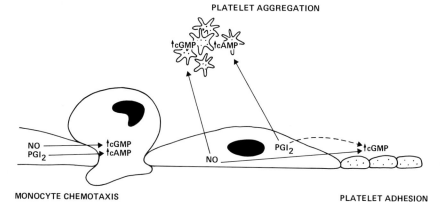

Fig. 4. Diagrammatic representation of the possible relationships among endothelial cell, prostacyclin, and nitric oxide production and their effects on the second messengers cAMP and cGMP in modulating platelet and monocyte behaviour. (See also Ch. 1, this volume.)

leased by the vessel wall during the initiation phase of early atherosclerotic development. However, other vasoactive substances, such as endothelin, and the mitogen PDGF do not appear to affect monocyte behaviour (47). Many more agents require further study. The development of in vitro tissue culture systems for the study of cell–cell interactions in response to many stimuli provide the foundation on which many cellular and biochemical relationships can be studied. Scientific innovation will be required to unravel the complex nature in which the endothelium may play a role in the maintenance of a nonthrombogenic surface and a semi-permeable barrier for cells and other blood-borne constituents.

REFERENCES

1. Jonasson L, Holm J, Skalli O, Bondjers G, Hansson GK. Regional accumulations of T-cells, macrophages and smooth muscle cells in the human atherosclerotic plaque. Atherosclerosis 1986;6:131–138.
2. Stary HC. Evolution and progression of atherosclerotic lesions in coronary arteries of children and young adults. Atherosclerosis 1989;9(1) (supplt 1) 1–19.
3. Ross R, Glomset JA. The pathogenesis of atherosclerosis. N Engl J Med 1976; 295:369–377.
4. Karino T, Asakura T, Mabuchi S. Vascular geometry, flow patterns and preferred site of atherosclerosis in human coronary and cerebral arteries. In: Crepaldi G, et al, eds. Atherosclerosis. Vol. VIII. Amsterdam: Excerpta Medica/Elsevier, 1989;417–424.
5. Ross R. The pathogenesis of atherosclerosis—An update. N Engl J Med 1986; 314:488–500.
6. Smith E. Human atherosclerotic lesions: An overview. In: Crepaldi G, et al., eds. Atherosclerosis. Vol. VIII: Amsterdam: Excerpta Medica/Elsevier, 1989; 13–20.
7. Benditt EP, Benditt JM. Evidence for a monoclonal origin of human atherosclerotic plaques. Proc Natl Acad Sci USA 1973;70:1753.
8. Melnick JL, Dreesman GR, McCollum CH, Petrie BL, Burek J, DeBakey ME. Cytomegalovirus antigen within human arterial smooth muscle cells. Lancet 1983;2:644–647.
9. Gutstein WH. The central nervous system and atherogenesis: Endothelial injury. Atherosclerosis 1988;70:145–154.
10. Virchow R. (1856). In: Gesamelte Abhandlungen zur wissenschaftlichten Medizin. Phlagose und Thrombose in Gefassystem. Frankfurt: Meidinger Sohn and Co., 1856;458–636.
11. Rokitansky C. In: A Manual of Pathological Anatomy. Vol. 4. London: The Sydenham Society, 1852;272.
12. Duguid RB. Thrombosis as a factor in the pathogenesis of coronary atherosclerosis. J Pathol 1946;58:207–220.
13. Reidy MA, Fingerle J, Majesky MW. Proliferation of vascular smooth muscle cells in vivo. In: Suckling KE, Groot PHE, eds. Hyperlipidaemia and Atherosclerosis. San Diego, California: Academic Press 1988;149–164.
14. Wissler RW, Vasselinovich D. Evaluation of animal models for the study of the pathogenesis of atherosclerosis. In: Hauss WH, et al, eds. State of Prevention and Therapy in Human Arteriosclerosis and in Animal Models. 1978.

15. Booth RFG, Martin JF, Honey AC, Hassall DG, Beesley JE, Moncada S. Rapid development of atherosclerotic lesions in the rabbit carotid artery induced by perivascular manipulation. Atherosclerosis 1989;76:257–268.

16. Gerrity RG. The role of the monocyte in atherogenesis I and II. Am J Pathol 1981;103:181–199.

17. Bevilacqua MP, Wheeler ME, Pober JS, Fiers W, Mendrick DC, Cotran RS, Gimbrone MA Endothelial dependent mechanisms of leukocyte adhesion: Regulation by interleukin-1 and tumour necrosis factor. In Movat HZ, ed. Leukocyte Emigration and Its Sequelae. Basel: S. Karger, 1987;79–93.

18. Heistad DD, Marcus ML, Martins JB. The effects of neural stimuli on blood flow through the vasa vasorum in dogs. Circ Res 1979;45:615–620.

19. Sakariassen KS, Powell JS, Raines EW, Ross R. Selective expression of platelet derived growth factor B chain mRNA by human endothelial cells and by human peripheral blood monocytes but not by smooth muscle cells. Thromb Haemost 1987;58:261–268.

20. Mukodani S, Ishiuawa Y, Miyazaki N, Taniguchi T, Watanabe N, Takano S, Okamoto R, Fukuzaki H. Hypoxia promotes the cholesteryl ester accumulation in cultured aortic smooth muscle cells by enhancement of acyl CoA: Cholesterol acyl transferase activity. Arteriosclerosis 1986;6:525 (abst)

21. Timperley WR, Ward JD, Preston FE, Duckworth T, O'Malley BC. Clinical and histological studies in diabetic neuropathy. A reassessment of vascular factors in relation to intravascular coagulation. Diabetologia 1976;12:237–243.

22. Ross R, Glomset J, Kariya B, Harker L. A platelet dependent serum factor that stimulates the proliferation of arterial smooth muscle cells in vitro. Proc Natl Acad Sci USA 1974;71:1207–1210.

23. Roberts WC, Ferrans VJ. The role of thrombosis in the etiology of atherosclerosis (a positive one) and in precipitating fatal ischaemic heart disease (a negative one). In Donoso E, Haft J, eds. Thrombosis, Platelets, Anticoagulation and Acetylsalicylic Acid. New York: Stratton, 1976;143–155.

24. Harker LA, Slichter SJ. Platelet and fibrinogen consumption in man. N Engl J Med 1972;28:999–1005.

25. Carvalho ACA, Colman RW, Lees RS. Platelet function in hyperlipoproteinaemia. N Engl J Med 1974;290:434–438.

26. Kannel WB, Castelli WP, Gordon T, McNamara PM. Serum cholesterol, lipoproteins and the risk of coronary heart disease. The Framingham Study. Ann Intern Med 1971;74:1–12.

27. Martin MJ, Hulley SB, Browner WS, Kuller LH, Wentworth D. Serum cholesterol, blood pressure and mortality: Implications from a cohort of 361662 men. Lancet 1986;2:933–936.

28. Hassall DG, Forrest LA, Bruckdorfer KR, Marenah CB, Turner P, Cortese C, Miller NE, Lewis B. Influence of plasma lipoproteins on platelet aggregation in a normal male population. Arteriosclerosis 1983;3:332–338.

29. Hassall DG, Owen JS, Bruckdorfer KR. The aggregation of isolated human platelets in the presence of lipoproteins and prostacyclin. Biochem J 1983;216:43–49.

30. Martin JF, Trowbridge EA, Salmon G, Plumb J. The biological significance of platelet volume: Its relationship to bleeding time, platelet thromboxane B_2

production and megakaryocyte nuclear DNA concentration. Thromb Res 1983; 32:443–460.

31. Corash L, Huei YC, Levin J, Baker G, Lu M, Mok Y. Regulation of thrombopoieisis: Effects of the degree of thrombocytopenia on megakaryocyte ploidy and platelet volume. Blood 1987;70:177–185.

32. Davies MJ, Thomas A. Thrombosis and acute coronary artery lesions in sudden cardiac ischaemic death. N Engl J Med 1984;310:1137–1140.

33. Martin JF, Plumb J, Kilby RS, Kishk YT. Changes in platelet volume and density in myocardial infarction. Br Med J [Clin Res] 1983;287:456–459.

34. Cameron HA, Philips R, Ibbotson RM, Carson PHM. Platelet size in myocardial infarction. Br Med J [Clin Res] 1983;287:449–451.

35. Kishk YT, Trowbridge EA, Martin JF. Platelet volume sub-populations in myocardial infarction: An investigation of their homogeneity for smoking, infarct size and site. Clin Sci 1985;68:419–425.

36. Milner PC, Martin JF. Shortened bleeding time in acute myocardial infarction and its relation to platelet mass. Br Med J [Clin Res] 1985;290:1767–1770.

37. Harker L, Slichter S. The bleeding time as a screening test for evaluation of platelet function. N Engl J Med 1972;287:155–159.

38. Kristensen SD, Bath PMW, Martin JF. The bleeding time is inversely related to megakaryocyte nuclear DNA content and size in man. Thromb Haemost 1988;59:357–359.

39. Martin JF, Slater DN, Kishk YT, Trowbridge EA. Platelet and megakaryocyte changes in cholesterol-induced experimental atherosclerosis. Arteriosclerosis 1985;5:604–612.

40. Schick BP, Schick PK. The effect of hypercholesterolaemia on guinea-pig platelets, erythrocytes and megakaryocytes. Biochem Biophys Acta 1985;833:291–302.

41. Fujitani B, Tsuboi T, Yoshida K, Shimizu M. Aggregation of gel-filtered guinea-pig platelets by lipoproteins. Thromb Haemost 41:416–424.

42. Kristensen SD, Roberts KM, Kishk YT, Martin JF. Accelerated atherogenesis occurs following platelet destruction and increases in megakaryocyte size and DNA content. Eur J Clin Invest. 1990; in press.

43. Curtiss LK, Black AS, Tagaki Y, Plow EF. New mechanism for foam cell generation in atherosclerotic lesions. J Clin Invest. 1989;80:367–373.

44. Fingerle J, Johnson R, Clowes AW, Majesky MW, Reidy MA. Role of platelets in smooth muscle cell proliferation and migration after vascular injury in rat carotid artery. Proc Natl Acad Sci USA 1989;86:8412–8416.

45. Hassall DG, Ward J, Moncada S, Martin JF, Booth RFG. Monocyte adherence and chemotaxis are inhibited by carbacyclin. In: Suckling KE, Groot PHE, eds. Hyperlipidaemia and Atherosclerosis. San Diego, California: Academic Press, 1988;212–213.

46. Bath PMW, Hassall DG, Booth RFG, Martin JF. Nitric oxide inhibits monocyte chemotaxis and adhesion to endothelial monolayers. Clin Sci 1989;76(Suppl. 20):25P.

47. Bath PMW, Mayston SA, Martin JF. Endothelin and PDGF do not stimulate peripheral blood monocyte chemotaxis, adhesion to endothelium or superoxide production. Exp Cell Res 1990; in press.

The Endothelium: An Introduction to Current Research, pages 107–117
© 1990 Wiley-Liss, Inc.

10
Coronary Vasomotion and the Endothelium: Possible Role in Ischemic Syndromes

JOHN CLARKE, SIMON LARKIN, GRAHAM DAVIES, AND
ATTILIO MASERI
*Department of Medicine, Cardiovascular Division, Hammersmith
Hospital, London W12 ONN, England*

VASOCONSTRICTION IN ISCHEMIC SYNDROMES

Angina pectoris and myocardial infarction occur in patients with a variable amount of coronary atherosclerosis and with variable severity of stenosis. Angina frequently occurs in patients with normal coronary arteries; indeed, as many as 20% of more than 20,000 patients entered in the CASS registry in the United States had no significant stenoses on coronary arteriography. Myocardial infarction occurs in patients with normal coronary arteries in about 5% of cases and in as many as 30% of infarcts occurring below the age of 35 years. Infarct-related arteries recanalized by thrombolytic therapy often show mild or moderate stenosis only (1). Thus, occlusive thrombosis frequently develops in the absence of a severe coronary stenosis.

Prinzmetal proposed that increased tonus at the site of an atherosclerotic plaque was the likely cause of a "variant" form of spontaneous angina characterized by ST-segment elevation (2). The hypothesis of spasm gained credence when it was invoked to explain the preserved exercise tolerance of patients with Prinzmetal's angina (3). Objective demonstration of spasm was first provided in isolated case reports (4,5) and subsequently by systematic studies (6,7).

Stimuli that are not sufficiently powerful to cause occlusive spasm in normal arteries may do so in arteries with severe atherosclerosis (8) because (i) the response to vasoactive stimuli may be altered by the disease process, and (ii) the presence of atheromatous plaques may magnify geometrically the extent of luminal narrowing for any given degree of smooth muscle shortening (9).

Effort angina is classically taken to occur because of an increase in myocardial oxygen demand in the presence of a fixed, reduced coronary reserve (10). Many patients have a threshold of exertion that cannot be exceeded without developing angina but have in addition episodes of angina at rest or at levels of exertion that are usually quite well tolerated (11). During unstable angina, transient repetitive opening and closing of the coronary artery has been described evidenced both angiographically and as ST-segment change on the electrocardiogram (ECG) (12).

It appears that acute stimuli occurring on a background of coronary atherosclerosis may cause transient or permanent impairment of regional coronary blood flow. These acute stimuli may be either coronary vasoconstriction or thrombosis, or both. A close interaction between thrombosis and vasoconstriction is suggested by the release of powerful constrictor substances from thrombus: 5-hydroxytryptamine (5-HT), thromboxane A_2 (TxA_2), and thrombin.

DISTINCTION BETWEEN PHYSIOLOGIC CONSTRICTION AND SPASM: HYPERREACTIVITY

The term *hyperreactivity,* when applied to the behaviour of coronary vessels, implies a greater than normal response in these vessels to a vasoactive stimulus (13). The term *coronary spasm* is now often used to indicate any form of coronary vasoconstriction associated with ischemic episodes, whether painful or silent (14). This generalization is incorrect, as the term spasm implies a sudden abnormal intense constriction of coronary vessels (15). In patients who do not have variant angina, the reduction in epicardial coronary artery diameter in response to cold pressor test, handgrip, and exercise is usually uniformly distributed and quite mild, ranging from 10–20%. The degree of constriction in response to ergonovine is also of the same order of magnitude (16). The question arises as to whether occlusive spasm, i.e., nonphysiological coronary vasoconstriction, is caused by exceptionally strong local constrictor stimuli or by an abnormal exaggerated local coronary artery response to common constrictor stimuli.

The mechanism by which the endothelium may contribute to coronary hyperreactivity is twofold, either through a loss of vasodilator capacity, resulting in unopposed vasoconstriction, or through an exaggerated effect of the constrictor mechanisms contained within the endothelium. The altered contribution of the endothelium to coronary vasomotion may be due to focal abnormality of endothelial morphology or function.

FACTORS INFLUENCING VESSEL RESPONSE

The response of the coronary circulation to vasoactive agents is highly dependent on species, site, and the concentration of agonist used. Changes that occur following receptor stimulation vary depending on whether the transmitter is released by nerve stimulation, arrives via the bloodstream or other humoral mechanism, or is given exogenously in an experimental situation. Responses obtained in vivo may differ from responses in vitro. Furthermore, the distribution of different receptor subtypes may vary in large versus small coronary vessels.

ROLE OF THE ENDOTHELIUM

The endothelium in atherosclerotic vessels may exhibit abnormal function. Intracoronary acetylcholine (ACh) produces contractions of coronary arteries in patients with coronary artery disease, whereas in patients with angiographically normal vessels coronary dilation is seen (17). Histamine is a vasodilator of the normal coronary circulation in vivo; it causes endothelium-dependent relaxations in isolated human coronary arteries (18,19) with intact endothelium but contractions when the endothelium is removed. Angiographically normal epicardial segments dilate during exercise, whereas stenotic coronary segments constrict reversibly (20). The two main vasodilator agents derived from the endothelium are prostacyclin, identified approximately twenty years ago, and, more recently, nitric oxide, an endothelium-dependent relaxant factor initially described by Furchgott in 1980. The physiological significance of these substance is not clear. While there is no known physiological mechanism of physiological release for prostacyclin, it has been shown that nitric oxide is released from vascular endothelial cells in culture by shear stress.

Dilator Agents

PGI$_2$. Endothelial cells produce 10–20 times more prostaglandin I_2 (PGI$_2$) than do vascular smooth muscle cells (21). Prostacyclin inhibits platelet aggregation and dilates coronary arteries. Its mode of action appears to be by increasing intracellular cyclic adenosine monophosphate (cAMP). Platelet inhibitor drugs, such as aspirin, which inhibit cyclo-oxygenase, reduce vascular prostacyclin production.

EDRF. Acetylcholine relaxes arteries in vitro via a diffusible endothelium-derived relaxant factor (EDRF) (22) subsequently characterized as nitric oxide. L-Arginine is the precursor substance from which nitric oxide is cleaved in endothelial cells. Haemoglobin, oxygen-derived free radicals, and antioxidants are potent inhibitors of EDRF (23,24). EDRF is a potent vasodilator and inhibitor of platelet aggregation and adhesion (25,26). Concentrations of either EDRF or PGI$_2$, which have no vasomotor action, enhance the vascular and antiaggregatory effects of other substances (27). EDRF has been shown to increase subendocardial blood flow preferentially (28). Inhibition of cyclic guanine monophosphate cGMP formation using methylene blue or LY83583 reduces endothelium-dependent relaxations. EDRF is released in response to flow (shear stress), platelet-derived products (ADP, thrombin, serotonin), hormones and autacoids (bradykinin (29), histamine, noradrenaline, substance P, vasopressin (30,31)).

Large coronary arteries may contract or relax to ACh in vitro. This may reflect species variation or differences in the techniques employed during tissue preparation (32). Canine epicardial coronary arteries consistently relax in the organ bath following the application of ACh, whereas constriction has been observed in experiments involving vessels from other animal species. Both constriction and relaxation to ACh (33) have been reported using human coronary artery. It is possible that differences in the degree of damage to the endothelial lining of the coronary vessels may cause variation in the amount of EDRF released. Also, where vessels are preconstricted prior to eliciting relaxant effects to ACh, the method of preconstriction used may be important.

The effects of intracoronary administration of ACh has been studied in man (17,34–37). These studies were conducted in patients with some coronary disease. At moderate doses, minor dilatation was seen, whereas at the highest dose (34) low oxygen saturation was observed when the epicardial segments were dilated. One explanation for these results is that the net effect of ACh on a particular site may depend on the local balance between ACh-induced release of EDRF and the direct vasoconstrictor effect of ACh on smooth muscle. This may reflect (i) variations in the local ratio between the number of functioning endothelial and smooth muscle cells, (ii) the distribution and affinity of muscarinic receptors on smooth muscle and endothelial cells, or (iii) the local concentration–response relationships between direct constriction and EDRF-mediated dilation. Ludmer et al. (17) observed that angiographically normal epicardial vessels dilate in response to intracoronary ACh, whereas those with angiographic evidence of atheroma constrict under the same conditions suggesting that the presence of atheroma may have profound effects on the response of epicardial vessels to ACh.

Substance P, the 11-amino acid vasodilator peptide, is widely distributed throughout the sensory nervous system (38), including the nerves supplying human epicardial coronary arteries and smaller arterioles (39). Substance P releases EDRF, causes a drop in the peripheral vascular resistance after intravenous infusion (40), and increases forearm blood flow following brachial artery infusion (41). It is a potent dose-dependent dilator of human epicardial coronary arteries, both normal and diseased, and induces a moderate increase in blood flow (42). Dilation of diseased segments implies preservation of endothelial function at that site.

Constrictor Agents

EDCF. Endothelin, the 21-amino acid peptide, was first isolated and sequenced in 1989 from porcine endothelial cells and was thought to be the endothelial constrictor factor first described by Hickey et al. in 1985 (43). Autoradiographic studies in human coronary arteries have shown the presence of binding sites for endothelin in the smooth muscle layer of these vessels but not within the endothelium itself (44). Endothelin binding sites were also demonstrated in perivascular nerves.

In vitro studies of the effects of endothelin in the presence and absence of nicardipine on isolated ring preparations of left anterior coronary arteries obtained from both animal tissue (45) and explanted human hearts (44) show that endothelin can constrict these vessels in a dose-related fashion. In the presence of nicardipine, the EC_{50} obtained with endothelin remained unaltered, while the maximal response was reduced. Organ bath studies have shown that the sensitivity of coronary artery from animals differed depending on the size of vessel studied, the smaller vessels being more sensitive (i.e., a lower EC_{50}) (44). Intracoronary infusions of picomolar doses of endothelin-1 into the left anterior descending coronary artery of the open-chest greyhound induced a dose-dependent reduction in flow in that vessel. The profound reduction of flow was exclusive to the infused vessel and was sufficient to cause transmural myocardial ischaemia (46). Using arteriographic and microsphere techniques, it was also demonstrated that the vasoconstriction observed was confined to the microcirculation. The in vivo constrictor effects are reversible by dihydropyridine calcium-channel antagonists (47). Endothelin is a potent constrictor of forearm vessels in human subjects with a long duration of action (48). In view of its great potency and long duration of action both in vivo and in vitro, it's likely possible physiological role is not clear.

EDHF. The endothelium also may release an endothelium-derived hyperpolarising factor (EDHF). Ouabain, a $Na^+K^+ATPase$ inhibitor, reduces endothelium-dependent relaxations to ACh in the canine femoral artery (49). It is possible that hyperpolarization of vascular smooth muscle cells may contribute to the sustained phase of endothelium-dependent relaxations and may render the cells less responsive to contractile stimuli.

Endothelial Absence

Using hyperlipidemic pigs in vivo, it has been shown that the application of histamine to vessels in which endothelial denudation has been performed can induce coronary vasospasm (50), although in this paper, the animals were studied 5 days after denudation, when it is likely that endothelium of the vessel under study had regenerated. A local increase in adventitial mast cells has been documented in a patient with coronary spasm (51). However, histamine is effective in provoking vasospasm only in some, but not all patients with variant angina (52).

Endothelin-dependent vasorelaxation of some vessels by calcitonin gene-related peptide has been described in certain species, but to date this does not include man. It is speculated that the action of this potent vasodilator peptide that coexists with substance P in perivascular sensory neurons may in part be dependent on endothelial cell function.

There are mixed reports as to whether the action of neuropeptide Y (NPY) is dependent on the endothelium (53). Certainly, NPY can cause myocardial ischaemia in patients with angiographically normal coronary arteries by acting predominantly on smaller coronary vessels (54). In the organ bath, epicardial coronary vessels do not react to NPY (55), whereas smaller vessels do (56). NPY can reduce coronary blood flow in anaesthetized greyhound dogs by acting on small vessels (57).

In normal dog coronary arteries, intracoronary infusion of serotonin in-vivo decreases epicardial vessel diameter. Ketanserin, an S_2-blocking agent, only partially prevents the contraction induced by serotonin in vitro in the canine coronary artery. A nonselective S_1 and S_2 serotonin receptor antagonist methiothepin does block the effect, suggesting that receptors other than S_2 receptors are involved (58). This may explain why ketanserin is ineffective in the prevention of attacks of variant angina (59). Removal of the endothelium potentiates the response to serotonin (60), suggesting that the effect of serotonin on epicardial coronary arteries is the net result of direct vasoconstriction and endothelium-mediated vasodilation. Where endothelial regeneration has occurred, e.g., following balloon injury in porcine coronary arteries, a defect of endothelium-dependent relaxations in response to serotonin and aggregating platelets may occur (61). Serotonin can produce marked constriction of compliant coronary stenoses in dogs in vivo, but this effect is mediated by non-S_2-serotonergic receptors (62). In normal human coronary arteries in vitro (63), serotonin caused contraction, which was markedly enhanced by removal of the endothelium, and not completely blocked by ketanserin. Activation of serotonin receptors by ergonovine causes constriction of canine epicardial coronary arteries in vitro (64).

ABNORMAL ENDOTHELIAL FUNCTION

Risk factors for coronary artery disease, such as hyperlipidemia, atherosclerosis, and hypertension, impair endothelium-dependent relaxations in experimental animals and in human coronary arteries. In the rabbit aorta, low-density lipoprotein (LDL), but not high-density lipoprotein (HDL), inhibits endothelium-dependent relaxations in response to ACh (65). The inhibitory concentration of the lipoprotein corresponds to that found in plasma of patients with severe hyperlipidaemias. LDL and atherosclerosis inhibit vascular prostacyclin production (66). In experimental hypertension, endothelium-dependent relaxations are reduced in most vascular beds (67,68).

Endothelial injury promotes platelet adhesion and aggregation in coronary artery disease (69). Aggregating platelets cause contraction of arteries denuded of endothelial cells in vitro, which is inhibited by serotonin antagonists (70). In patients with coronary artery disease, endothelial dysfunction appears to occur both in stenotic sites (17) and in angiographically normal coronary segments (71).

CONCLUSION

The precise role that any or all of these factors plays in the normal regulation of coronary blood flow is unclear, but a currently favoured hypothesis is that endothelial abnormalities, both structural and functional, may contribute to the pathophysiology of ischaemic cardiac syndromes.

REFERENCES

1. Hackett D, Davies G, Chierchia S, Maseri A. Intermittent coronary occlusion in acute myocardial infarction. N Engl J Med 1987;317:1057–1059.
2. Prinzmetal M, Kennamer R, Merliss R, Wade T, Bor N. Angina pectoris: A variant form of angina pectoris. Am J Med 1959;27:375–384.
3. MacAlpin RN, Kattus AA, Alvaro AB. Angina pectoris at rest with preservation of exercise capacity: Prinzmetal's variant angina. Circulation 1973;47:946–958.
4. Oliva PB, Potts DE, Pluss RG. Coronary arterial spasm in Prinzmetal's angina: documentation by coronary arteriography. N Engl J Med 1973;288:745–751.
5. Maseri A, Mimmo R, Chierchia S, Marchesi C, Pesola A, L'Abbate A. Coronary spams as a cause of acute myocardial ischaemia in man. Chest 1975;68: 625–632.
6. Maseri A, Parodi O, Severi S, Pesola A. Transient transmural reduction of myocardial blood flow, demonstrated by thallium-201 scintigraphy, a cause of variant angina. Circulation 1976;54:280–288.
7. Maseri A, L'Abbate A, Pesola A, Ballestra AM, Marzilli M, Maltini G, Severi S, De Nes DM, Parodi O, Biagini A. Coronary vasospasm in angina pectoris. Lancet 1977;1:713–717.
8. Brown BG. Response of normal and diseased epicardial coronary arteries to vasoactive drugs: Quantitative arteriographic studies. Am J Cardiol 1985; 56:23E–29E.
9. MacAlpin RN, Kattus AA, Alvaro AB. Angina pectoris at rest with preservation of exercise capacity: Prinzmetal's variant angina. Circulation 1973;47:946–958.
10. Maseri A. Pathogenetic mechanisms of angina pectoris: Expanding views. Br Heart J 1980;43:648–660.
11. Maseri A, Chierchia S. A new rationale for the clinical approach to the patient with angina pectoris. Am J Med 1981;71:639–644.
12. Davies GJ, Chierchia S, Maseri A. Prevention of myocardial infarction by very early treatment with intracoronary streptokinase. N Engl J Med 1984;23:1488–1492.
13. Crea F, Davies G, Romeo F, Chierchia S, Bugiardini R, Maseri A. Myocardial ischaemia during ergonovine testing: Different susceptibility to coronary vasoconstriction in patients with exertional and variant angina. Circulation 1984; 69:690–694.
14. Maseri A, The role of coronary artery spasm in symptomatic and silent myocardial ischaemia. J Am Coll Cardiol 1987;9:249–262.

15. Hackett D, Larkin S, Chierchia S, Davies G, Kaski J, Maseri, A. Induction of coronary artery spasm by a direct local action of ergonovine. Circulation 1987; 75:577–580.

16. Curry RC, Pepine CJ, Sabom MB, Feldman RL, Christie LG, Conti R. Effects of ergonovine in patients with and without coronary artery disease. Circulation 1977;56:803–809.

17. Ludmer PL, Selwyn AP, Shook TL, Wayne RR, Mudge GH, Alexander RW, Ganz P. Paradoxical vasoconstriction induced by acetylcholine in atherosclerotic coronary arteries. N Engl J Med 1986;315:1046–1051.

18. Vigorito C, Giordano A, DeCaprio L, Vitale D, Ferrara N, Tuccillo B, Maurea N, Rispoli M, Rengo F. Direct coronary vasodilator effects of intracoronary histamine administration in humans. J Cardiovasc Pharmacol 1986;8:933–939.

19. Toda N. Mechanism of histamine actions in human coronary arteries. Circ Res 1987;61:280–286.

20. Gage JE, Hess OM, Murakami T, Ritter M, Grimm J, Krayenbuehl HP. Vasoconstriction of stenotic coronary arteries during dynamic exercise in patients with classic angina pectoris: Reversibility by nitroglycerin. Circulation 1986; 73:865–876.

21. Moncada S, Vane JR. Pharmacology and endogenous roles of prostaglandin endoperoxides, thromboxane A_2 and prostacyclin. Pharmacol Rev 1979;30:293–331.

22. Furchgott RF, Zawadzki JV. The obligatory role of endothelial cells in the relaxation of arterial smooth muscle by acetylcholine. Nature (Lond) 1980;299:373–376.

23. Luscher TF, Diederich D, Siebenmann R, Lehmann K, Stulz P, Von Segesser L, Yang Z, Turina M, Gradel E, Weber E, Buhler FR. Difference between endothelium-dependent relaxation in arterial and in venous coronary bypass grafts. N Engl J Med 1988;319:462–467.

24. Rubanyi GM, Vanhoutte PM. Superoxide anions and hyperoxia inactivate endothelium-derived relaxing factor. Am J Physiol 1986;250:H822–827.

25. Radomski MW, Palmer RMJ, Moncada S. The antiaggregating properties of vascular endothelium: Interactions between prostacyclin and nitric oxide. Br J Pharmacol 1987;92:639–646.

26. Radomski MW, Palmer RMJ, Moncada S. Endogenous nitric oxide inhibits human platelet adhesion to vascular endothelium. Lancet 1987;2:1057–1068.

27. Shimokawa H, Flahavan NA, Lorenz RR, Vanhoutte PM. Prostacyclin releases endothelium-derived relaxing factor and potentiates its action in porcine coronary arteries. Br J Pharmacol 1988;95:1197–1203.

28. Pelc LR, Gross GJ, Warltier DC. Preferential increase in subendocardial perfusion produced by endothelium-dependent vasodilators. Circulation 1987;76: 191–200.

29. Palmer RMJ, Ferrige AG, Moncada S. Nitric oxide release accounts for the biological activity of endothelium-derived relaxing factor. Nature (Lond) 1987; 327:524–526.

30. Luscher TF. Endothelial Vasoactive Substances and Cardiovascular Disease. Basel: S. Karger, 1988.

31. Luckhoff A, Busse R, Winter I, Bassenge E. Characterization of vascular relaxant factor released from cultured endothelial cells. Hypertension 1987;9:295–303.
32. Kalsner S. Cholinergic mechanisms in human coronary artery preparations: Implications of species differences. J Physiol (Lond) 1985;358:509–526.
33. Bossaller C, Habib GB, Yamamoto H, Williams C, Wells S, Henry PD. Impaired muscarinic endothelium-dependent relaxation and cyclic guanosine 5'-monophosphate formation in atherosclerotic human coronary artery and rabit aorta. J Clin Invest 1987;79:170–174.
34. Newman CM, Hackett DR, Fryer M, El-Tamimi HM, Davies GJ, Maseri A. Dual effects of acetylcholine on angiographically normal human coronary arteries in vivo. Circulation 1987;76(4):56.
35. Horio Y, Yasue H, Rokutanda M, Nakamura N, Ogawa H, Takaoka K, Matsuyama K, Kimura T. Effects of intracoronary injection of acetylcholine on coronary arterial diameter. Am J Cardiol 1986;57:984–989.
36. Yasue H, Yutaka H, Nakamura N, Fumi H, Imoto N, Sonoda R, Kugiyama K, Obata K, Morikami Y, Kimura T. Induction of coronary artery spasm by acetylcholine in patients with variant angina: Possible role of the parasympathetic nervous system in the pathogenesis of coronary artery spasm. Circulation 1986; 74:955–963.
37. Fish RD, Nabel EG, Selwyn AP, Ludmer PL, Mudge GH, Kirshenbaum JM, Schoen FJ, Alexander RW, Ganz P. Responses of coronary arteries of cardiac transplant patients to acetylcholine. J Clin Invest 1987;81:21–31.
38. Pernow B. Substance P. Pharmacol Rev 1983;35:85–141.
39. Weihe E, Reinecke M, Opherk D, Forssmann WG. Peptidergic innervation (substance P) in the human heart. J Mol Cell Cardiol 1981;13:331–333.
40. Fuller RW, Maxwell DL, Dixon CMS, McGregor GP, Barnes VF, Bloom SR, Barnes PJ. Effect of substance P on cardiovascular and respiratory function in subjects. J Appl Physiol 1987;62:1473–1479.
41. McEwan JR, Benjamin N, Fuller RW, Larkin S, Dollery CT, MacIntyre I. Vasodilation by calcitonin gene-related peptide and by substance P. A comparison of their effects on resistance and capacitance vessels of the human forearm. Circulation 1988;77:1072–1080.
42. Crossman DC, Larkin SW, Fuller RW, Davies GJ, Maseri A. Substance P dilates epicardial coronary arteries and increases coronary blood flow in humans. Circulation 1989;80:475–484.
43. Hickey KA, Rubanyi G, Paul RJ, Highsmith RF. Characterization of a coronary vasoconstrictor produced by cultured endothelial cells. Am J Physiol (Lond) 1985;248:C550–C556.
44. Chester AH, Dashwood MR, Clarke JG, Larkin SW, Tadjkarimi S, Davies GJ, Maseri A, Yacoub M. Influence of endothelin on human coronary arteries and localization of its binding sites. Am J Cardiol 1989;63:1395–1398.
45. Tippins JR, Antoniw JW, Maseri A. Endothelin-1 is a potent constrictor in conductive and resistive coronary arteries. J Cardiovasc Pharmacol 1989;13(5):S177–S179.
46. Larkin S, Clarke J, Keogh B, Araujo L, Rhodes C, Brannan J, Taylor K, Davies GJ, Maseri A. Intracoronary endothelin infusion induces transmural myocardial ischaemia in the dog. J Am Coll Cardiol 1989;13(2):84a (abst).

47. Clarke JG, Larkin S, Keogh B, Taylor K, Maseri A, Davies GJ. Endothelin induced vasoconstriction is reversible by calcium antagonists and endogenous vasodilators in the dog hindlimb vasculature. J Cardiovasc Pharmacol 1989; 13(5):211–212.

48. Clarke JG, Benjamin N, Larkin SW, Webb DJ, Davies GJ, Maseri A. Endothelin is a potent long-lasting vasoconstrictor in man. Am J Physiol 1989;257:H2033–H2035.

49. DeMey J, Vanhoutte PM. Role of Na$^+$·K$^+$-ATPase in the vasodilator response to acetylcholine. In: Vanhoutte PM, Leusen I, eds. Vasodilatation. New York: Raven Press. 1981;331–337.

50. Shimokawa H, Tomoike H, Nabeyama S, Yamamoto H, Arake H, Nakamura M. Coronary artery spasm induced in atherosclerotic miniature swine. Science 1983;221:560–562.

51. Forman MB, Oates JA, Robertson D, Robertson RM, Roberts LJ, Virmani R. Increased adventitial mast cells in a patient with coronary spasm. N Engl J Med 1985;313:1138–1141.

52. Kaski JC, Crea F, Meran D, Rodriguez L, Araujo L, Chierchia S, Davies G, Maseri A. Local coronary supersensitivity to diverse vasoconstrictive stimuli in patients with variant angina. Circulation 1986;74:1255–1265.

53. Daly RN, Hieble JP. Neuropeptide Y modulates adrenergic neurotransmission by an endothelium-dependent mechanism. Eur J Pharmacol 1987;138:445–446.

54. Clarke JG, Davies GJ, Kerwin R, Hackett D, Larkin S, Dawbarn D, Lee Y, Bloom SR, Yacoub M, Maseri A. Neuropeptide Y reproduces angina pectoris and myocardial ischaemia in patients. Lancet 1987;1:1057–1059.

55. Tippins JR, Clarke J, Larkin S, Yacoub M, Maseri A. Investigation of the action of neuropeptide Y in the isolated human coronary artery. Br J Pharmacol 1988;94:244 (abst).

56. Franco-Cereceda A, Lundberg JM: Potent effects of neuropeptide Y and calcitonin gene-related peptide on human coronary vascular tone in-vitro. Acta Physiol Scand 1987;131:159–160.

57. Clarke J, Larkin S, Osinawa O, Davies GJ, Taylor K, Maseri A. Neuropeptide Y reduces dog coronary blood flow by increased small vessel resistance. Clin Sci 1987;73(17):6 (abst).

58. Cohen RA. Contractions of isolated canine coronary arteries resistant to S$_2$-serotonergic blockade. J Pharmacol Exp Ther 1986;237:548–552.

59. Freedman SB, Chierchia S, Rodriguez-Plaza L, Bugiardini R, Smith G, Maseri A. Ergonovine induced myocardial ischaemia: No role for serotonergic receptors? Circulation 1984;70:178–183.

60. Lamping KG, Marcus ML, Dole WP. Removal of the endothelium potentiates canine large coronary artery constrictor responses to 5-hydroxytryptamine in vivo. Circ Res 1985;57:46–54.

61. Shimokawa H, Aarhus L, Vanhoutte PM. Porcine coronary arteries with regenerated endothelium have a reduced endothelium-dependent responsiveness to aggregating platelets and serotonin. Circ Res 1987;64:256–270.

62. Ichikawa Y, Yokoyama M, Akita H, Fukuzaki H. Constriction of a large coronary artery contributes to serotonin-induced myocardial ischaemia in the dog with pliable coronary arteries. J Am Coll Cardiol 1989;14:449–459.

63. Berkenboom G, Unger P, Fang Z, Degre S, Fontaine J. Comparison of the responses to acetylcholine and serotonin on isolated canine and human coronary arteries. Circ Res 1990; in press.
64. Brazenor RM, Angus JA. Ergometrine contracts isolated canine coronary arteries by a serotonergic mechanism: No role for alpha adrenoceptors. J Pharmacol Exp Ther 1981;218:530–534.
65. Andrews HE, Bruckdorfer KR, Dunn RC, Jacobs M. Low density lipoproteins inhibit endothelium-dependent relaxations in rabbit aorta. Nature (Lond) 1987;327:237–239.
66. Nordoy A, Svensson B, Wiebe D, Hoak JC. Lipoprotein and the inhibitory effect of human endothelial cells on platelet function. Circ Res 1978;43:527–534.
67. Luscher TF, Diederich D, Weber E, Vanhoutte PM, Buhler FR. Endothelium-dependent responses in the common carotid and renal artery of normotensive and spontaneously hypertensive rats. Hypertension 1988;11:573–578.
68. Lamping KD, Dole WP. Acute hypertension selectively potentiates constrictor responses of large coronary arteries to serotonin by altering endothelial function in vivo. Circ Res 1987;61:904–913.
69. Vanhoutte PM, Houston DS. Platelets, endothelium and vasospasm. Circulation 1985;72:728–734.
70. Houston DS, Shepherd JT, Vanhoutte PM. Aggregating human platelets cause direct contraction and endothelium-dependent relaxation of isolated canine coronary arteries. J Clin Invest 1986;78:539–544.
71. Werns SW, Walton JA, Hsia HH, Nabel EG, Sanz ML, Pitt B. Evidence of endothelial dysfunction in angiographically normal coronary arteries of patients with coronary artery disease. Circulation 1989;79:287–291.

The Endothelium: An Introduction to Current Research, pages 119–128
© 1990 Wiley-Liss, Inc.

11
Procoagulant Functions of Endothelium

D.C. CROSSMAN AND E.D.G. TUDDENHAM
Haemostasis Research Group, Clinical Research Centre, Harrow, Middlesex HA1 3UJ, England

INTRODUCTION

The vascular endothelium, situated as it is at the interface between the blood and vessel wall, must, necessarily, be an anticoagulant surface under basal conditions. This is achieved by a number of functions characteristic of this cell, including prostacyclin production, which prevents platelet aggregation (1); nitric oxide, which prevents platelet aggregation (2) and adhesion (3); protein C activation by thrombin/thrombomodulin (4,5); the binding of thrombin to endothelium-associated heparin-like molecules (6,7); and tissue plasminogen activator (tPA) expression (8,9), which promotes the lysis of any fibrin formed. The procoagulant functions of endothelium may be divided into three interrelated groups. It is clear that the endothelium may provide a facilitatory role for coagulation, expressing binding sites for factors IX and X and platelet adhesion molecules. These are presumably more than adequately balanced under basal conditions by the anticoagulant mechanisms described above. Down-regulation of these, which is known to occur in response to a number of agents, is therefore a second procoagulant mechanism of the vascular endothelium. The third, and potentially most powerful, is the ability of the endothelium to express an initiator of coagulation, tissue factor (TF), which will activate the extrinsic pathway of coagulation upon exposure to factor VII/VIIa in the blood.

The division of the second and third of these procoagulant mechanisms, is now perhaps artificial. It will be shown that up-regulation of initiatory TF expression can occur in response to the same stimuli that cause down-regulation of the anticoagulant mechanisms. The mechanisms by which these opposite responses (towards a common end) to the same stimulus occur are still unclear, but they demonstrate a highly specialised cell, which possesses multiple mechanisms to pass from its natural anticoagulant state to a powerfully prothrombotic state.

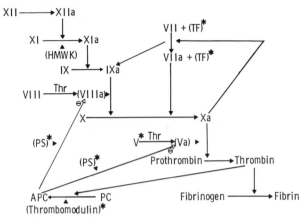

Fig. 1. The coagulation cascade showing the intrinsic (factor XII) and the extrinsic pathway (VII + TF), converging on Xa generation. Constituents that are made by vascular endothelium are marked with an asterisk (*). Cofactors are shown in brackets. Feedback of the natural anticoagulant system is shown with open arrowheads. PC, protein C; APC, activated protein C; PS, protein S.

COAGULATION

Figure 1 shows the cascades of coagulation factors that lead to the formation of thrombin by the intrinsic and extrinsic pathways. Thrombin has various functions, in addition to its first described role in the formation of fibrin. Formation of thrombin causes coagulation; thrombin generation is therefore the focal point of the coagulation cascades. Direct effects of thrombin on endothelium are shown in Table I.

Each unit of the coagulation cascade is the activation of a zymogen protein by an active serine protease. With one exception (XIa → IX), these reactions require the presence of a cofactor (HMWK, V, VIII, or TF), which may itself need to be activated by thrombin (V and VIII) (Fig. 1). In the case

TABLE I. Thrombin Effects on Vascular Endothelium

Plasminogen activator inhibitor synthesis and release (10,12)
Tissue plasminogen activator synthesis and release (11,12)
Prostacyclin release (13)
Platelet activating factor release (14)
von Willebrand factor release (15)
Tissue factor expression (16)
Binds to thrombomodulin (4,5)
Nucleotide release (17)
Neutrophil adhesion (18)
Shape change (19)
Endothelin synthesis and release (20)

of the extrinsic pathway of coagulation since factor VII circulates, the point of control is exclusively at the level of TF expression, as both factor VII and VIIa are devoid of activity in the absence of TF (see Fig. 5).

FACILITATORY ROLES OF ENDOTHELIUM IN COAGULATION

Figure 1 shows components of the coagulation synthesised by the endothelium. In addition, the endothelium may act as a template for the propagation of coagulation. The key roles of factors IX and X, standing sentinel between intrinsic and extrinsic pathways, led to the search for receptors for IX and X on endothelium. Scatchard analysis by Heimark and Schwartz (21) demonstrated high-affinity sites for IX and X with K_d values of 4.9 nM and 21 nM, respectively. Saturation and displacement binding studies by Stern et al. (22) demonstrated binding of IX and IXa to a possible receptor on bovine aortic endothelium (BAE), which also had a K_d value of $\sim$ 4 nM. The functional relevance of such a binding site had to be viewed in the light of the normal plasma level of IX at 70–100 nmol/L. This would predict any such site being fully occupied by the inactive zymogen. Since coagulation reactions seldom reach completion, a substantially lower concentration of active enzyme is predicted than that of zymogen. Furthermore, from kinetic studies, the half-maximal concentration of IXa to effect Xa generation with saturating levels of X and VIII was only 150 pM. Hence, the observations of Stern et al. (23) that factor IXa binding was facilitated by the assembly of a VIII–X complex on the endothelial cell membrane was critical to the thesis of a supportive role for endothelium in coagulation. Stern and co-workers showed the ability of BAE to support activation of X in the presence of added IXa and VIII. Figure 2 demonstrates the increase in IXa binding to BAE in the presence of either saturating concentrations of X and an increasing concentration of VIII or saturating concentrations of VIII and an increasing concentration of X. Their experiments demonstrated the acquisition of a high-affinity status for the IXa binding site with a K_d value of 127 pM, coinciding with the kinetic data.

These elaborate studies demonstrate that the endothelium is capable of sustaining the activation of X and that binding of the enzyme IXa is augmented by the addition of cofactor (VIII) and substrate (X). However, to date no factor IX receptor has been characterised, although a candidate protein has been purified (24). Nonetheless, the supportive role of endothelium in this reaction has been demonstrated whatever the nature of the binding site.

The assembly of prothrombin Va and Xa on a membrane-bound complex (the prothrombinase complex) is well documented in the platelet. This key reaction may also be sustained on the surface of BAE, in contrast to nonvascular cells, as shown by Rodgers and Shuman (25). The moiety contributed by the BAE in this reaction appeared to be factor V, since the

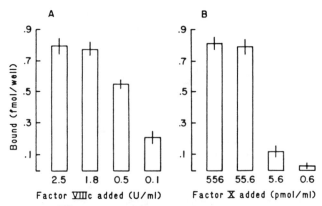

Fig. 2. Binding of ^{125}I factor IXa to bovine endothelial cells in the presence of factors VIII and X. **A:** Increase in ^{125}I IXa binding with increasing concentrations of factor VIII in the presence of 300 pmol/ml factor X. **B:** Increase in ^{125}I IXa binding with increasing concentrations of factor X in the presence of 2.4 U/ml factor VIII. Reproduced from Stern et al. (23), with permission of the publishers.

thrombin generation could be inhibited by anti-V antibody. The possibility that V was in fact synthesised by the BAE was raised in this paper, since thrombin generation by the cells could still be seen when they had been cultured in serum free medium. ^{35}S-methionine pulse studies by Cerveny et al. (26) support this notion since labelled V could be isolated from those cells and, in addition, could be activated by thrombin to form the two characteristic cleavage products.

In the overall generation of thrombin, the most important source quantitatively is the platelet, which upon activation provides the surface for assembly of the prothrombinase complex. However, the potential for endothelium to form small amounts of thrombin at its surface could prime the platelet system by causing the release reaction in platelets (which are triggered to release by small amounts of thrombin), permitting the propagation of much greater amounts of thrombin. Under basal conditions, however (Fig. 3) and in the absence of the initiating stimulus of TF expression, the small amounts of thrombin that are generated will be either inactivated by membrane bound antithrombin III or bound by thrombomodulin. The thrombomodulin–thrombin complex causes activation of protein C, which, in the presence of protein S (its cofactor), causes the inactivation of factors Va and VIIIa. In this situation, the facilitatory mechanisms of coagulation that exist on the endothelial surface are held in check. By contrast, should TF expression occur in the presence of downregulation of the thrombin inactivation systems (Fig. 4), the procoagulant reactions will predominate.

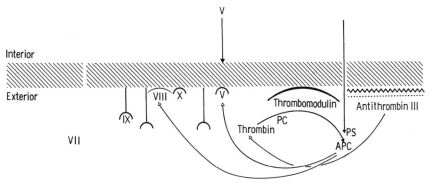

Fig. 3. The anticoagulant state of the endothelial cell under basal conditions. Thrombin formation is not favoured because of the absence of an initiator of coagulation. Should a small amount of thrombin be generated, this will complex with cell surface-bound thrombomodulin and activate protein C (APC), which by inactivation of factor VIII and V blocks further thrombin generation. In addition, antithrombin III, bound to endothelial cell surface by heparin-like molecules, will inactivate thrombin. Protein S, the cofactor for APC, is also synthesised by the endothelium.

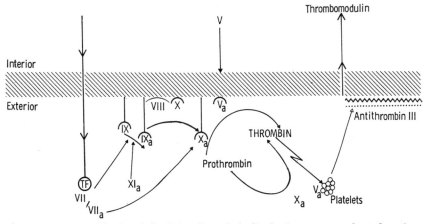

Fig. 4. The perturbed endothelial cell surface displaying procoagulant function. The perturbation (cytokines or bacterial lipopolysaccharide) has caused down-regulation of thrombomodulin and expression of tissue factor (TF). The latter now has a catastrophic effect. Interaction with circulating factor VII or VIIa (see text) interacts with factor IX, which is bound to the endothelial surface. Coagulation is rapidly propogated and results in thrombin formation. The restraining effect of thrombomodulin has been removed, and activation of platelets occurs. More thrombin can then be generated at their surface. Platelet factor 4 may dissociate antithrombin III from the endothelial cell surface. Thrombin will back-activate the pro-cofactors VIII and V to their active forms.

TISSUE FACTOR EXPRESSION

Tissue factor is a 47-kDa membrane-bound glycoprotein that is widely distributed at extravascular sites (27). TF is the cofactor for factor VIIa, which in its absence is devoid of activity. No activation of the TF is required once expressed at a cell membrane surface. TF and VIIa cause the activation of factors IX and X (Fig. 5), producing IXa or Xa, which themselves may back-activate VII to VIIa. The absolute initiator of this circular amplification system is unclear. According to one view (27), it may reside in the observation that the TF–VII complex has a low, but sufficient, activity on X to cause the generation of Xa and thereby initiate the system. If this is the case, TF expression is the key control point of the extrinsic pathway. Alternatively, subliminal amounts of factor Xa or VIIa may be present in the circulation, which are normally undetectable but sufficient on binding to TF to begin the generation of factor VIIa or Xa (28,29).

Within the vasculature, the only cells with direct contact with the blood and the ability to express TF are the monocyte and the endothelium. A variety of agents have been shown to cause TF expression by endothelium, including bacterial lipopolysaccharide, cytokines (IL-1, TNF), as well as phorbol esters and histamine [an exhaustive list can be found in Prydz and Pettersen (30)]. Under basal conditions, TF is not expressed by endothelium in culture, but induction is rapid, with cell surface activity detectable by 2 hr following stimulation. This is maximal by 6 hr and declines to low levels at 24 hr (31). This brisk induction of TF expression is also seen in vivo (32). When rabbits are infused with IL-1 and the aorta excised, the luminal surface demonstrates TF activity in a time course similar to the tissue culture results.

The rapid time course of induction is characteristic for TF. Inducible changes of other properties in endothelium, such as PA1, occur over considerably longer times in response to the same agonist (33). Analysis of the TFmRNA in BAE exposed to TNF demonstrates that a stimulated rise in TFmRNA does not require protein synthesis and is presumably not the

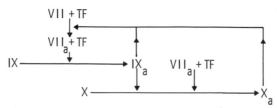

Fig. 5. The activation of the extrinsic pathway. Factor VIIa + TF may activate both X and IX. These are capable of back-activating VII to VIIa, amplifying the system. The TF–VII complex may itself have a small degree of activity and be capable of activating enough Xa to sustain VIIa generation by the feedback loop (see text).

result of the generation of further cytokines (e.g., IL-1), which might feed back on the cell in an autocrine manner (34). The exact control of TF in the endothelial cells has yet to be clarified, but the recent publication of the TF gene organisation shows a number of potential control points (35). In the 5' flanking region are found the consensus sequence for phorbol response elements. In addition, the 3' untranslated region contains sequences that would code for a message rich in AU sequences. This repeated motif is known to confer mRNA instability (36), raising the possibility that TF control may also be at the level of RNA breakdown (36a).

DOWN-REGULATION OF THROMBOMODULIN

Thrombomodulin is the membrane-bound cofactor that, in the presence of thrombin, causes the activation of protein C to activated protein C (APC). APC itself requires a cofactor (protein S) to exert its inhibitory role upon coagulation, by cleaving factors VIIIa and Va, and destroying the activity of these cofactors. Protein S is a vitamin K-dependent protein made by the liver as well as by endothelial cells (37). The control mechanisms for protein S synthesis by endothelium are unknown.

There is now increasing evidence that endothelial cell perturbation by cytokines and bacterial lipopolysaccharide reduces thrombomodulin activity (32, 38). This removes a powerful force that holds prothrombin activation in check via the generation of APC. The rabbit IL-1 infusion experiment previously described showed that, after a lag of 5 hr, there was a substantial reduction in thrombomodulin activity (21). Conway and Rosenberg (39) have gone a long way to unravel the mechanism of this effect. Upon stimulation of endothelium in culture with TNF, these investigators found clear reduction in thrombomodulin mRNA, declining to a sustained low level at 5 hr. The results of nuclear run-on experiments revealed almost complete abolition of transcription of this gene in response to the TNF. Clearly, the cytokine is able to induce the formation of a powerful repressor for this gene (38), while at the same time and in the same cell promoting a positive TF response (34).

CONCLUSION

The endothelial cell has multiple mechanisms for controlling its coagulant status. These are under tight control, with the cell being capable of sustaining reciprocal changes in function that work synergistically. Within the setting of its environment, the endothelial cell, being in contact with the blood, resides in an anticoagulant state, which hinders the formation of thrombin and inactivates it if formed. The cell can rapidly change its state, however, and, with the facilitatory mechanisms of coagulation at its surface, provide a potent template for the generation of thrombin. The internal workings of the cell that elaborate these effects are undoubtedly complex and their unravelling presents an exciting challenge for the cell biologist interested in the vascular endothelium.

ACKNOWLEDGMENTS

D.C.C. is an MRC Clinical Training Fellow. E.G.D.T. is a member of MRC Clinical Scientific Staff.

REFERENCES

1. Moncada S. Biological importance of prostacyclin. Br J Pharmacol 1982; 76:3–31.
2. Radomski MW, Palmer RMJ, Moncada S. The anti-aggregating properties of vascular endothelium: Interaction between prostacyclin and nitric oxide. Br J Pharmacol 1987;92:639–646.
3. Radomski MW, Palmer RMJ, Moncada S. The role of nitric oxide and cGMP in platelet adhesion to vascular endothelium. Biochem Biophys Res Commun 1987;148:1482–1489.
4. Esmon CT, Owen WG. Identification of an endothelial cell cofactor for thrombin-catalysed activation of protein C. Proc Natl Acad Sci USA 1981;78:2249–2252.
5. Osmon NL, Owen WG, Esmon CT. Isolation of a membrane-bound cofactor for thrombin-catalysed activation of protein C. J Biol Chem 1982;257:859–864.
6. Marcum JA, McKenney JB, Rosenburg RD. The acceleration of thrombin–antithrombin complex formation in rat hind quarters via naturally occurring heparin-like molecules bound to endothelium. J Clin Invest 1984;74:341–350.
7. Colburn P, Buonassisi V. Anti-clotting activity of endothelial cell cultures and heparin sulfate proteoglycans. Biochem Biophys Res Commun 1982;104:220–227.
8. Backmann F, Kruithof EKO. Tissue plasminogen activation : chemical and physiological aspects. Semin Thrombos Haemost 1984;10(1):6–17.
9. Loskutoff DJ. The fibrinolytic system of cultured endothelial cells: Insights into the role of endothelum in thrombolysis. In: Gimbrone MA, ed. Vascular Endothelium in Haemostasis and Thrombosis. New York: Churchill Livingston, 1986.
10. Gelehrter TD, Senyecer-Laszuk R. Thrombin induction of plasminogen activator in cultured human endothelial cells. J Clin Invest 1986;77:165–169.
11. Levin EG, Marzec U, Anderson J, Harker LA. Thrombin stimulates tissue plasminogen activator release from cultured endothelial cells. J Clin Invest 1984;74:1988–1995.
12. Dicheck D, Quartermous T. Thrombin regulation of mRNA levels of tissue plasminogen activator and plasminogen activator inhibitor 1 in cultured umbilical vein endothelial cells. Blood 1989;222–228.
13. Weksler BB, Ley CW, Jaffe EA. Stimulation of endothelial cell prostacyclin production by thrombin, trypsin and the ionophore A23187. J Clin Invest 1978; 62:923–930.
14. Prescott SM, Zimmerman GA, McIntyre TM. Human endothelial cells in culture produce platelet activating factor (1-alkyl-2 acetyl-sn-glycero-3 phosphocholine) when stimulated with thrombin. Proc Natl Acad Sci USA 1986:81:3534–3538.

15. Levine JD, Harlan JM, Harker LA, Joseph ML, Counts RB. Thrombin-mediated release of factor VIII related antigen from human umbilical vein endothelial cells in culture. Blood 1982;60:531–534.
16. Galdal KS, Lyborg T, Evansen SA, Nilsen E, Prydz H. Thrombin induces thromboplastin synthesis in cultured vascular endothelial cells. Thromb Haemost 1985;54:373–376.
17. Pearson JD, Gordon JL. Vascular endothelial and smooth muscle cells in culture selectively release adenine nucleotides. Nature (Lond) 1979;281:384–386.
18. Zimmerman GA, McIntyre TM, Prescott SM. Thrombin stimulates the adherence of neutrophils to human endothelial cells in vitro. J Clin Invest 1985;76:2235–2246.
19. Galdal KS, Evensen SA, Brosstad F. Effects of thrombin on the integrity of monolayers of cultured human endothelial cells. Thrombos Res 1982;27:575–584.
20. Yanagisawa M, Kurihara H, Kimura S. A novel potent vasoconstrictor produced by endothelial cells. Nature (Lond) 1988;332:411–415.
21. Heimark RL, Schwartz SM. Binding of coagulation factors IX and X to the endothelial cell surface. Biochem Biophys Res Commun 1983;111:723–731.
22. Stern DM, Drillings M, Nossel HL, Jensen A, La Gamma KS, Owen J. Binding factors IX and IXa to cultured vascular endothelial cells. Proc Natl Acad Sci USA 1983;80:4119–4123.
23. Stern DM, Nawroth PP, Kisiel W, Vehar G, Esmon CT. The binding of factor IXa to cultured bovine aortic endothelial cells. J Biol Chem 1985;260:6717–6722.
24. Rimon S, Melamed R, Savion N, Scott T, Nawroth PP, Stern DM. Identification of a factor IX/IXa binding protein on the endothelial cell surface. J Biol Chem 1987;262:6023–6031.
25. Rodgers GM, Shuman MA. Prothrombin is activated on vascular endothelial cells by factor Xa and calcium. Proc Natl Acad Sci USA 1983;80:7001–7005.
26. Cerveny TJ, Fass DN, Mann KG. Synthesis of coagulation factor V by cultured aortic endothelium. Blood 1984;63:1467–1474.
27. Nemerson Y. Tissue factor and haemostasis. Blood 1988;71:1–8.
28. Rapaport SI. Inhibition of factor VIIa/tissue factor-induced blood coagulation: with particular emphasis upon a factor Xa-dependent inhibitory mechanism. Blood 1989;73:359–365.
29. Rao LVM, Rapaport SI. Activation of factor VII bound to tissue factor. A key step in the tissue factor pathway of coagulation. Proc Natl Acad Sci USA 1988;85:6687–6691.
30. Prydz H, Pettersen KS. Synthesis of thromboplastin tissue factor by endothelial cells. Haemostasis 1988;18:215–223.
31. Bevilacqua MP, Pober JS, Majeau GR, Fiers W, Cotran RS, Gimbrone MA Jr. Recombinant tumor necrosis factor induces procoagulant activity in cultured human vascular endothelium: Characterisation and comparison with the actions of interleukin 1. Proc Natl Acad Sci USA 1986;86:4533–4537.
32. Nawroth PP, Handley DA, Esmon CT, Stern DM. Interleukin 1 induces endothelial cell procoagulant while suppressing cell-surface anticoagulant activity. Proc Natl Acad Sci USA 1986;83:3460–3464.
33. Sawdey M, Podor TJ, Loskutoff DJ. Regulation of Type 1 plasminogen activator inhibitor gene expression in cultured bovine aortic endothelial cells. J Biol Chem 1989;264:10396–10401.

34. Conway EM, Back R, Rosenberg RD, Konigsberg WH. Tumour necrosis factor enhances expression of tissue factor mRNA in endothelial cells. Thrombos Res 1989;53:231–241.
35. Mackman N, Morrissey JH, Fowler B, Edgington TS. Complete sequence of the human tissue factor gene, a highly regulated cellular receptor that initiates the coagulation protease cascade. Biochemistry 1989;28:1755–1762.
36. Shaw G, Kamem R. A conserved AU sequence from the 3' untranslated region of GM–CSF mRNA mediates selective mRNA degradation. Cell 1986;46:659–667.
36a. Crossman DC, Carr DP, Tuddenham EDG, Pearson JD, McVey JH. The regulation of tissue factor mRNA in human endothelial cells in response to endotoxin or phorbol ester. J Biol Chem 1990 (in press).
37. Stern DJ, Brett K, Harris K, Nawroth P. Participation of endothelial cells in the protein C–protein S anti-coagulant pathway: The synthesis and release of protein S. J Cell Biol 1986;102:1971–1978.
38. Esmon CT. The regulation of natural anticoagulant pathways. Science 1987;-235:1348–1352.
39. Conway EM, Rosenberg RD. Tumour necrosis factor suppresses transcription of the thrombomodulin gene in endothelial cells. Mol Cell Biol 1989;8:5588–5592.

The Endothelium: An Introduction to Current Research, pages 129–139

12
Endothelium as a Source of Tissue-Type Plasminogen Activator (t-PA) for Fibrinolysis

C. KLUFT

Gaubius Institute TNO, 2313 AD Leiden, The Netherlands

INTRODUCTION TO t-PA

Tissue-type plasminogen activator is a very specific serine protease. The enzyme catalyses the conversion of plasminogen to active plasmin by hydrolysis of the peptide bond between Arg 560 and Val 561 in the plasminogen molecule. Another very specific interaction occurs between t-PA and the plasminogen activator inhibitor 1, PAI-1.

t-PA is produced as a single polypeptide chain of 527 amino acid residues, in two variants in about equal amounts with either two or three carbohydrate antennae. N-glycosylation at Asp-184 (complex type of oligosaccharide) is optional, at Asp-117 (high mannose-type) and Asp-448 (complex type) it is always present.

The amino acid sequence of t-PA shows homology with parts of other proteins (domains) and consequently t-PA is considered to be built up from five domains (starting from the N-terminus): a finger domain (homologous to a similar structure in fibronectin), a growth factor domain (homologous to epidermal growth factor), two kringle domains (originally discovered in prothrombin) and a protease domain (resembling trypsin).

Structure and function studies on t-PA using protein chemistry as well as molecular biology have shown the involvement of kringle 2 and the finger domain in fibrin binding and stimulation by fibrin of the t-PA/plasminogen reaction. There is involvement of the high mannose antennae in clearance via the mannose receptor on liver endothelium and involvement of the loop between the kringle 2 and protease domain in the interaction with PAI-1. Lysine 416 is also important in that single-chain t-PA has already considerable activity as a pro-enzyme (1). A second clearance site in the liver on hepatocytes seems to involve the three-dimensional structure of the t-PA protein core. The role of the growth factor and kringle 1 domains is not clear (2).

The size of the t-PA gene from the site of initiation of transcription to the polyadenylation site is 32,720 bp (3). The gene is located on chromosome 8, bands 8p.12–q.11.2 (4), located near a chromosomal breakpoint in myeloproliferative disorders (5). In the genomic DNA, 14 coding regions are intervened by 13 introns. Regulatory elements that have been recognized (3,4,6) include a TATA box, a CAAT box, activator proteins (AP-1) sites, AP-2 binding motifs, and a cyclic adenosine monophosphate (cAMP) regulating element. Further 28 Alu repeats and a single Kpn I repeat are found. An interesting homology with the genomic DNA sequence of PAI-1 has been found, showing 81% homology between the PAI-1 noncoding strand and the t-PA coding strand (7). A computer search on the 5'-flanking DNA of the t-PA gene showed a number of sequences differing only in one or two nucleotides from the consensus sequences for the glucocorticoid, progesterone and estrogen response elements (8). Regulation of t-PA synthesis appears possible via protein kinase C, cAMP, and steroids and may be coordinated with the regulation of PAI-1 synthesis.

ENDOTHELIUM-DERIVED t-PA

The endothelium releases t-PA both continuously and also acutely in response to triggering factors.

Continuous Production of t-PA by the Endothelium

The normal plasma concentration of t-PA of $\sim$ 5 ng/ml, represents a balance between the synthesis of t-PA by endothelial cells and the clearance of t-PA by the liver (the plasma half-life of t-PA is $\sim$ 5 minutes). It can be calculated that the endothelium produces a few milligrams of t-PA per day, which can be compared with $\sim$ 70 mg/day of its substrate, plasminogen, produced by the liver.

The plasma level shows a broad interindividual variation but is stable in each individual for weeks (9). There is a clear increase in plasma level with age (10) and a slight difference between sexes (11). In healthy persons, both oral contraceptives (12) and anabolic steroids (13) can cause a clear decrease in t-PA antigen levels. Furthermore, there is a moderate diurnal rhythm (amplitude 2.5 ng/ml) in the continuous blood level (14). It has been suggested that endothelial cells exhibit a circadian fluctuation in metabolism, possibly explaining the circadian fluctuations in both t-PA and PAI-1 (which can also be produced by the endothelium) (9). A circadian fluctuation in clearance capacity of the liver is not excluded, however.

In accordance with the above assumption that endothelial cells continuously produce t-PA, all cultured endothelial cells have so far been shown to produce t-PA (15). It has been shown that cells of different origin have different production levels of t-PA and different ratios of t-PA versus mRNA levels (16). Microvascular endothelium makes up the largest part of the total surface area of endothelial cells exposed to blood in the body. These cells produce in culture approximately 4 ng/ml/day in discs of 0.2 ml/cm^2 (15), which would suggest that this microvascular endothelial surface in the body, estimated to 600 m^2 (17), can contribute milligram quantities per day. This amount compares well with the turnover of t-PA in blood (see above).

It remains to be established exactly how in vivo each vascular bed contributes to the blood level of t-PA. Some information about local variations in t-PA production comes from the use of the Todd slide technique, a fibrin zymographic technique employed on tissue sections. In principle, the data obtained by this activity assay are modulated by the presence of inhibitors such as PAI-1 and plasmin inhibitors (18). It is striking, however, that the distribution of activity recorded with the Todd method shows a resemblance to preliminary data on in situ hybridization (19). As a summary, Todd slide data show negative results for endothelium in large arteries and focal spots of activity in large veins. Positive results are found in smaller veins and venules, in the vaso vasorum of larger veins and arteries, and in the pulmonary arteries and arterioles (20). The data on in situ hybridization in a panel of 14 tissues from rhesus monkey show negative results for arterial endothelium of aorta, carotid artery, coronary artery and kidney intralobular arterioles. Positive results were found in the endothelial cells of small venules and in the adventitia of larger vessels (19).

In situ hybridization provides information about the occurrence of messenger RNA (mRNA) in different vessels. The variability in the ratio of t-PA versus mRNA levels in cells cultured from endothelium of different origin (see above) indicates that in situ hybridization data do not definitely indicate the quantitative contribution of each type of endothelium to blood levels of t-PA. The results suggest, nevertheless, an emphasis on t-PA production by the small blood vessels.

Two other approaches to discern where the continuous synthesis of t-PA occurs are the use of catheters to sample at specific locations in the body (21) and the venous occlusion test. The latter is usually performed on the arm, and results in accumulation of secreted t-PA in the occluded segment. From experiments on residual blood flow and calculations of theoretical accumulations, Keber (22) concluded that, during venous occlusion, the accumulation of t-PA can be explained merely by continuously produced t-PA, and there is no need to postulate increased t-PA release. This implies that t-PA is continuously secreted at least in the arm. Similar experiments of occlusion of the leg showed little or no increase in t-PA in the occluded segment, suggesting that in the leg no continuous release of t-PA occurred (22). Interestingly, the leg venous occlusion test can show accumulation of t-PA after fourteen days bed rest. It has been suggested that the high venous pressure in the legs usually shuts off t-PA production (22). In addition, t-PA release in the leg can normally be induced by infusion of dDAVP, indicating that induced release remains possible.

These data indicate that the local, continuous production of t-PA will presumably be variable along the vascular tree. The circulating levels of t-PA can be viewed as averaged information about this production. Plasma t-PA levels show large interindividual variation, either because of a variation in production rate by the endothelium or a variation in the sites of the vascular endothelium involved in continuous production.

Acute Release of t-PA from Endothelium

In the whole organism, and in isolated vascular beds, acute release of t-PA has been demonstrated in response to a variety of stimuli. These substances also include reaction products from platelet and coagulation activation, thus linking these processes to fibrinolysis activation (23). A common denominator appears to be the activation of a calcium-, phospholipase-, and lipoxygenase-dependent mechanism that closely resembles the activation mechanism for endothelial cell dependent vasorelaxation (23). Although some leukotrienes (LTC4 and LTD4) are capable of releasing t-PA, they do not provide the only pathway in the above said mechanism (24). The response shows tachyphylaxis for each individual stimulus, but not for the subsequent effects of other stimuli (23,25).

The cellular mechanism of acute increase of t-PA has not been elucidated so far. That it occurs with isolated endothelial cells (26) suggests that direct stimulation of endothelial cells is involved. Attempts to identify a t-PA storage pool, similar to Weibel–Palade bodies for von Willebrand factor, have so far not been successful, only diffuse immunohistochemical staining has been obtained (23,27).

Recent data indicate that protein synthesis is not required for either the release or storage of t-PA (28). That there is a significant pool of t-PA can also be inferred from extractions of tissues, which have been found to yield between 0.24–1.6 mg t-PA per kilogram tissue (in heart and uterus (29)). The perfusion of vascular beds of human cadavers has also been shown to yield significant amounts of t-PA (30). The potency of the acute release mechanism and its triggering by coagulation activation was strikingly demonstrated following infusion of activated factor X with phospholipid vesicles in primates (31); a peak level of 0.9 µg/ml of t-PA was observed 10 min after the start of the infusion. This level approaches the plasma concentration of t-PA observed during thrombolytic treatment of acute myocardial infarction and clearly exceeds levels seen after venous occlusion, maximal exercise, and administration of the vasopressin analogue dDAVP, where increases of the order of tenth's of nanograms of t-PA usually occur.

Besides an intracellular pool of t-PA, there may be an extracellular pool, notably on binding sites on the endothelium. Several reports indicate the occurrence of such sites, although no clear consensus has yet been reached concerning the characteristics and identity of these sites. Reports show 3,600–12,000,000 (32–35) sites per cell and binding constants ranging from 0.03 to 4,200 nM (32,34,35). Among the reported sites, some require the active site of t-PA (34,35) suggesting binding to PAI-1, as shown recently to be possible (34).

For three of the described binding sites, t-PA is protected from inhibition by PAI-1 and/or can be dissociated in an active form (32,34). The capacity of these sites is different, showing 3,700 (32), 815,000 (32), and $1.5.10^6$ (34) sites/cell, indicating a capacity for 0.20, 45, and 85 mg t-PA respectively, when all endothelial cells in vivo have these amounts of sites exposed (assuming 700 m^2 endothelium and on average 7.10^4 cells/cm^2). The occupation of these sites is only partial, however, as judged by the reported dissociation constants of 28.7 pM, 18.1 nM, and 170 nM, respectively (32,34). Receptor occupation can be calculated from the equilibrium: free t-PA + binding site $\rightleftarrows$ t-PA*Site, where the t-PA concentration (a pM) is constant despite binding, because of the continuous synthesis with rapid turnover. The total concentration of sites is b pM, and at equilibrium there will be b-x unoccupied sites, x being the concentration of bound t-PA. The fraction of occupied sites can be calculated to be $x/b = (K_d/a + 1)^{-1}$ where K_d is the dissociation constant. For the site with K_d 28.7 pM (32), the occupation will be 47% for a blood baseline concentration of t-PA of 25 pM harbouring $\sim$100 μg t-PA; for the site with K_d 170 nM, this will be 0.015% and will concern 13 μg t-PA. It is interesting to note that the two low-affinity sites (K_d 18.1 and 170 nM) (32,34) might be able to participate significantly in the biodistribution of t-PA during thrombolytic treatment. It can be calculated that when blood levels are 1 μg/ml, these sites can harbour approximately 20 mg and 6 mg t-PA, respectively. The amount of t-PA calculated to be bound to endothelial sites in baseline conditions (t-PA = 25 pM) seems insufficient to account for the t-PA found upon tissue extraction or after acute release. This suggests either the existence of another pool of t-PA, or that the above extrapolation of data from cultured cells to the in vivo situation is not correct with respect to the quantity and/or quality of the binding sites. The latter is a possibility when we consider that these sites might be subject to modulation in quantity and/or quality when involved in the acute release process.

Besides a role of the endothelial binding sites in biodistribution of t-PA for fibrinolysis, it is also possible that the bound t-PA plays a role in focal proteolysis of extracellular matrix as reported for urokinase (36).

SYSTEMIC VERSUS LOCAL SUPPLY

When comparing the relative importance of circulating t-PA, locally bound t-PA, and acutely released t-PA, it is necessary to consider the size of the blood vessel involved. In large blood vessels (diameter 1 mm), the cell surface to blood volume ratio is 100 times lower than the ratio in small vessels (diameter 10 μM). In this respect, in vitro studies of cell culture discs are comparable to the situation in large vessels. In a large vessel the acute release of t-PA from a fixed amount of cells is a hundred times less effective in raising the local blood level than the same quantity released per cell in a small vessel. Therefore, the circulating amount of t-PA will be more relevant to larger vessels than to smaller ones.

This reasoning only applies when all endothelial cells show a similar potency of reaction to triggers of acute release. It would be of interest to know whether cells from larger vessels show a phenotype with a compensatory increased potential for acute release.

If, as reasoned, the larger vessels have to rely more upon distantly produced, circulating t-PA, the effects of the inhibitor PAI-1 on the survival of t-PA becomes more important for these vessels, than compared to the microcirculation.

CIRCULATING INHIBITORS OF t-PA

t-PA is secreted as a single chain pro-enzyme. This pro-enzyme however, already has activities closely resembling those of the two-chain form that can be generated by plasmin action. The fact that the single chain form is already active has been ascribed to the existence of a charge relay system between the active site amino acids of the serine protease with a positive charge on lysine-416 (1). Usually this charge relay system is created by the split of a peptide bond in the pro-enzyme, rendering the two-chain enzyme active while the single chain is inactive. In t-PA, the charge relay system is already uniquely present in the single-chain form due to interaction with an in-chain positive charge.

As a consequence of this feature of single-chain t-PA, it can continuously interact with the specific inhibitor plasminogen activator inhibitor 1. This reaction with circulating PAI-1, which is normally in excess, is dependent upon the level of PAI-1. The reaction between t-PA and PAI-1 is second order with a rate constant of 10^7 $M^{-1}s^{-1}$ (37). In normal individuals, usually PAI-1 levels are such that they reduce the t-PA activity to one half in about 5–10 min. This inactivation of t-PA is competitive with the disappearance of t-PA by liver clearance with a half-life of about 5 min. In traumatic conditions, however, PAI-I levels can be increased temporarily 10- to a 1,000-fold (38), and the action radius of circulating t-PA becomes greatly reduced. With a 10-fold increase, the time to reduce t-PA activity by one-half becomes $\sim$30 sec; with a 100-fold increase, this falls to just a few seconds. Under such conditions, the reduction of t-PA activity by reaction with PAI-1 can overshadow liver clearance. In such cases of high PAI-1, the local supply of t-PA will be more important than the supply via circulating blood. Data of Colucci et al. (39) suggest that tissue-derived components can reduce the above calculated influence of PAI-1.

ROLE OF THE TIMING OF SUPPLY

In the case of fibrin formation, the triggers for acute release derived from activation of the coagulation system can release t-PA not only locally but also downstream of the site of fibrin formation. The downstream processes have the disadvantage of dilution of the triggers. The t-PA released there is diluted and delayed by the circulation time when it reaches the site again. In the case of high PAI-1, the t-PA released at the site of fibrin formation also has the shortest time of exposure to this inhibitor before it becomes bound to fibrin.

Of special importance is the timing of the t-PA supply relative to the formation of the fibrin matrix. t-PA becomes nearly totally incorporated into a forming clot but only slowly binds and penetrates an existing fibrin clot, which becomes a separate compartment after the matrix formation. The difference in effectiveness of t-PA in lysing the fibrin is large (40) and may involve a factor of 100–1,000 (41) for t-PA available before clot formation as compared to after clot formation.

This mechanism emphasizes the importance of the timing of the release of t-PA, the most rapidly available supply being from the endothelium locally. Although many studies have measured t-PA release in response to a fixed stimulus, practically no data are available concerning the variability in the time profile of the acute release.

ABNORMALITIES IN t-PA IN BLOOD

It might be expected that a reduced availability of t-PA will predispose to a thrombotic diathesis, whereas increased availability will cause a tendency to bleed. Indeed it has, been observed that among patients with recurrent venous thrombosis, the t-PA antigen response to venous occlusion is abnormally reduced in 10–12% of cases (42–44). These cases have a significantly higher incidence of recurrence (43). Evidence for familial clustering of the abnormality has also been reported (44). In some cases low t-PA antigen values and a poor response may be caused by a genetic defect (45). In other reports, a bleeding tendency has been ascribed to a high t-PA level in blood (46,47) or a reduced PAI-1 (48,49). Abnormalities in individual patients are difficult to define because of the large normal range in both basal and stimulated t-PA blood concentrations.

CONCLUDING REMARKS

Fibrinolysis depends not only on the supply of t-PA by the circulation, but also on the local activity of t-PA released by the endothelium in response to various stimuli, such as reaction products from coagulation. The importance and potency of a coagulation dependent t-PA release has recently been clearly illustrated in primates (31).

This local release provides high concentrations of active t-PA at the site of the forming fibrin. The specific timing, as well as the magnitude, of this acute release is of importance relative to the speed of fibrin formation. Only t-PA incorporated during fibrin formation becomes an efficient fibrinolysis activator; t-PA is relatively poorly active on a pre-existing fibrin clot (40,41). It can be concluded that the endothelium plays a major role and a predominantly local dynamic role in the supply of t-PA for fibrinolysis.

REFERENCES

1. Petersen LC, Boel E, Johannessen M, Foster D. Possible involvement of a lysine residue in establishing the charge-relay system responsible for one-chain t-PA (1ch-t-PA). Thromb Haemost 1989;62:322 (abst SY-XVI-4).
2. Krause J, Tanswell P. Properties of molecular variants of tissue-type plasminogen activator. Arzneim Forsch/Drug Res 1989;39:632–637.
3. Degen SJF, Rajput B, Reich E. The human tissue plasminogen activator gene. J Biol Chem 1986;261:6972–6985.
4. Ny T, Ohlsson M, Strandberg L. The gene for t-PA. In: Kluft C, ed. Tissue-Type Plasminogen Activator (t-PA): Physiological and Clinical Aspects. Vol. 1. Boca Raton, Florida: CRC Press, 1988;83–100.
5. Yang-Feng TL, Opdenakker G, Volckaert G, Francke U. Human tissue-type plasminogen activator gene located near chromosomal break point in myeloproliferative disorder. Am J Hum Genet 1986;39:79–87.
6. Medcalf RL, Ruegg M, Schleuning W-D. Tissue-type plasminogen activator (t-PA) and c-JUN/activator protein-1 (AP-1) gene promotors contain an identical regulatory Cis-acting DNA element. Thromb Haemost 1989;62:38 (abst 81).
7. Bosma PJ, Van den Berg EA, Kooistra T, Siemieniak DR, Slightom JL. Human plasminogen activator inhibitor-1 gene. Promoter and structural gene nucleotide sequences. J Biol Chem 1988;263:9129–9141.
8. Kooistra T, Bosma PJ, Jespersen J, Kluft C. Studies on the mechanism of action of oral contraceptives with regard to fibrinolytic variables. Am J Gynecol Obstet 1990; in press.
9. Kluft C, Jie AFH, Rijken DC, Verheijen JH. Daytime fluctuations in blood of tissue-type plasminogen activator (t-PA) and its fast-acting inhibitor (PAI-1). Thromb Haemost 1988;59:329–332.
10. Rånby M, Bergsdorf N, Nilsson T, Mellbring G, Winblad B, Bucht G. Age dependence of tissue plasminogen activator concentrations in plasma as studied by an improved enzyme-linked immunosorbent assay. Clin Chem 1986;32:2160–2165.
11. Stegnar M, Keber D, Pentek M, Vene N, Kluft C. Age and sex differences in resting and postocclusion values of tissue plasminogen activator in a healthy population. Fibrinolysis 1988;2:121–122.
12. Gevers Leuven JA, Kluft C, Bertina RM, Hessel LW. Effects of two low-dose oral contraceptives on circulating components of the coagulation and fibrinolytic systems. J Lab Clin Med 1987;109:631–636.
13. Verheijen JH, Rijken DC, Chang GTG, Preston FE, Kluft C. Modulation of rapid plasminogen activator inhibitor in plasma by stanozolol. Thromb Haemost 1984;51:396–397.

14. Andreotti F, Davies GJ, Hackett D, Khan MI, De Bart A, Dooijewaard G, Maseri A, Kluft C. Circadian variation of fibrinolytic factors in normal human plasma. Fibrinolysis 1988;2:90–92.
15. Van Hinsbergh VWM. Regulation of the synthesis and secretion of plasminogen activators by endothelial cells. Haemostasis 1988;18:307–327.
16. Van Zonneveld A-J, Chang GTG, Van den Berg J, Kooistra T, Verheijen JH, Pannekoek H, Kluft C. Quantification of tissue-type plasminogen activator (t-PA) mRNA in human endothelial-cell cultures by hybridization with a t-PA cDNA probe. Biochem J 1986;235:385–390.
17. Wolinsky H. A proposal linking clearance of circulating lipoproteins to tissue metabolic activity as basis for understanding atherogenesis. Circ Res 1980;47: 301–311.
18. Noordhoek Hegt V, Brakman P. Histochemical study of an inhibitor of fibrinolysis in the human arterial wall. Nature (Lond) 1974;248:75–76.
19. Gordon D, Augustine AJ, Smith KM, Schwartz SM, Wilcox JN. Localization of cells expressing t-PA, PAI-1, and urokinase by in situ hybridization in human atherosclerotic plaques and in the normal rhesus monkey. Thromb Haemost 1989;62:131 (abst 419).
20. Van Hinsbergh VWM. Synthesis and secretion of plasminogen activators and plasminogen activator inhibitor by endothelial cells. In: Kluft C, ed. Tissue-Type Plasminogen Activator (t-PA): Physiological and Clinical Aspects. Vol. 2. Boca Raton, Florida: CRC Press, 1988; 3–20.
21. Brommer EJP, Derkx FHM, Schalekamp MADH, Dooijewaard G, Van der Klaauw MM. Renal and hepatic handling of endogenous tissue-type plasminogen activator (t-PA) and its inhibitor in man. Thromb Haemost 1988;59:404–411.
22. Keber D. Mechanism of tissue plasminogen activator release during venous occlusion. Fibrinolysis 1988;2:96–103.
23. Emeis JJ. Mechanisms involved in short-term changes in blood levels of t-PA. In: Kluft C, ed. Tissue-Type Plasminogen Activator (t-PA): Physiological and Clinical Aspects. Vol. 2. Boca Raton, Florida: CRC Press, 1988;21–35.
24. Tranquille N, Emeis JJ. Release of tissue-type plasminogen activator is induced in rats by leukotrienes C4 and D4, but not by prostaglandins E_1, E_2 and I_2. Br J Pharmacol 1988;93:156–164.
25. Smith D, Gilbert M, Owen WG. Tissue plasminogen activator release in vivo in response to vasoactive agents. Blood 1985;66:835–839.
26. Booyse FM, Bruce R, Dolenak D, Grover M, Casey LC. Rapid release and deactivation of plasminogen activators in human endothelial cell cultures in the presence of thrombin and ionophore A 23187. Semin Thromb Haemost 1986;12: 228–230.
27. Kristensen P, Larsson LI, Nielsen LS, Grøndahl-Hansen J, Andreasen PA, Danø K. Human endothelial cells contain one type of plasminogen activator. FEBS Lett 1984;168:33–37.
28. Tranquille N, Emeis JJ. Protein synthesis inhibition by cycloheximide does not affect the acute release of tissue-type plasminogen activator. Thromb Haemost 1989;61:442–447.
29. Rijken DC, Wijngaards G, Collen D. Tissue-type plasminogen activator from human tissue and cell cultures and its occurrence in plasma. In: Collen D,

Lijnen HR, Verstraete M, eds. Thrombolysis: Biological and Therapeutic Properties of New Thrombolytic Agents. Edinburg: Churchill Livingstone, 1985;15–30.

30. Aoki N. Preparation of plasminogen activator from vascular trees of human cadavers. J. Biochem 1974;75:731–741.

31. Giles AR, Hoogendoorn H, Herring S, Nesheim ME, Stump DC, Helderbrandt C. The fibrinolytic response in primates following the co-infusion of activated factor X (F.Xa) and phosphatidylcholine/phosphatidylserine vesicles (PCPS). Thromb Haemost 1989;62:307 (abst 990).

32. Hajjar KA, Hamel NM, Harpel PC, Nachman RL. Binding of tissue plasminogen activator to cultured human endothelial cells. J Clin Invest 1987;80:1712–1719.

33. Liu CY, Wallén P, Handley DA. Preparation of active iodinated and gold-labeled tissue plasminogen activator and their binding to fibrin and endothelial cells. Thromb Haemost 1985;54:60 (abst 0356).

34. Barnathan ES, Kuo A, Van der Keyl H, McCrae KR, Larsen GR, Cines DB. Tissue type plasminogen activator binding to human endothelial cells. Evidence for two distinct binding sites. J Biol Chem 1988;263:7792–7799.

35. Beebe DP. Binding of tissue plasminogen activator to human umbilical vein endothelial cells. Thromb Res 1987;46:241–254.

36. Danø K, Andreasen PA, Grøndahl-Hansen J, Kristensen P, Nielsen LS, Skriver L. Plasminogen activators, tissue degradation and cancer. Adv Cancer Res 1985;44:139–266.

37. Sprengers ED, Kluft C. Plasminogen activator inhibitors. Blood 1987;69:381–387.

38. Kluft C, De Bart ACW, Barthels M, Sturm J, Moller W. Short term extreme increases in plasminogen activator inhibitor 1 (PAI-1) in plasma of polytrauma patients. Fibrinolysis 1988;2:221–226.

39. Colucci M, Paramo JA, Stassen JM, Collen D. Influence of the fast-acting inhibitor of plasminogen activator on in vivo thrombolysis induced by tissue-type plasminogen activator in rabbits. Interference of tissue-derived components. J Clin Invest 1986;78:138–144.

40. Brommer EJP. The level of extrinsic plasminogen activator (t-PA) during clotting as a determinant of the rate of fibrinolysis; inefficiency of activators added afterwards. Thromb Res 1984;34:109–115.

41. Fox KAA, Robison AK, Knabb RM, Rosamond TL, Sobel BE, Bergmann SR. Prevention of coronary thrombosis with sub-thrombolytic doses of tissue-type plasminogen activator. Circulation 1985;72:1346–1354.

42. Nilsson IM, Ljungner H, Tengborn L. Two different mechanisms in patients with venous thrombosis and defective fibrinolysis: Low concentration of plasminogen activator or increased concentration of plasminogen activator inhibitor. Br Med J 1985; 290:1453–1455.

43. Juhan-Vague I, Valadier J, Alessi MC, Aillaud MF, Ansaldi J, Philip-Joet C, Holvoet P, Serradimigni A, Collen D. Deficient t-PA release and elevated PA inhibitor levels in patients with spontaneous or recurrent deep vein thrombosis. Thromb Haemost 1987;57:67–72.

44. Petäjä J, Myllylä G, Rasi V. Familial clustering of defective release of t-PA. Thromb Haemost 1989;62:442 (abst 1422).

45. Phillips G, Kaufman RE, Pizzo SV. Tissue plasminogen activator deficiency: A molecular analysis. In Lowe GDO, Douglas JT, Forbes CD, Henschen A, eds. Fibrinogen, Vol. 2: Biochemistry, Physiology and Clinical Relevance. Amsterdam: Elsevier Science Publishers BV, 1987;281–284.
46. Booth NA, Bennett B, Wijngaards G, Grieve JHK. A new life-long hemorrhagic disorder due to excess plasminogen activator. Blood 1983;61:267–275.
47. Aznar J, Estellés A, Vila V, Regañón E, España F, Villa P. Inherited fibrinolytic disorder due to an enhanced plasminogen activator level. Thromb Haemost 1984;52:196–200.
48. Schleef RR, Higgins DL, Pillemer E, Levitt LJ. Bleeding diathesis due to decreased functional activity of type 1 plasminogen activator inhibitor. J Clin Invest 1989;83:1747–1752.
49. Dieval J, Gross S, Nguyen G, Kruithof EKO, Delobel J. Bleeding diathesis related to a deficiency in plasminogen activator inhibitor type 1 in a young patient. Thromb Haemost 1989;62:474 (abst 1485).

13
Cytokines and Thrombomodulin

J.C. GIDDINGS
Haematology Department, University of Wales College of Medicine, Cardiff CF4 4XN, Wales

INTRODUCTION

Other chapters in this book have amply demonstrated that endothelial cells, lining the luminal surface of blood vessels, actively contribute to the thromboresistant nature of the intact vessel wall. It is especially pertinent in this respect that endothelial cells synthesise and secrete a number of physiogically important substances, including a variety of proteins involved in haemostasis, angiotensin 1 converting enzyme, prostaglandin metabolites, and endothelium-derived relaxing factor (Table I).

ENDOTHELIAL CONTROL OF COAGULATION AND FIBRINOLYSIS

The localisation and production of von Willebrand factor (vWF), in particular, has been investigated widely in recent years. vWF is known to be a vital component of platelet–endothelial reactions, especially under conditions of high sheer stress, and the identification of von Willebrand factor antigen (vWFAg) in normal plasma, platelets, endothelial cells, and subendothelial matrices emphasises that this protein plays a pivotal role in primary haemostatic mechanisms (1). In addition, the release of vWFAg from endothelial cells is believed to be mediated by two essential pathways: (i) a constitutive pathway, in which the synthesised protein is secreted directly to the external environment; and (ii) a regulated pathway, in which vWFAg is initially stored in Weibel–Palade bodies and subsequently released upon stimulation of the endothelium with agents such as thrombin and the calcium ionophore, A23187.

Endothelial cells also produce and secrete both urokinase (uPA) and tissue type plasminogen activators (tPA). Furthermore, the presence of a fast-acting inhibitor of plasminogen activation, appropriately termed plasminogen activator inhibitor 1 (PAI-1), has been demonstrated in endothelial cells, and the process of fibrinolysis in vivo is understood to be controlled by a balanced reaction of these biosynthetic products. Signifi-

TABLE I.   Examples of Substances Synthesised or
Released by Vascular Endothelial Cells

von Willebrand factor antigen (factor VIII related antigen)
Fibronectin
Plasminogen activator (tPA)
Plasminogen activator inhibitor
Tissue factor thromboplastin
Collagen (especially types III and IV)
Elastin and microfibrils
Glycosaminoglycans
Heparin
Angiotensin 1 converting enzyme
Prostaglandin metabolites
Endothelium-derived relaxing factors
Endothelin

cantly, thrombin, the serine protease that converts fibrinogen to fibrin, enhances the release of plasminogen activators and PAI-1 from endothelial cells; thus, the enzyme not only promotes blood coagulation but also influences the mechanisms that are responsible for the subsequent dissolution of the fibrin clot. Indeed, relatively recent studies have shown that thrombin catalyses several other endothelial activities, including the formation of prostacyclin and the synthesis or release of endothelial proteins such as fibronectin and vWFAg. (Table II). Moreover, thrombin is generated on the surface of endothelial cells in response to activation of the coagulation cascade (2,3), and it seems highly likely that the enzyme produced in this manner modulates a diverse range of stimulus-induced reactions at localised sites of endothelial damage.

ENDOTHELIAL-DERIVED THROMBOMODULIN

A major contributor to these properties of the vascular intima is the endothelial cell-bound ligand for thrombin, termed thrombomodulin (TM) (4). This substance is a high-affinity receptor for thrombin and forms a stoichiometric complex with the enzyme. In this manner, TM is central to the endogenous anticoagulant activities of the endothelium, especially

TABLE II.   Thrombin and Endothelial Cell Function

Stimulated release of plasminogen activator (tPA); ? also inactivation of tPA by increased PAI-1

Enhanced synthesis of prostacyclin

Increased synthesis and release of fibronectin

Stimulated release of von Willebrand factor (vWf)

Decreased expression of cell-surface thrombomodulin (degradation and endocytosis)

those involving the vitamin K dependent serine esterase named protein C (Fig. 1). Activated protein C destroys the activity of thrombin-modified coagulation factors V and VIII, severely restricting the ability of these cofactors to participate in the formation of active enzyme–phospholipid complexes in the clotting mechanism. Thrombin is the only known physiological activator of protein C, but in solution this activation process is slow, probably too slow to be of biological relevance. In the presence of TM, however, the rate of activation is enhanced ∿ 20,000 fold, and on the surface of the vascular lumen potent anticoagulant activity is believed to develop very rapidly.

Moreover, the well-known procoagulant properties of thrombin, such as the ability to clot fibrinogen, activate factors V and VIII, and stimulate platelets are neutralised by the formation of the complex with TM. It is clear that TM manifests direct as well as indirect anticoagulant activity.

Under normal circumstances, TM has been identified only on vascular endothelial cells and perhaps in very small quantities in human platelets. It is not found on fibroblasts and smooth muscle cells, and it appears to be absent from the microvasculature of human brain. The syncytiotrophoblast of human placenta, a cell with endothelial characteristics, expresses relatively large amounts of the antigen and one report suggests that the ligand is present on serosal surfaces and on synovial membranes. In addition, TM is detected on transformed cell lines such as cultured human lung carcinoma cells (A459). By challenge, Ishii and Majerus (5) detected trace quantities of TM in normal human plasma and urine. These investigators demonstrated that some of the biochemical properties of this soluble material were different from those of the solid-phase substance; they postulated that the circulating antigen could exist as a specific secretory product for the humoral activation of protein C or could be derived from proteolysis

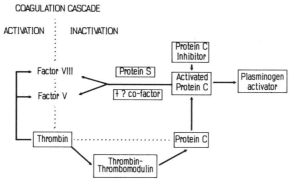

Fig. 1. Modulating effect of thrombomodulin, protein C, and protein S on coagulation and fibrinolysis.

of endothelial-bound TM, either as a result of normal turnover or due to endothelial injury.

Since the original descriptions of the mechanisms associated with TM, additional studies have shown that the function of protein C is optimum only in the presence of a further vitamin K dependent protein called protein S. The precise details of these reactions are not fully clarified but their physiological relevance is strongly justified by many reports indicating that inherited defects of protein C and protein S predispose to familial thromboembolic disease (6). Furthermore, several lines of research indicate that protein C-related mechanisms also regulate fibrinolysis and might be involved in the pathogenesis of septic shock (7). In particular, coordinate binding of protein C and protein S onto phospholipid membranes appears to accelerate fibrin-clot lysis in vitro maximally, and infusion of activated protein C efficiently prevents intravascular coagulation, tissue injury, and death in baboons given lethal doses of *Escherichia coli*. The molecular basis for these phenomena remain to be established, but the data provide compelling evidence to support the hypothesis that there is a close relationship among inflammation, coagulation, and fibrinolysis in vivo.

EFFECTS OF INFLAMMATORY MEDIATORS ON VASCULAR ENDOTHELIUM

Indeed, some of the most important studies regarding the nature of the blood vessel wall have centred on the interaction of endothelial cells with various soluble products of lymphocytes and activated macrophages (8–15). For example, several of these cytokines, which are known principally to mediate inflammatory reactions, have been shown to enhance the synthesis of prostacyclin in endothelial cells, and have been shown to stimulate the activity of cell-associated platelet activating factor (PAF). They markedly increase the adhesive properties of the vascular surface, especially enhancing the adhesion of neutrophil leukocytes, and stimulate the production of PAI-1. They regulate the release of vWF from its Weibel Palade storage compartment (Table III).

TABLE III. Inflammatory Mediators and the Endothelium

Enhanced synthesis of prostacyclin

Stimulation of cell-associated platelet activating factor (PAF)

Markedly increased adhesion of neutrophil leukocytes

Increased production of plasminogen activator inhibitor (PAI-1)

Stimulated release of von Willebrand factor (vWf)

Enhanced biosynthesis and cell-surface expression of tissue factor

Depressed expression of cell-surface anticoagulant activity (protein C–protein S mechanisms)

Suppression of thrombomodulin activity (degradation and internalisation)

We have confirmed several of these findings in studies of cultured endothelial cells derived from human umbilical veins and from human foreskin. Primary cultures of endothelial cells were grown in medium containing either recombinant human interleukin 1 (IL-1) or recombinant tumour necrosis factor (TNF), and confluent endothelial cells, grown initially in the absence of additives, were subsequently incubated for up to 36 hr in serum-free medium containing these monokines. Control cultures were maintained in the absence of cytokines or in the presence of interleukin 2 (IL-2). The results demonstrated that secretion of vWF and PAI-1 was significantly enhanced in the presence of IL-1 and TNF, while the release of tPA was not affected by these agents (Figs. 2 and 3). The findings indicate that these regulatory pathways may be independently controlled and are not necessarily linked.

In addition, cultures of confluent endothelial cells were incubated in serum-free medium containing calcium ionophore, thrombin, thrombin treated with diisopropyl fluorophosphate (DIP thrombin) or thrombin preincubated with thrombomodulin (Table IV). As expected, the results showed that the release of vWFAg was stimulated by calcium ionophore and thrombin but was not affected by DIP thrombin. DIP inhibits the active site of thrombin but does not prevent binding to the endothelial surface. The findings are thus consistent with the view that thrombin-induced secretion of vWFAg is directed by the active site of the enzyme. It is especially noteworthy, however, that the release of vWFAg in these experiments was markedly inhibited by preincubation of thrombin with TM. These data emphasise that TM restricts the ability of thrombin to participate in primary haemostasis as well as neutralising its coagulant activity.

EFFECTS OF INFLAMMATORY MEDIATORS ON THE ENDOTHELIAL EXPRESSION OF THROMBOMODULIN

In this context, it may be particularly relevant that several studies have shown that the biosynthesis and surface expression of endothelial cell tissue factor is enhanced by thrombin, IL-1, and TNF, while at the same time TM activity is depressed (14–16). It has been suggested that this latter function is mediated by the degradation and internalisation of the surface-bound TM molecule. We have extended our studies on endothelial cells in culture to examine the effects of thrombin, IL-1, and TNF on this expression of TM. An immunoradiometric assay (IRMA) for human TM has been established and has been used to measure the concentration of TM antigen in detergent-solubilised endothelial cells and culture supernatants. Initially, the results showed that the level of TM in cells obtained at intervals during primary culture is proportional to the number of cells harvested for assay (Fig. 4). In these experiments, we also confirmed that treatment of endothelial cells with purified α thrombin for 30 min in serum-free medium resulted in approximately 30% reduction in TM antigen measured

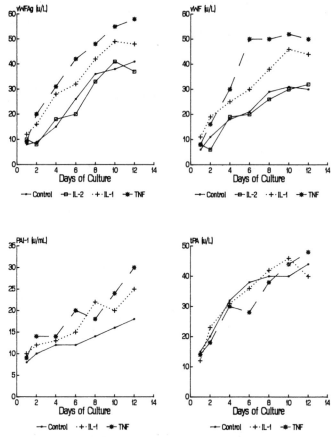

Fig. 2. Release of von Willebrand factor antigen (vWFAg), von Willebrand factor activity (vWF), plasminogen activator inhibitor activity (PAI-1), and tissue-type plasminogen activator (tPA) from primary cultures of human umbilical vein endothelial cells. Cells were grown in medium 199 and 10% newborn calf serum in the presence of 1 U/ml interleukin 1 (IL-1), 1 U/ml interleukin 2 (IL-2), or 10 ng/ml tumour necrosis factor (TNF). Aliquots of supernatant culture medium were removed at intervals and were assayed for vWFAg by immunoradiometric assay, for vWf by ristocetin co-factor activity, and for PAI-1 and tPA by the respective chromogenic assays (Kabi).

subsequently in the solubilised cells (Fig. 5). Similarly, the levels of TM antigen were reduced in endothelial cells treated with recombinant TNF or recombinant IL-1. In all these instances, there were no significant differences between the results of cells derived from umbilical vein and those derived from foreskin microvessels.

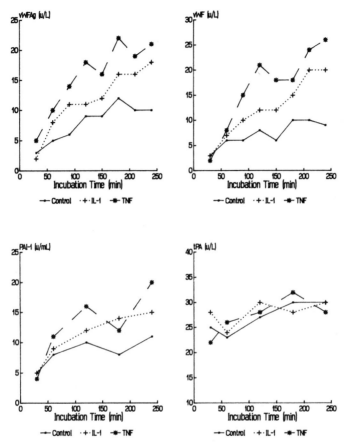

Fig. 3. Confluent control endothelial cells were washed briefly with serum-free medium and were then incubated in serum-free medium containing the cytokines at the concentrations indicated in Figure 2. Aliquots of supernatant medium were removed at intervals and assayed as above.

These preliminary experiments were expanded so that parallel cultures of confluent cells derived from the same source were incubated in serum-free medium in multiwell dishes with (i) buffer, (ii) α-thrombin at 1 U/ml, (iii) DIP thrombin, (iv) recombinant human IL-1 at 1 U/ml, (v) an admixture of interleukin and thrombin, (vi) recombinant TNF-α at 10 ng/ml, and (vii) an admixture of TNF and thrombin.

The results (Table V) showed that, in a series of twelve experiments, the mean concentration of TM in the control cells was 9.7 ng/ml. In cultures incubated with medium containing α-thrombin, the concentration of TM was 6.8 ng, and in cells incubated with IL-1 or TNF the concentration of

TABLE IV. Induced Release of
vWFAg from Endothelial Cells

Agonist	vWFAg (U/L)
A23187	58.4 $\pm$ 9.8
Thrombin	33.6 $\pm$ 6.2
DIP thrombin	3.8 $\pm$ 0.6
Thrombin/TM	4.4 $\pm$ 0.6
Control	2.8 $\pm$ 0.5

TM was 7.6 ng and 7.1 ng/ml, respectively. The concentration of TM in cells treated with DIP thrombin was not significantly different from that in untreated cells. Moreover, confluent cells incubated in medium containing both α-thrombin and IL-1 or α-thrombin and TNF contained significantly lower amounts of TM than when the reagents were used alone. It is noteworthy that in these instances the effect of the combined mixtures appeared to be additive rather than synergistic.

Measurements of soluble TM in concentrated culture medium obtained from each of these experiments demonstrated that the reduction in cellular TM was accompanied by an increase in the TM antigen in solution. It appeared, however, that not all of the loss of cellular TM could be accounted for by release of the ligand into solution, and the molecular structure of the TM found in the culture supernatant remains to be determined. Nevertheless, the results strongly suggest that thrombin, IL-1, and TNF might cleave TM from its bound, endothelial site. It may be important to note at this stage that marked morphological changes were induced by treatment of the endothelial cells with recombinant TNF, and similar but less pronounced changes were induced by IL-1. No damage was observed by treatment of the cells with thrombin.

MEASUREMENT OF THROMBOMODULIN IN PLASMA IN VARIOUS DISEASES

These results are very much in keeping with earlier reports that thrombin and inflammatory cytokines modulate protein C-related mechanisms at the endothelial surface. Moreover, they tend to confirm that the presence of soluble TM in normal human plasma might reflect endothelial damage in vivo. This finding might be especially useful in view of the current difficulties that are encountered in attempting to identify endothelial injury in clinical practice. The classification of patients with vasculitis in particular is not straightforward, and the diagnosis is usually based on clinical judgment supported by invasive histological biopsies (17). Some reports have indicated that a number of immunological features might be typical of specific disorders, but in general there are no laboratory tests currently available that consistently reflect disease activity.

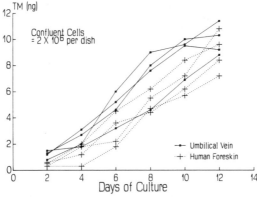

Fig. 4. Increase in thrombomodulin antigen (TM) in cultured endothelial cells. The cells were solubilised by freezing and thawing three times in buffer pH 7.2 containing 1% (v/v) Triton X 100.

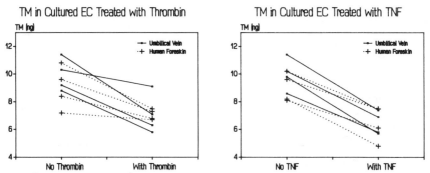

Fig. 5. Effects of thrombin and TNF on thrombomodulin antigen in solubilised endothelial cells.

Within the last few years, vWFAg has been suggested as a marker of vascular disease (18–22), and levels of this protein are raised in plasma in a variety of patients with vasculitic lesions (Table VI). The interpretation of immunoassays for vWf is complicated, however. Large amounts of the antigen are present in normal human plasma, and it is also localised and secreted by megakaryocytes and platelets. Sensitive IRMA for vWFAg give nonparallel dose–response curves with some plasma samples and with antigen prepared from endothelial cells; conventional immunoprecipitin assays for vWFAg are relatively insensitive and do not adequately detect subtle changes in antigen concentration. By contrast, thrombomodulin is normally present in very low concentrations in plasma and its cellular origin is very predominantly endothelial in nature. Furthermore, parallel dose–response curves have been obtained with all plasma samples and

TABLE V. Thrombomodulin in Solubilised
Endothelial Cells and Culture Supernatant

Confluent cells incubated with:	Thrombomodulin (ng/ml)	
	Cells	Supernatant
Buffer control	9.7	<0.1
α-Thrombin	6.8	1.4
DIP thrombin	9.5	<0.1
Interleukin 1 (IL-1)	7.6	1.3
Tumor necrosis factor	7.1	1.2
α-Thrombin + IL-1	5.0	2.1
α-Thrombin + TNF	6.1	1.8

TABLE VI. vWFAg as a Marker of Vascular Disease

Synthesised and secreted by endothelial cells (and by megakaryocytes and platelets)

Enhanced release induced by various agonists

Raised levels in:
  Homocystinaemia
  Diabetic angiopathy
  Myocardial infarction
  Giant cell arteritis
  Systemic lupus erythematosus (SLE)
  Primary necrotising arteritis
  Scleroderma
  Systemic sclerosis
  Behçet syndrome
  Rheumatoid arthritis

endothelial cell preparations so far examined in the IRMA (Fig. 6). It was reasonable to propose, therefore, that increased levels of circulating thrombomodulin might reflect endothelial injury, and the development of the IRMA for TM prompted a comparison of the levels of TM and vWFAg in the plasma of patients with a variety of clinical disorders.

Overall, the results on the different patient groups indicated that the levels of vWFAg and TM were elevated to a broadly similar extent (Table VII). In particular, high average levels of both the antigens were detected in patients with temporal arteritis, leukaemia, and glomerular nephritis. In some instances, however (e.g., in glomerular nephritis), the increased levels of TM seemed to be proportionally greater than those of vWF, while in other cases (e.g., in systemic sclerosis), the increases of vWF appeared to be greater than those of TM.

In addition, unusual results were observed in some individual patients within these groups (Table VIII). High levels of vWFAg were seen in the presence of normal amounts of TM, and conversely, increased levels of TM were noted in the presence of normal quantities of vWFAg.

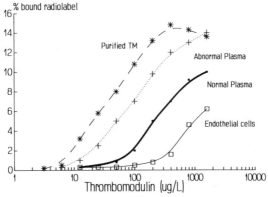

Fig. 6. Dose–response curves for the immunoradiometric assay for human thrombomodulin. Purified thrombomodulin was fractionated from human placenta. Endothelial cells were obtained from primary cultures of human umbilical vein cells and were solubilised as above. The abnormal plasma sample was obtained from a patient with acute leukaemia treated with cyclosporin A after bone marrow transplant.

Furthermore, it was not possible on the basis of these assays to identify consistent differences between those patients with and without clinical and histological evidence of vasculitis (Fig. 7). For example, there was a tendency for vWFAg to be higher in patients with vascultis, but the differences were not statistically significant, except in those with underlying rheumatoid arthritis. The measurements of TM were slightly raised in all these patients, but again there were no significant differences between those patients reported with and those without clinical vasculitis.

In several cases the highest levels of both vWFAg and TM appeared to be present in patients with the most severe clinical symptoms. This seemed to be especially evident in patients with systemic lupus erythematosus

TABLE VII. Comparison of von Willebrand Factor Antigen (vWFAg) and Thrombomodulin Antigen (TM) in Patients with Various Diseases

Condition	N	vWFAg (U/dl)	TM (μg/L)
Normal	40	94 + 31	165 + 42
Systemic lupus erythematosus (SLE)	30	268 + 125	200 + 89
Behçet syndrome	4	163 + 26	170 + 50
Rheumatoid arthritis	18	193 + 85	201 + 47
Diabetes	14	184 + 32	201 + 50
Temp. Art.	6	480 + 160	400 + 167
Glomerular Nephritis	10	190 + 45	406 + 115
Systemic sclerosis	6	240 + 145	185 + 63
Leukaemia	29	235 + 140	310 + 101

TABLE VIII. Comparison of von Willebrand Factor Antigen
(vWFAg) and Thrombomodulin Antigen (TM) in Some Patients

Patient	Condition	vWFAg (U/dl)	TM (μg/L)
	Rheumatoid arthritis		
1		180	135
2		235	160
3		290	145
4		315	170
	Systemic sclerosis		
1		360	185
2		295	175
3		385	200
	Glomerular nephritis		
1		165	405
2		135	365
3		120	280
	Normal		
		94 + 31	165 + 42

(SLE), rheumatoid arthritis, and polyarteritis nodosa. Moreover, three patients with polyarteritis nodosa, three patients with rheumatoid arthritis, and two patients with SLE were monitored during treatment. Five of these patients demonstrated a good clinical response to treatment, and there was a significant fall in the measurements of vWFAg and TM. Three patients, however, one from each group, showed a very poor response to therapy, and the circulating levels of vWFAg and TM tended to rise in the follow up period in these instances (Fig. 8).

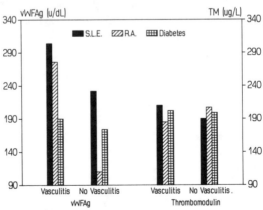

Fig. 7. Comparison of vWFAg and TM antigen in plasma from patients with and without clinical or histological evidence of vasculitis.

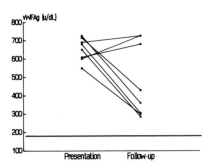 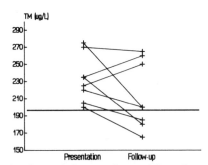

Fig. 8. Levels of vWFAg and TM antigen in three patients polyarteritis nodosa, in three patients with rheumatoid arthritis, and in two patients with SLE prior to treatment and during the follow-up period.

Some of the highest levels of plasma vWFAg and TM were found in plasma of leukaemic patients after bone marrow transplant (Table IX). To date 29 patients have been monitored, 18 allogeneic and 11 autologous transplants. In our unit, the current policy is to include cyclosporin A in the treatment regime for allogeneic transplant but not to use this drug for autologous transplant. In all other respects, the treatment of these patients is usually identical. The levels of both vWFAg and TM in these patients before transplant were increased and there were no significant differences between the allogeneic and autologous groups. After transplant, however, the concentration of vWFAg and TM increased dramatically in those patients treated with cyclosporin but changed to a much lesser degree in those patients not given the drug.

Furthermore, examination of five of these patients treated with cyclosporin indicated that the concentration of vWFAg and TM remained elevated for several months whilst the patients were on cyclosporin therapy. Figure 9 illustrates the levels of vWFAg and TM in plasma samples taken at intervals of approximately 2 months after transplant. Levels returned close to the normal range when the cyclosporin was discontinued.

Overall, therefore, increased levels of both vWf antigen and thrombomodulin were found in patients with disorders known to be associated

TABLE IX. von Willebrand Factor Antigen (vWFAg) and Thrombomodulin Antigen (TM) in Patients After Bone Marrow Transplant

	N	vWFAg (U/dl)	(TM μg/L)
Allogeneic	18	247 + 128	295 + 106
Autologous	11	223 + 140	325 + 120
Cyclosporin A	18	610 + 192	895 + 185
No cyclosporin	9	306 + 125	350 + 135
Normal	40	94 + 31	165 + 42

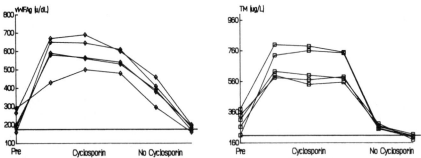

Fig. 9. Levels of vWFAg and TM antigen in five patients treated with cyclosporin A following bone marrow transplant. Plasma samples were obtained at approximately 2-month intervals.

with vascular disturbances. The highest levels were observed in patients with severe disease and persistently high levels seemed to be associated with poor prognosis. Very high levels were seen in patients with leukaemia treated with cyclosporin A after bone marrow transplant.

However, abnormalities of vWFAg and TM were not consistently found in patients with vasculitis and these measurements did not help to classify the disorders. Nevertheless, the present results supported the suggestion that cyclosporin A induced damage to the blood vessel wall (23), and the data indicate that increased levels of vWFAg and TM in plasma might reflect endothelial injury in vivo in some important circumstances.

CONCLUSIONS

There can be little doubt that thrombin and various natural products of inflammatory reactions mediate profound changes in the properties of the endothelium. Many of these modifications directly stimulate the biosynthesis or secretion of proteins involved in haemostasis and fibrinolysis, including vWF, plasminogen activators, and plasminogen activator inhibitors. Studies using thrombin and purified thrombomodulin indicated that the release of vWFAg from endothelial cells was inhibited by preincubation of the thrombin with thrombomodulin. These results were in keeping with the hypothesis that formation of a complex between thrombin and thrombomodulin neutralises the haemostatic capacity of the enzyme. In addition, thrombin, IL-1 and TNF clearly modulated the balance between procoagulant and anticoagulant functions of the endothelial surface, including the expression of cell-bound thrombomodulin. Experiments using endothelial cells in culture suggested that thrombin and these particular cytokines depressed the levels of cell associated thrombomodulin and at least partly induced release of the ligand into solution. The most marked affects were observed when thrombin and IL-1 or thrombin and TNF were used in combination. The data supported the suggestion that the presence of circulating thrombomodulin in plasma might reflect proteolysis of the endothelial bound material.

Measurements of vWFAg and thrombomodulin in plasma from patients with a variety of clinical disorders did not confirm consistently, however, that circulating thrombomodulin was the product of endothelial injury. Abnormalities of vWFAg and thrombomodulin were not reliably found in patients with vasculitis, and assays of these proteins did not help to classify vascular disorders. Nevertheless, persistently elevated levels seemed to be associated with poor prognosis in some instances, and very high levels were seen in patients with leukaemia treated with cyclosporin A after bone marrow transplant. These data were consistent with the view that cyclosporin A induced damage to the blood vessel wall, and it is possible that further development of these assays might provide an index of endothelial injury in vivo.

In general there is now a substantial amount of evidence to show that thrombin and inflammatory cytokines modulate protein C-related mechanisms at the endothelial surface. The data emphasise the dynamic role of these substances in vascular biology and provide further proof for the close association among inflammation, blood coagulation, and fibrinolysis.

REFERENCES

1. Handin RI, Wagner DD. Molecular and cellular biology of von Willebrand factor. In: Coller BS, ed. Progress in Hemostasis and Thrombosis. Philadelphia: WB Saunders Co., 1989;233–259.
2. Nawroth PP, Stern DM. Endothelial cells as active participants in procoagulant reactions. In Gimbrone MA, ed. Vascular Endothelium in Hemostasis and Thrombosis. New York: Churchill Livingstone, 1986; 14–39.
3. Tracy PB. Regulation of thrombin generation at cell surfaces. Semin Thromb Hemost 1988;14:227–232.
4. Esmon NL. Thrombomodulin. In: Collar BS, ed. Progress in Hemostasis and Thrombosis. Philadelphia: WB Saunders Co., 1989;29–55.
5. Ishii H, Majerus PW Thrombomodulin is present in human plasma and urine. J Clin Invest 1985;76:2178–2181.
6. Giddings JC. Molecular Genetics and Immunoanalysis in Blood Coagulation. Chichester: VCH/Ellis Horwood, 1988;143–162.
7. Taylor FB Jr, Chang A, Esmon CT, D'Angelo A, Vigano-D'Angelo S, Bick KE. Protein C prevents the coagulopathic and lethal effects of E. coli infusion in the baboon. J Clin Invest 1987;79:918–925.
8. Nawrorth PP, Stern DM. Modulation of endothelial cell hemostatic properties by tumor necrosis factor. J Exp Med 1986;163:740–745.
9. Bevilacqua MP, Pober JS, Wheeler ME, Cotran RS, Gimbrone MA Jr. Interleukin-1 activation of vascular endothelium. Effects on procoagulant activity and leukocyte adhesion. Am J Pathol 1985;121:394–403.
10. van Hinsbergh VWM, Kooistra T, van den Berg EA, Princen HMG, Fiers W, Emeis JJ. Tumor necrosis factor increases production of plasminogen activator

inhibitor in human endothelial cells in vitro and in rats in vivo. Blood 1988; 72:1467–1473.

11. Dejana E, Breviario F, Erroi A, Bussolino F, Mussoni L, Gramse M, Pintucci G, Casali B, Dinarello CA, van Damme J, Mantovani A. Modulation of endothelial cell functions by different molecular species of interleukin 1. Blood 1987;69:695–699.

12. Moore KI, Esmon CT, Esmon NL. Tumor necrosis factor leads to internalisation and degradation of thrombomodulin from the surface of bovine aortic endothelial cells in culture. Blood 1989;73:159–165.

13. Moore KL, Andreoli SP, Esmon NL, Esmon CT, Bang NU. Endotoxin enhances tissue factor and suppresses thrombomodulin expression of human vascular endothelium in vitro. J Clin Invest 1987;79:124–130.

14. Nawroth PP, Handley DA, Esmon CT, Stern DM. Interleukin 1 induces endothelial cell procoagulant whilst suppressing cell-surface anticoagulant activity. Proc Natl Acad Sci USA 1986;83:3460–3464.

15. Hanss M, Collen D. Secretion of tissue-type plasminogen activator and plasminogen activator inhibitor by cultured human endothelial cells: Modulation by thrombin, endotoxin and histamine. J Lab Clin Med 1987;109:97–104.

16. Maruyama I, Majerus PW. The turnover of thrombin-thrombomodulin complex in cultured human umbilical vein endothelial cells and A549 lung cancer cells. Endocytosis and degradation of thrombin. J Biol Chem 1985;260:15432–15438.

17. Lie JT. Editorial. Classification and immunodiagnosis of vasculitis: A new solution or promises unfulfilled. J Rheumatol 1988;15:728–732.

18. Nusinow SR, Federici AB, Zimmerman TS, Curd JC. Increased von Willebrand factor antigen in the plasma of patients with vasculitis. Arthritis Rheum 1984; 27:1405–1410.

19. Editorial. Factor VIII-related antigen and vasculitis. Lancet 1988;1:1203–1204.

20. Yazici H, Hekim N, Ozbakir F, Yurdakul S, Tuzun T, Pazarli H, Muftuoglu A. von Willebrand factor in Behçet's syndrome. J Rheumatol 1987;14:305–306.

21. Lufkin EG, Fass DN, O'Fallon WM, Bowie EJW. Increased von Willebrand factor in diabetes mellitus. Metabolism 1979;28:63–66.

22. Woolfe AD, Wakerley G, Wallington TB, Scott DGI, Dieppe PA. Factor VIII related antigen in the assessment of vasculitis. Ann Rheum Dis 1987;46:441–447.

23. Brown Z, Neild GH, Willoughby JJ, Somia NV, Cameron SJ. Increased factor VIII as an index of vascular injury in cyclosporine nephrotoxicity. Transplantation 1986;42:150–153.

The Endothelium: An Introduction to Current Research, pages 157–170

14
Endothelial Damage During Angioplasty

A.J.B. BRADY AND J.B. WARREN

Departments of Medicine (Division of Cardiology) (A.J.B.B.) and Clinical Pharmacology (J.B.W.), Royal Postgraduate Medical School, Hammersmith Hospital, London W12 OHS, England

INTRODUCTION

During the 25 years since its introduction by Dotter and Judkins as a transluminal method of treating atherosclerotic obstruction, angioplasty has gained wide acceptance (1). The earliest uses were for arteriosclerotic lesions in the lower limb, but the use of intra arterial balloon dilatation of localized stenoses was soon applied to other sites. The use of balloon angioplasty was extended to cerebral, renal and other peripheral sites of arterial obstruction (2). The first application of angioplasty to disease of the coronary arteries was described by Gruentzig in 1977 and since then percutaneous transluminal coronary angioplasty (PTCA) has assumed an increasingly prominent position in cardiological clinical practice. The attraction of the technique is that it offers the opportunity to open narrowed arteries by means of a relatively simple catheter approach, thereby obviating the need for major cardiac surgery. During 1987, more than 200,000 PTCAs were performed worldwide (3). Increased experience and advances in technology have combined to give a primary success rate for coronary balloon angioplasty of 90–95% (i.e., initial success in relief of the arterial obstruction). These advances have been accompanied by a fall in the complication rate to 4–5% (4).

From the outset, it has been apparent that relief of arterial obstruction was not always sustained, and restenosis within months, days or even hours sometimes occurs. In coronary arteries, restenosis occurs in 16–45% of initially successful angioplasties (5–8), and this figure has changed little since the introduction of PTCA, despite intensive investigation. The vast majority of restenoses occur early, within the first six months following angioplasty (9). Data on restenosis rates for various sites in the arterial tree are sparse. As an example, in renal artery angioplasty there are no large studies available. The determination of the presence of restenosis usually requires invasive radiological procedures. The recurrence of stenosis may not be apparent clinically and repeat angiography in asymptomatic patients is not usually pursued. Only for coronary angioplasty is there a large body of data relating to the incidence of restenosis.

The major drawback to angioplasty is that it necessarily involves endothelial damage and this may underlie the mechanisms of restenosis or acute closure of vessels. This chapter describes the consequences of endothelial and intimal damage during angioplasty and discusses how the interactions among endothelium, other constituent cells of the vessel wall, and the coagulation system relate to the problems of restenosis seen in clinical practice. The relevance of these observations to new developments in angioplasty technique that aim to minimise intimal damage is discussed. Most of the research into the role of endothelium and endothelial damage as a result of angioplasty described in this review will relate to PTCA for atheromatous obstruction, because much of the published work in this area, both clinical and experimental, has addressed mechanisms related to coronary artery disease.

MECHANICS OF DILATATION BY BALLOON ANGIOPLASTY IN ATHEROMATOUS DISEASE

In the original description of angioplasty, success was ascribed to the redistribution and compression of the composite material of the atherosclerotic plaque (1). It was suggested that atheroma could be "moulded" by the balloon, and moreover that existing normal intima could be stretched without harm. It was soon shown, however, by post mortem and animal studies that balloon expansion of an artery caused endothelial desquamation and neointimal tears with a variable degree of intimal perforation (10,11). Furthermore, atheroma in coronary arteries is usually composed of dense, inelastic fibre-collagen tissue with variable amounts of calcium within the plaque. Such material could not be moulded so plaque compression probably plays a minor role in human PTCA.

In animal models, experimental atherosclerosis is much softer, and in these situations compression of atheromatous tissue can occur. It is now accepted that the major mechanism of balloon dilatation of human atherosclerotic arteries is by fracture or cracking of the atheromatous plaque. In some cases, additional localised medial dissection, leading to the formation of intimal flaps can occur (12). Furthermore, when the atheromatous plaque is eccentric (i.e., not concentric atherosclerotic narrowing), stretching of the plaque-free wall may occur (12,13), with a variable degree of plaque compression or cracking. These mechanisms are not mutually independent, and it is likely that during PTCA in patients, each of these explanations will contribute to some degree.

CELLULAR CONSEQUENCES OF ANGIOPLASTY

It is readily demonstrated in vascular preparations in vitro that the endothelium is a tissue exquisitely sensitive to trauma. Moreover, the established methods for deendothelialisation of an artery include such techniques as the gentle rubbing of the vessel with a wooden stick or forceps tip or insufflation of a jet of air. It is therefore not surprising that forcing a balloon against the intima results in efficient endothelial cell loss. In order to try to explain the limitations of angioplasty, it is necessary to examine the consequences of endothelial denudation that occurs as an unavoidable effect. The technique of angioplasty had been applied to patients before the importance of the endothelium as a source of dilator and antithrombogenic factors was appreciated. Intact endothelium acts as an antithrombotic, selectively permeable vascular lining, each cell producing a number of agents protecting against thrombus formation and local vasoconstriction, as well as concealing thrombogenic subendothelial tissues. Stripping the endothelium exposes these thrombogenic surfaces to the blood, permitting platelet adhesion.

Endothelial cell turnover and regeneration are enhanced by both hypertension and hypercholesterolaemia. The atherosclerotic process has been shown experimentally to start during the period of endothelial regeneration and therefore endothelial injury may be particularly harmful in the presence of other risk factors. Unfortunately, patients who undergo angioplasty tend to have a higher incidence of risk factors, such as smoking, hypertension, hyperlipidaemia, and diabetes.

IMPLICATIONS OF EDRF LOSS

When the intima is damaged by an angioplasty balloon, the endothelium-dependent responses of blood vessels to vasoactive agents may be reversed. For example, in intact arteries the platelet products ADP, serotonin, and thromboxane A_2 (TxA_2) all have mild relaxant effects, but in endothelium-denuded vessels they have strong vasoconstrictive actions (14). Serotonin has been shown to have an augmented vasospastic effect in deendothelialised dog coronary arteries, and thus activated platelets may predispose to coronary spasm at the site of endothelial denudation (15). Interestingly, studies in which acetylcholine (ACh) has been injected into human coronary arteries suggest that atheromatous arteries contract to ACh, whereas normal vessels dilate (16,17). This agrees with data from animal experiments (18), and implies that endothelium-mediated vasodilatation may be lost in atherosclerotic areas of the vessel wall.

CHANGES IN COAGULATION STATUS FOLLOWING ANGIOPLASTY

Intact endothelial lining presents a nonthrombogenic surface, maintained by cell production of prostacyclin, EDRF, tissue plasminogen activator (tPA), and antithrombotic cell-surface proteins. Endothelial cells normally produce von Willenbrand factor (vWF), one of the components of the coagulation cascade. Endothelial-derived vWF is found not only in blood but also passes into the intimal extracellular matrix (19). In the event of deendothelialisation the loss of prostacyclin, EDRF, and tPA plus the revelation of thrombogenic subendothelial collagen and vWF allows platelet adhesion. Furthermore, the endothelium produces not only the anticoagulants prostacyclin and tissue plaminogen activator but also thrombomodulin, the cell-bound thrombin-binding protein required as a cofactor for the activation of protein C at the endothelial cell surface (20). This additional anticoagulant protection from the normal endothelial lining is lost during balloon dilatation, although smooth muscle cells are capable of producing thrombomodulin. The importance of thrombomodulin in limiting the platelet response to endothelial loss has not yet been determined.

Recent work has shown the products of platelet aggregation, platelet-derived growth factor (PDGF) and epidermal growth factor (EGF), both have vasoconstrictive actions that may augment the vasoconstriction produced by serotonin at the site of thrombus formation (21). These platelet products might conceivably be important in the vascular response to angioplasty and in atherogenesis, and pharmacological intervention affecting both the vasoactive and mitogenic actions may be important in future therapies of these conditions.

It may be asked why all angioplastied arteries do not restenose or thrombose after balloon dilatation. A minority do, but establishing the mechanisms by which arteries subjected to similar stresses in different patients have different responses has not yet been achieved. In vitro experiments can show individual actions, each of which may contribute to some degree in the thrombotic response of angioplastied blood vessels. The degree to which each of these reactions contributes to the overall balance of thrombosis and anticoagulation remains to be established.

PLATELETS AND THE PROLIFERATIVE RESPONSE

In animal models of balloon angioplasty, mild intimal injury with no disruption of tissue below the internal elastic lamina causes deposition of a thin, laminar layer of platelets without macroscopic thrombus formation (22). When deeper structures are injured, the media is exposed to flowing arterial blood, and macroscopic mural thrombus is formed. The progression of these lesions has been studied; 1 hr after experimental balloon angioplasty, there was extensive platelet deposition. By 4 days, platelet deposition was considerably reduced, and endothelial repair, manifest by endothelial proliferation, was present. After 7 days, this repair was nearly complete, but smooth muscle cell proliferation had developed. By 14 days, there was circumferential smooth muscle cell proliferation involving the intima, which was unchanged 30 and 60 days later (23).

The response to injury hypothesis as an explanation for atherosclerosis (24) states that vascular endothelial injury results in denudation, platelet adhesion, and thrombus formation. The subsequent monocyte infiltration can lead to smooth muscle cell proliferation, partly due to PDGF and possibly to other, including monocyte-derived, growth factors.

Endothelial cells themselves can release PDGF if damaged (25). This may augment the vasospasm which can occur after angioplasty, since PDGF does have a direct vasoconstrictor effect (25). Endothelial cells produce heparin-like proteoaminoglycans, which inhibit both platelet aggregation and smooth muscle cell growth. Heparin and heparan sulphate thus form normal components of the extracellular matrix. There may be a dynamic equilibrium state between mitogenic growth factors and heparin-like products, which is disturbed when the endothelial lining is damaged (26). Adhering platelets also release platelet factor 4, which is an antiheparin (27), thus tending to neutralize any remaining endothelium-derived heparin which would normally be expected to suppress smooth muscle hyperplasia. This equilibrium which is presumably central to vessel wall repair may if disturbed be important in both atherogenesis and restenosis after angioplasty.

ENDOTHELIAL REGROWTH

The time course of recovery of the endothelium after deendothelialisation has been studied in both normal and in atherosclerotic animal models. In pigs, a full endothelial lining had regrown by 8 days following balloon injury, but at 4 weeks the endothelial cells were still morphologically different and irregularly oriented (28). Smooth muscle cell migration from the media was observed at 8 days postangioplasty, and by 4 weeks intimal thickening with stratified layers of smooth muscle cells and interstitial tissue was well established.

In atherosclerotic rabbits there is also a major early platelet response to endothelial injury by balloon angioplasty. At 4 weeks there was restenosis and considerable fibrocellular proliferation (29). In experiments in which there has been extensive endothelial cell loss over a large area of intima, complete regrowth of the endothelium may not occur, even within a 3-year follow-up period (25). Why this does not permit unrestricted smooth muscle cell growth is not clear. It has been demonstrated that one year after balloon deendothelialisation the medial response was no greater at 12 months than at 6 weeks, in normocholesterolaemic animals (25).

All the above animal experiments suggest that mild, localised superficial endothelial injury has as its repair mechanism an early platelet response followed by endothelial cell migration and division to effect repair. If more severe damage occurs, with subintimal exposure, the response involves a further smooth muscle cellular proliferative stage, with consequent arterial wall thickening.

The endothelial response to platelet aggregation has been examined in vascular strips taken from porcine coronary arteries after balloon deendothelialisation and subsequent regrowth (28). After 8 days a full endothelial lining could be observed and normal endothelium-dependent relaxation to aggregating platelets could be demonstrated. By 4 weeks eccentric myointimal thickening had occurred, but relaxations to aggregating platelets were markedly depressed. This appeared to be due to a lack of responsiveness to serotonin. Moreover, endothelium-dependent relaxation to aggregating platelets has been shown to be impaired in hypercholesterolaemic pigs (30). These findings have far-reaching implications if human coronary endothelium behaves in a similar manner, since loss of the dilator response by intact endothelium to aggregating platelets may predispose to mural thrombosis at the site of regenerated endothelium.

ENDOTHELIAL DAMAGE AND ATHEROMATOUS CHANGE

The entire vasculature is normally lined with a contiguous endothelial cell monolayer, but in experimental atheroma there is focal endothelial cell loss. These denuded areas are associated with smooth muscle proliferation and infiltration of lipid-filled macrophages, with platelet adhesion to the luminal surface. It has been shown in animals that areas of focal endothelial cell loss can be demonstrated in association with coronary atheroma (31). This association between endothelial loss and atheroma does not imply cause and effect, although direct endothelial trauma can cause atheromatous change in animal models (24).

A recent histological study of both normal arterial and atherosclerotic tissue taken from coronary arteries from patients undergoing heart transplantation has been performed (32). Areas of the intima with no atherosclerosis had a normal endothelial lining, the cells being aligned with their long axes in the direction of blood flow. Where atheroma was present, endothelial cells were haphazardly arranged, with a variable degree of demonstrable leucocyte adhesion. In all the coronary arteries studied, there were gaps in the endothelial cell lining over plaques. Endothelial denudation was frequently, although not invariably, associated with platelet aggregates on the damaged intima. Importantly, it was observed that gaps in the endothelial lining did not always correspond to those areas with atherosclerotic narrowing, but could also be seen in segments of unobstructed artery. Whether such endothelial cells overlying areas of atheroma act in similar fashion to endothelial cells in their normal environment has yet to be fully determined in human studies.

Recently a rabbit model has been described whereby a nonocclusive adventitial cuff is placed around the artery (33). Within 7 days, smooth muscle cell and macrophage infitration can be demonstrated, with preservation of the endothelial lining. This has been interpreted as evidence that endothelial damage is not a prerequisite for the development of atheroma. However, such an external occlusion may have induced turbulent flow within the vessel with increased shear stress and possible alteration in endothelial function.

In rabbits made hypercholesterolaemic, additional foam cells could be observed in the new plaques. It was considered by the authors that obstruction of the vasa vasorum with consequent medial ischaemia was the likely etiology in this model (33). Whether this mechanism is important in human atherogenesis or the cellular response to balloon angioplasty (e.g., obstruction of the vasa vasorum by redistributed medial material) remains to be explored.

CLINICAL CONSEQUENCES OF ANGIOPLASTY

In most cases of angioplasty, the vessel remains patent after dilatation. However, abrupt closure of coronary arteries immediately following dilatation occurs in 2–6% of patients treated, despite advances in equipment and technique (12). This occurs as a result of occlusion by formation of an intimal flap in 56% of cases, coronary dissection in 34%, localized thrombus in 8%, and coronary artery spasm in 2% (4) and is usually clinically and angiographically obvious. Late closure or restenosis occurs in 16–45% of initially successful coronary angioplasties (5–8). Data for renal artery angioplasty are much more scarce. In our experience, and in published reports (34), early successful dilatation can usually be achieved with approximately one third of cases being cured of renovascular hypertension, one third gaining an improvement in their hypertensive control, and one third remaining unchanged over 6 months. However, of 65 angioplasties performed for renal artery stenosis at our hospital, the early benefits in blood pressure control have not been sustained. The efficacy of renal angioplasty for atheromatous disease has never been tested in a randomised, controlled trial.

Published figures for restenosis rates after renal artery angioplasty vary from as low as 2 of 27 patients (35) to 7 of 16 patients (36). For PTCA, many variables have been analysed in relation to restenosis, but there is little unified opinion on the significance and predictability of individual clinical, angiographic, or pharmacological factors.

CHARACTERISTICS OF RESTENOSIS IN MAN

The major drawback of PTCA is the development in about one third of patients of recurrent luminal narrowing, usually within the first 3 months. Moreover, it is difficult to predict those lesions that will stay dilated and those that will restenose. Early exercise electrocardiographic (ECG) testing can sometimes help (37). There are no large clinical series published of pathological features of restenosis in human coronary arteries and available data are limited to case reports. Animal experiments describe myointimal thickening as a response to endothelial denudation and clinical case reports have found intimal fibrous proliferation at the site of angioplasty. The fibrocellular hyperplasia often corresponds in dimensions to the angioplasty balloon (12). Some studies reporting intimal fibrous proliferation (12) have described fibrocellular growth at areas related not only to the fractured plaque but to surrounding portions of atherosclerotic plaque. One of the mechanisms by which angioplasty increases flow is the formation of channels which can subsequently become filled by fibrocellular tissue, thus greatly narrowing the luminal diameter (10).

In the few small studies published, a degree of fibrocellular proliferation has been demonstrated in most cases at sites of angiographically successful angioplasty (12). The reasons such lesions progress to frank stenotic narrowings in some patients and not in others have yet to be elucidated. The instrumentation required to guide the angioplasty balloon to the site of the narrowing might itself cause intimal damage and subsequent atheroma in the proximal coronary artery (38). Other reports have not found this to be the case (39), and the relevance of proximal arterial damage as a mechanism for accelerated atheroma has not yet been prospectively tested.

PREVENTION OF RESTENOSIS

The effects of angioplasty may be viewed as a balance between the benefits of dilation of the stenoses and the detrimental effects of endothelial damage. Loss of functioning endothelium increases the possibility of vasospasm by reducing EDRF and prostacyclin production and converts a nonthrombogenic surface to a procoagulant surface. Animal experiments show that angioplasty permits the proliferation of smooth muscle cells. This proliferation also occurs in patients with restenosis after angioplasty, and may predispose later to local and possibly even proximal vessel atheroma formation. Improving the long-term (i.e., >3 months) success rate of PTCA will depend on the development of new approaches to minimize the consequences of endothelial damage, since preservation of endothelium is impossible if balloon dilatation is to be performed.

RISK FACTORS FOR RESTENOSIS

Some studies have described clinical or technical factors associated with a higher incidence of restenosis [for review, see Blackshear et al. (40)]. Angioplasties attempted on totally occluded or $>90\%$ stenosed vessels have a greater chance of renarrowing, and the left anterior descending coronary artery seems for some reason to be more susceptible than other coronary arteries. The presence of diabetes mellitus may also confer a higher risk of restenosis. These studies cannot explain whether the mechanisms of renarrowing are different, or just accelerated, in these clinical groups.

PHARMACOLOGICAL APPROACHES TO RESTENOSIS

Numerous clinical trials have attempted to demonstrate agents that will improve the outcome after PTCA. Data from animal experiments have shown that pharmacological agents can modify the cellular response to experimental balloon angioplasty. These agents have subsequently been tested in clinical trials; the results are described below.

Antiplatelet Agents

Antiplatelet agents have been shown in both animal models of balloon endothelial injury and in clinical trials to reduce the platelet adhesion that inevitably occurs after dilatation (22,29,40–42). The successful maintenance of patency of coronary artery bypass grafts with such drugs has also been found in clinical trials. A recent large randomised trial of alternate-day low-dose aspirin to prevent stroke and myocardial infarction in American physicians demonstrated unequivocally that inhibition of platelet function was associated with a reduced rate of cardiovascular events (43). However, another recent clinical trial of aspirin and dipyridamole versus placebo examining restenosis after angioplasty showed no beneficial effect on restenosis in the treated group (44), although the incidence of transmural myocardial infarction during or soon after PTCA was markedly reduced (1.6% in the treated group versus 6.9% in the placebo group).

Anticoagulants

In experimental preparations, heparin given within 12 hr of deendothelialisation decreased intimal proliferation (45), but when given 48 hr after injury it had no such protective effect. Heparin can reverse atheroma in experimental hypercholesterolaemic animal models, when given long-term. Unfortunately, heparin causes osteoporosis if given in prolonged dosage, which contraindicates its antiatheromatous use in man, although low-dose inhalation might circumvent this problem (46).

Heparin has been used since the introduction of angioplasty as a perioperative intravenous infusion to inhibit thrombosis, but not until 1989 did a randomised controlled trial report the effects of an 18 to 24-hr infusion of heparin after PTCA (47). However, as with other hypotheses successfully tested in animal studies, when applied to clinical angioplasty, no reduction could be demonstrated in the restenosis rate in the group receiving heparin. Encouragingly, however, it has been demonstrated in a rat model that 3 days of heparin therapy after balloon injury suppresses neointimal formation, with up to 50% inhibition of cellular hyperplasia (48). Such a prolonged infusion of heparin has not yet been studied in patients undergoing PTCA. The use of warfarin has been examined post angioplasty but 6 months of therapy had no effect on restenosis rates (42,49).

Glyceryltrinitrate

GTN (Nitroglycerin) has been used for over a century to treat cardiac ischaemia. As well as relaxing epicardial coronary arteries GTN can also decrease platelet deposition in experimental animal models (50). GTN is sometimes used routinely to inhibit coronary spasm during PTCA, but evidence that long-term nitrate therapy has any effect on restenosis is lacking.

Calcium Antagonists

Calcium-channel blockers in animal models inhibit smooth muscle cell hyperplasia after balloon intimal injury, although this benefit has not been confirmed in clinical studies. Calcium antagonists can reduce coronary artery spasm and so are often prescribed postangioplasty, but no beneficial action against restenosis has yet been demonstrated in patients (51).

Glucocorticoids

Immunological mechanisms are important in atherogenesis, and the endogenous steroid dehydroepiandrosterone (DHEA) causes reduction of atherogenesis in hypercholesterolaemic rabbits (52). Pharmacological doses of glucocorticoids have potent anti-inflammatory effects, and this might modulate the cellular response to angioplasty (53). This hypothesis is being tested in a prospective clinical trial of intravenous methylprednisolone, which has yet to report its findings (53). There are as yet no trials of steroids to reduce atheroma in man. A major drawback to the use of steroids is not only their broad spectrum of side effects, but also the association between accelerated atheroma and Cushing's syndrome.

Fish Oils and HMG-CoA Reductase Inhibitors

Fish oil dietary supplements have been given to prevent restenosis after coronary angioplasty, the rationale being that N-3 (omega-3) fatty acids are potent inhibitors of platelet function. In animal models these acids seem to have a direct antiatherosclerotic effect. Excitement was caused by an uncontrolled clinical trial of fish oil given before and for a prolonged period after angioplasty which seemed to result in a reduced restenosis rate (54). A second, randomised, double-blind, placebo-controlled trial of fish oil unfortunately failed to confirm the beneficial effect demonstrated in the earlier trial (55). A prospective clinical trial of the cholesterol-synthesis pathway blocking drug, simvastatin, to try and reverse atheromatous lesions is being conducted. This approach has not yet been tried in angioplasty-induced stenoses.

Angiotensin-Converting Enzyme Inhibitors

Exciting new work has thrown light on the role of local angiotensin II activity in the cellular response to endothelial injury (see Chapter 8). It has been found that the administration of an angiotensin-converting enzyme inhibitor (ACE inhibitor) to rats subjected to carotid artery de-endothelialisation during the postoperative period resulted in an 80% decrease in the neointimal response to injury (56). The free compound had no effect on cell proliferation in vitro, confirming that its mode of action was due to inhibition of ACE. This has to date not yet been tested in PTCA but raises exciting prospects regarding the limitation of restenosis following angioplasty. Whether other growth factors such as insulin, platelet-derived growth factor (PDGF), or epidermal growth factor (EGF) have similar actions has not to date been examined.

TECHNICAL APPROACHES

Physical interventions to modify the vascular response to balloon dilation include thermal balloon angioplasty, which is used to "smooth off" the dilated segment of artery (12). The heat is generated by a laser, radiofrequency, chemical or ultrasound energy source either in the balloon or directed to it along the catheter. Such ingenious methods have yet to become established in clinical practice and they are unlikely to cause less endothelial damage. However, intravascular expandable stents that "hold open" the dilated artery show promise in both experimental and small clinical series (12,57). The direct intraluminal observation of coronary arteries by angioscopy is a new research tool that provides exciting opportunities to observe the morphological changes following angioplasty (58).

CONCLUSION

The dramatic increase in our knowledge of the importance of the endothelium to the control of local vessel calibre and coagulation has helped to explain why the impressive immediate correction of atheromatous stenoses is not always sustained. The consequences of endothelial damage have also dogged other techniques such as laser therapy and bypass grafting. Our understanding of how the endothelium influences smooth muscle cell growth is still limited, but this has become a very active research area.

To improve the long-term outcome of angioplasty will require a combined pharmacological approach to the vasospasm, thrombosis, and smooth muscle cell proliferation that occur as a result of endothelial damage. Future trials will need to evaluate not only improvements in vasodilator and anticoagulant therapy, but also drugs that might modify vascular smooth muscle growth.

REFERENCES

1. Dotter CT, Judkins MP. Transluminal treatment of arteriosclerotic obstruction. Circulation 1964;30:654–670.
2. Gruentzig A, Rentrop K, Bussman WD (eds). Transluminal Coronary Angioplasty and Intracoronary Thrombolysis. Berlin: Springer-Verlag 1982;1–41, 197–229.

3. Bourassa MG, Alderman EL, Bertrand M, et al. Report of the joint ISFC/WHO task force on coronary angioplasty. Circulation 1988;78:780–789.
4. Baim DS (ed). A symposium: Interventional cardiology-1987. Am J Cardiol 1988;61:1G–117G.
5. Gruentzig AR, King SB III, Schlumpf M, Siegenthaler W. Long term follow-up after percutaneous transluminal coronary angioplasty: The early Zurich experience. N Engl J Med 1987;316:1127–1132.
6. Guiteras Val P, Bourassa MG, David PR, et al. Restenosis after successful percutaneous transluminal coronary angioplasty: The Montreal Heart Institute experience. Am J Cardiol 1987;60:50B–60B.
7. Levine S, Ewwls CJ, Rosing DR, Kent KM. Coronary angioplasty: Clinical and angiographic follow-up. Am J Cardiol 1984;53:77C–81C.
8. Holmes DRJ, Vlietstra RE, Smith HC, et al. Restenosis after percutaneous transluminal coronary angioplasty (PTCA): A report from the PTCA registry of the National Heart, Lung and Blood Institute. Am J Cardiol 1984;53:77C–81C.
9. Faxon DP, Sanborn TA, Haudenschild CC. Mechanism of angioplasty and its relation to restenosis. Am J Cardiol 1987;60:5B–9B.
10. Block PC, Myler RK, Sterzer S, Fallon JT. Morphology after transluminal angioplasty in human beings. N Engl J Med 1981;305:382–385.
11. Waller BF. Pathology of transluminal balloon angioplasty used in the treatment of coronary heart disease. Hum Pathol 1987;18:476–484.
12. Waller BF. Crackers, stretchers, drillers, scrapers, shavers, burners, welders, melters—The future treatment of coronary artery disease? A clinical–morphologic assessment. J Am Coll Cardiol 1989;13:969–987.
13. Saner HE, Gobel FL, Salomonowitz E, Erlien DA, Edwards JE. The disease-free wall in coronary atherosclerosis: Its relation to degree of obstruction. J Am Coll Cardiol 1985;6:1096–1099.
14. Forstermann U, Mugge A, Bode S, Frohlich J. Response of human coronary arteries to aggregating platelets: Importance of endothelium-derived relaxing factor and prostanoids. Circ Res 1988;63:306–312.
15. Dole WP, Lamping KG, Marcus ML. Endothelium and responses of large coronary arteries to serotonin in vivo. In: Vasodilation. Vanhoutte PM, ed. New York: Raven Press, 1988.
16. Newman CM, Hackett Dr, Fryer M, El-Tamimi HM, Davies GJ, Maseri A. Dual effects of acetylcholine on angiographically normal human coronary arteries. Circulation 1987;76(suppl IV):56.
17. Werns SW, Walton JA, Hsia HH, Nabel EG, Sanz ML, Pitt B. Evidence of endothelial dysfunction in angiographically normal coronary arteries of patients with coronary artery disease. Circulation 1989;79:287–291.
18. Verbeuren TJ, Herman AG. Endothelium-dependent relaxations are inhibited in atheromatous blood vessels. In: Vasodilation. Vanhoutte PM, ed. New York: Raven Press, 1988.
19. Jaffe EA. Synthesis of von Willenbrand factor by endothelial cells. In: Ryan US, ed. Endothelial Cells. Vol. I. Boca Raton, Florida: CRC Press, 1988;119–126.
20. Esmon CT. The roles of protein C and thrombomodulin in the regulation of blood coagulation. J Biol Chem 1989;264:4743–4746.
21. Berk BC, Alexander RW. Vasoactive effects of growth factors. Biochem Pharmacol 1989;38:219–225.

22. Chesebro JH, Lam JYT, Badimon L, Fuster V. Restenosis after arterial angioplasty: A hemorrheologic response to injury. Am J Cardiol 1987;60:10B–16B.

23. Steele PM, Chesebro JH, Stanson AW, Holmes DR, Denwanjee MK, Badimon L, Fuster V. Balloon angioplasty—Natural history of the pathophysiological response to injury in a pig model. Circ Res 1985;57:105–112.

24. Ross R. The pathogenesis of atherosclerosis- an update. N Engl J Med 1986;314: 488–500.

25. Reidy MA. A reassessment of endothelial injury and arterial lesion formation. Lab Invest 1985;53:513–520.

26. Scott-Burden T, Buhler FR. Regulation of smooth muscle proliferative phenotype by heparinoid-matrix interactions. TIPS 1988;9:94–98.

27. Harker LA, Ross R, Glomset JA. The role of endothelial cell injury and platelet response in atherogenesis. Thromb Haemost 1978;39:312–321.

28. Shimokawa H, Aarhus LL, Vanhoutte PM. Porcine coronary arteries with regenerated endothelium have a reduced endothelium-dependent responsiveness to aggregating platelets and serotonin. Circ Res 1987;61:256–270.

29. Faxon DP, Sanborn TA, Haudenschild CC, Ryan TJ. Effect of antiplatelet therapy on restenosis after experimental angioplasty. Am J Cardiol 1984;53:72C–76C.

30. Shimokowa H, Kim P, Vanhoutte PM. Endothelium-dependent relaxation to aggregating platelets in isolated basilar arteries of control and hypercholesterolaemic pigs. Circ Res 1988;63:604–612.

31. Kim DN, Scott RF, Schmee J, Thomas WA. Endothelial cell denudation, labelling indices and monocyte attachment in advanced coronary artery lesions. Atherosclerosis 1988;73:247–257.

32. Davies MJ, Woolf N, Rowles PM, Pepper J. Morphology of the endothelium over atherosclerotic plaques in human coronary arteries. Br Heart J 1988;60:459–464.

33. Booth RFG, Martin JF, Honey AC, Hassall DG, Beesley JE, Moncada S. Rapid development of atherosclerotic lesions in the rabbit carotid artery induced by perivascular manipulation. Atherosclerosis 1989;75:257–268.

34. Brawn LA, Ramsay LE. Is improvement real with percutaneous transluminal angioplasty in the management of renovascular hypertension? Lancet 1987;2: 1313–1316.

35. Arlart IP, von Dewitz H, Bargon G. Transvenous digital subtraction angiography (DSA) for diagnostic control following percutaneous transluminal angioplasty (PTA) in patients with renovascular hypertension. Eur J Radiol 1985;5:115.

36. Grim CE, Luft FC, Yune HY, Klatte EC, Weinberger MH. Percutaneous transluminal dilatation in the treatment of renal vascular hypertension. An Intern Med 1981;95:439.

37. El-Tamimi H, Davies GJ, Hackett D, Fragasso G, Crea P, Maseri A. Very early prediction of restenosis after successful coronary angioplasty: Anatomical and functional assessment. J Am Coll Cardiol 1990;15:259–264.

38. Waller BF, Pinkerton CA, Foster LN. Morphologic evidence of accelerated left main coronary artery stenosis: A late complication of percutaneous transluminal balloon angioplasty of the proximal left anterior descending coronary artery. J Am Coll Cardiol 1987;9:1019–1023.

39. Cequier A, Bonan R, Crepeau J, et al. Restenosis and progression of coronary atherosclerosis after coronary angioplasty. J Am Coll Cardiol 1988;12:49–55.
40. Blackshear JL, O'Callaghan WG, Califf RM. Medical approaches to prevention after coronary angioplasty. J Am Coll Cardiol 1987;9:834–838.
41. Faxon DP, Sanborn TA, Haudenschild CC, Ryan TJ. Effect of antiplatelet therapy on restenosis after experimental angioplasty. Am J Cardiol 1984;53:72C–76C.
42. McBride W, Lange RA, Hillis LD. Restenosis after successful coronary angioplasty. N Engl J Med 1988;318:1734–1737.
43. Steering Committee of the Physicians' Health Study Research Group. Preliminary report: Findings from the aspirin component of the ongoing physicians' health study. N Engl J Med 1988;318:262–264.
44. Schwartz LS, Bourassa MG, Lesperance J, et al. Aspirin and dipyridamole in the prevention of restenosis after percutaneous transluminal coronary angioplasty. N Engl J Med 1988;318:1714–1719.
45. Clowes AW, Clowes MM. Heparin inhibits injury-induced arterial smooth muscle migration and proliferation. Fed Proc 1983;44:1138–1142.
46. Engelberg H. Heparin and the atherosclerotic process. Pharmacol Rev 1984;36:91–100.
47. Ellis SG, Roubin GS, Wilentz J, Lin S, Douglas JS, King SB. Effect of 18–24-hour heparin administration for prevention of restenosis after uncomplicated coronary angioplasty. Am Heart J 1989;117:777–782.
48. Clowes AW, Clowes MM. Kinetics of cellular proliferation after arterial injury. II. Inhibition of smooth muscle growth by heparin. Lab Invest 1985;52:611–616.
49. Thornton MA, Gruentzig AR, Hollman J, King SB III. Coumadin and aspirin inprevention of recurrence after transluminal coronary angioplasty: A randomised study. Circulation 1984;69:721–727.
50. Lam JYT, Chesebro JH, Fuster V. Platelets, vasoconstriction and nitroglycerin during arterial wall injury. Circulation 1988;78:712–716.
51. White CW, Knudson M, Schmidt D, et al. Neither ticlopidine nor aspirin-dipyridamole prevents restenosis post PTCA: Results from a randomised placebo-controlled multicentre trial. Circulation 1987;76(Suppl IV):213.
52. Gordon GB, Bush DE, Weisman HF. Reduction of atherosclerosis by administration of dehydroepiandrosterone. J Clin Invest 1988;82:712–720.
53. MacDonald RG, Panush RS, Pepine CJ. Rationale for use of glucocorticoids in modification of restenosis after PTCA. Am J Cardiol 1987;60:56B–60B.
54. Dehmer GJ, Popma JJ, Van den Berg EK, et al. Reduction in the rate of early restenosis after coronary angioplasty by a diet supplemented with n-3 fatty acids. N Engl J Med 1988;319:733–740.
55. Reis GJ, Sipperly ME, Boucher TM, et al. Randomised trial of fish oil for prevention of restenosis after coronary angioplasty. Lancet 1989;2:178–181.
56. Powell JS, Clozel JP, Muller RKM, Kuhn H, Hefti F, Hosang M, Baumgartner HR. Inhibitors of angiotensin-converting enzyme prevent myointimal proliferation after vascular injury. Science 1989;245:186–188.
57. Robinson KA, Roubin GS, Siegel RJ, et al. Intra-arterial stenting in the atherosclerotic rabbit. Circulation 1988;78:646–653.
58. Uchida Y, Hasegawa K, Kawamura K, Shibuya I. Angioscopic observation of the luminal changes induced by PTCA. Am Heart J 1989;117:769–776.

The Endothelium: An Introduction to Current Research, pages 171–186
© 1990 Wiley-Liss, Inc.

15
Neutrophil–Endothelial Cell Interactions In Vivo

S. NOURSHARGH and T.J. WILLIAMS
Department of Applied Pharmacology, National Heart and Lung Institute, London SW3 6LY, England

INTRODUCTION

A characteristic feature of the acute inflammatory response is the local accumulation of neutrophilic leukocytes. The essential function of this process is the recruitment of blood cells capable of phagocytosis and microbial killing to a site of infection or injury.

As first observed by Dutrochet in 1824, the mechanisms involved in neutrophil accumulation in vivo are complex and dependent on an interaction between neutrophils and microvascular endothelial cells. This interaction is triggered by chemical signals generated in the tissue at inflammatory sites. This chapter discusses in sequence the steps involved in this complex process which have been investigated using both in vivo and in vitro studies.

CHEMICAL SIGNALS INVOLVED IN NEUTROPHIL ACCUMULATION IN VIVO

Invading microbes, other foreign organisms or particles, and damaged tissue cells can stimulate the release of chemical signals that act as mediators of the inflammatory process. This section will discuss the well-characterised mediators of neutrophil accumulation in vivo.

Bacteria-Derived Factors

Two categories of mediators can be derived from bacteria, namely, formylated chemotactic peptides and endotoxins. It has long been known that bacteria, such as *Escherichia coli,* can release potent chemotactic substances in cell culture medium (1,2). However, it was not until 1975 that Schiffmann and colleagues characterised the neutrophil chemotactic property of a partially purified bacterial product (3). That same year, they published their first report on the potent leukocyte chemotactic properties of synthetic N-formylmethionyl peptides (4). Since bacteria initiate protein synthesis with N-formylmethionine, Schiffmann et al. suggested that the synthetic chemotactic peptides may be analogous to peptides released by bacteria. Nearly a decade later, it was shown that the formyl peptides are indeed the natural chemotactic products of bacteria and that N-formyl-methionyl-leucyl-phenylalanine (FMLP), the most potent of the synthetic peptides, is the major peptide neutrophil chemotactic factor produced by *E. coli* (5). In vitro, these chemotactic peptides activate all neutrophil responses following an interaction with specific and saturable cell surface receptors (6). In vivo, intradermal injection of formyl peptides induces neutrophil accumulation and neutrophil-dependent edema formation (7,8). The potency of these peptides in vivo suggests that they may well contribute to the process of neutrophil accumulation at infected sites.

Endotoxins are lipopolysaccharide molecules released from gram-negative bacteria. In vitro, these molecules are not chemotactic for neutrophils but are very potent in inducing neutrophil accumulation in vivo (9). This may be related to the in vitro observation that endotoxins render endothelial cells adhesive for neutrophils (10) and stimulate the generation and release of interleukin 1 (IL-1) and interleukin 8 (IL-8) by monocytes/macrophages (see below) (11). Furthermore, although endotoxins have no apparent stimulatory effect on neutrophils, they are capable of enhancing the responses of these cells to a wide variety of stimuli (priming) (12).

C5a

The complement system in tissue fluid plays an important role in certain immune and inflammatory reactions. An invading microbe can activate the complement system by two pathways (13). The "classical pathway" is activated by immunoglobulin IgG or IgM antibodies, once they have formed a complex with antigens on the microbe or its products. The "alternative pathway" is typically activated, in the absence of antibody, by polysaccharides such as those in yeast cell walls (zymosan). The central event in complement activation is cleavage of the third component, C3, into two primary fragments C3a and C3b. The formation of C3b facilitates a similar cleavage of C5 to C5a and C5b, which is the last recognised enzymatic step in the complement cascade. The larger fragment, C5b, combines spontaneously with the later components, C6-C9, to form a macromolecular complex capable of inducing cell lysis.

C3b and iC3b, produced by the action of the enzyme C3b inactivator or factor I, bind covalently to microbes (opsonisation) and promote their subsequent phagocytosis by neutrophils having C3b and iC3b receptors on their cell surface. The biological activities of C3a include mast cell activation and consequently histamine-induced increased microvascular permeability. In addition to C3a, several other protein cleavage by-products are produced as a consequence of complement activation. However, probably the most important as a trigger for neutrophil accumulation in vivo is C5a (13).

C5a, a 74-amino acid polypeptide, is a potent neutrophil stimulating agent in vitro and was the first neutrophil chemoattractant to be fully characterised (14). Its effects on neutrophils are believed to be mediated by specific and saturable cell surface receptors (15). In vivo, C5a is metabolised to C5a des Arg by a carboxypeptidase N found in plasma and extravascular tissue fluid. C5a des Arg is less potent than C5a in assays in vitro, and it has been suggested that for optimal activity it requires the presence of a "helper factor" (16). However, C5a des Arg, detected in high concentrations in inflammatory exudates (17–19), is potent in inducing neutrophil accumulation and neutrophil-dependent edema in vivo (7,17,20,21). Furthermore, the chemotactic activities generated in a number of allergic and nonallergic inflammatory reactions have been ascribed, at least partly, to C5a or its des Arg metabolite (17,18). There is also evidence suggesting that C5a and C5a des Arg may contribute to the acute, neutrophil-dominated phases of inflammation in the rheumatoid joint (22).

Lipid Mediators

Lipids, released on stimulation of cells at inflammatory sites, can induce neutrophil–endothelial cell interaction in vitro and may have important roles as mediators of acute inflammatory reactions in vivo. Leukotrienes are lipids that result from the oxygenation of arachidonic acid and related fatty acids by specific lipoxygenases. The major products of this enzyme cascade are monohydroxy acids (e.g., 5-HETE and 12-HETE); dihydroxy acids such as LTB_4, and the sulfidopeptide leukotrienes LTC_4, LTD_4, and LTE_4 (23).

In addition to the lipoxygenase pathway, arachidonic acid is the substrate for the cyclo-oxygenase pathway responsible for the biosynthesis of prostaglandins (24). Although it is generally believed that cyclo-oxygenase products do not induce neutrophil accumulation in vivo, they do have important modulatory effects (25).

In neutrophils, the major pathway of arachidonic acid metabolism, originally described by Borgeat and Samuelsson in 1979, involves oxygenation at the 5-position by a 5-lipoxygenase, whereas in platelets, the major pathway involves a 12-lipoxygenase (23). Stimulated neutrophils release LTB_4 but only release very low levels of the cyclo-oxygenase products, prostaglandins and thromboxanes (26).

The most potent neutrophil-stimulating agent generated from the above cascade is LTB_4, although the monohydroxy acids are also weakly chemotactic for neutrophils (27). In vitro, in addition to being a potent chemoattractant, LTB_4 stimulates neutrophil adherence and aggregation (27). As found with C5a and the formylated chemotactic peptides, LTB_4 induces its effects on neutrophils via specific and saturable plasma membrane receptors (27). In vivo, LTB_4 induces neutrophil accumulation and neutrophil-dependent edema formation (24). There is also evidence suggesting that LTB_4 may be involved as a mediator of various inflammatory conditions such as psoriasis (28) and myocardial ischemia (29).

Although the sulfidopeptide leukotrienes do not directly activate neutrophils, they are reported to enhance the adherence of neutrophils to cultured endothelial cells (30). This effect correlates with the ability of these agents to stimulate the generation of a phospholipid, platelet activating factor, from endothelial cells.

Platelet activating factor (PAF) is a biologically active phospholipid synthesised on stimulation by several cell types, including neutrophils and endothelial cells (31). However, unlike the leukotrienes, a large proportion of the newly generated PAF remains intracellular and its exact role remains to be elucidated (32). Exogenous PAF stimulates neutrophil aggregation, neutrophil adherence to endothelial cells, and adherence to cell-free surfaces (31). In addition, PAF stimulates the release of LTB_4 from neutrophils. These effects are reportedly mediated via specific plasma membrane receptors for this phospholipid (31). In vivo, intradermal injection of PAF induces neutrophil accumulation (8,33). Furthermore, there is evidence suggesting that endogenously formed PAF contributes to the influx of neutrophils in an IgG-mediated allergic inflammatory reaction in the rabbit (34). The interactive nature of these lipid mediators in vitro, strongly suggests that, in vivo, leukotrienes and PAF can act in concert to mediate inflammatory processes.

Cytokines

Cytokines are a family of regulatory proteins synthesised and released by many cell types, but primarily by leukocytes, in response to various stimuli (35). IL-1, tumour necrosis factor (TNF), granulocyte–macrophage colony stimulating factor (GM-CSF), and IL-8 are members of this family of proteins and have been implicated in several aspects of the inflammatory process.

Interleukin 1, originally described as a stimulator of thymocyte proliferation, is now known to possess a broad range of biological activities (36). In vitro, IL-1 does not stimulate neutrophils, but among its target cells is the endothelial cell. IL-1 stimulates cultured endothelial cells to generate PAF and to become more adhesive for neutrophils, the latter response being associated with the induction of cell surface adhesive glycoproteins (37) (see below). In vivo, intradermally administered IL-1 induces neutrophil accumulation that is slow in onset and is protein synthesis dependent (21). There is evidence suggesting that IL-1 is the principal mediator of endotoxin-induced neutrophil accumulation (38). Other mediators such as IL-8 may also be involved, however. This is supported by in vitro studies showing endotoxin to be a potent stimulator of IL-1 and IL-8 release from macrophages (11,36).

Tumour necrosis factor, originally described as a cytotoxic mediator acting on certain tumour cells, acts on endothelial cells to enhance neutrophil–endothelial cell interaction in a similar manner to IL-1 (37). However, in contrast to IL-1, TNF may also directly activate neutrophils. It has been reported that TNF can stimulate neutrophil chemotaxis via interaction with specific cell surface receptors (39,40). However, other studies have failed to detect such chemotactic activity (41). In vivo, TNF has potent pro-inflammatory properties (38,42). TNF induces neutrophil accumulation and edema formation in rabbit skin. These responses are rapid in onset and short in duration. Interestingly, IL-1 and TNF act synergistically in eliciting neutrophil accumulation and inducing a local response similar to a Schwartzman reaction (38).

Granulocyte–macrophage colony stimulating factor is a glycoprotein produced by activated T lymphocytes, endothelial cells, fibroblasts, and macrophages that stimulates the proliferation and differentiation of granulocyte and monocyte hematopoietic precursor cells (43). In addition to this role, GM-CSF directly activates neutrophils and is capable of enhancing neutrophil responses to other stimuli (44,45). GM-CSF can also stimulate neutrophil accumulation in rabbit skin (46).

Recently, several groups have independently detected and characterised a novel neutrophil-activating protein released from stimulated macrophages/monocytes in vitro (11). This protein, for which the name IL-8 has been proposed, can also be released from fibroblasts and endothelial cells stimulated by other cytokines (11). A similar substance has been extracted from psoriatic scale (11). IL-8 may prove to be a component of the neutrophil chemotactic activity detected after injection of endotoxin into the rat peritoneal cavity (47) and the rabbit pleural cavity (48). Purified IL-8 is also a potent inducer of neutrophil accumulation in vivo (11).

MECHANISM OF NEUTROPHIL–ENDOTHELIAL CELL INTERACTION

Adherence of neutrophils to vascular endothelium is a prerequisite for extravascular accumulation of neutrophils at sites of inflammation. The factors involved in this interaction are of considerable experimental interest and potential clinical relevance. However, despite much research, the precise mechanisms involved in localised neutrophil accumulation remain unclear and to some extent controversial. In this section, the questions addressed are the site of mediator action and the role of adhesive glycoproteins.

Site of Mediator Action

At sites of inflammation, chemoattractants in the extravascular tissue induce the adherence of neutrophils to venular endothelial cells, followed by neutrophil emigration across the vessel wall. A fundamental question that remains open is whether chemoattractants act on the endothelial cell or the neutrophil to initiate this process. In most tissues, neutrophil–endothelial cell interaction takes place selectively in venules (in the lung, capillaries are involved) (49). This selectivity of adherence site implies either an active change in the surface of specialised endothelial cells induced by the chemoattractant, or a favoured site for the adherence of activated neutrophils. With respect to the former, it is not clear whether such a change in the endothelial cell surface can occur in response to chemoattractants. In vitro, the expression of high-affinity chemoattractant receptors on neutrophils has been well characterised, but their presence on endothelial cells is contentious. It has been suggested that cultured endothelial cells show increased adhesive properties in response to chemoattractants and that this is associated with the presence of specific chemoattractant receptors (50). However, other studies have failed to detect such effects (51). As these experiments are normally carried out with cultured cells from major vessels rather than microvessels, they may not reflect the conditions in vivo. To answer whether chemoattractants act on the endothelial cell or the neutrophil to induce attachment in situ will depend on experiments carried out in vivo. To investigate the latter we carried out a study using pertussis toxin as the pharmacological tool. Pretreatment of radiolabelled neutrophils with pertussis toxin, which inhibits all receptor-mediated responses induced by chemoattractants in vitro, inhibited neutrophil accumulation in vivo (52). The results of this study indicate that a receptor-mediated event on the neutrophil is crucial in neutrophil accumulation in response to chemoattractants such as C5a, FMLP, and LTB_4. These findings are supported by the recent study of Katori et al. (53). Katori and colleagues reported that in the hamster cheek pouch injection of LTB_4 or FMLP by a glass capillary pipette into the interstitial space close to capillaries results in neutrophil adhesion to venules downstream (53). Furthermore, a similar injection of these stimuli close to the venule did not cause adhesion of leukocytes, suggesting that, in vivo, chemoattractants act on the neutrophil and not on the endothelium to induce neutrophil–endothelial cell interaction. However, the above reports are apparently in conflict with the observations of Colditz and Movat, who demonstrated that skin sites in the rabbit can be specifically desensitised to particular chemoattractants by a previous intradermal injection of that substance (54). This study offers the intriguing possibility that receptors for chemoattractants may be present on endothelial cells or adjacent tissue cells. A possible explanation for these results is that chemoattractant receptors on the ablumenal surface of capillary endothelial cells may mediate the translocation of chemoattractant molecules across the capillary wall (55). Such a mechanism, for which there is now in vitro evidence (56), supports the possibility for an active role of vascular endothelial cells in chemoattractant-induced neutrophil accumulation in vivo.

Adhesion Molecules Mediating Neutrophil–Endothelial Cell Interaction

Recent experimental and clinical observations have begun to define the molecules on the surface of neutrophils and endothelial cells involved in the adhesive component of neutrophil–endothelial cell interaction. With respect to the neutrophil, valuable evidence was obtained following the recognition of a rare and inheritable disorder now known as the leukocyte adherence deficiency syndrome (LAD) (57). The clinical symptoms of this disease are characterised by recurrent bacterial infections, and impaired pus formation and wound healing (57). These clinical features appear to reflect a severe impairment of leukocyte mobilisation into extravascular inflammatory sites (57). Furthermore, in vitro, neutrophils from these patients are defective with respect to adherence-dependent responses such as chemotaxis, aggregation, adherence, and phagocytosis of iC3b-opsonised particles (57). These in vivo and in vitro features of the LAD syndrome are attributable to a severe or total deficiency of a family of leukocyte cell surface glycoproteins now known collectively as the CD11/CD18 antigen complex (57). This complex is composed of three heterodimers CD11a/CD18 (LFA-1), CD11b/CD18 (Mac-1 or CR3), and CD11c/CD18 (p150,95 or CR4) (Table I). Each glycoprotein is composed of a distinct α-subunit non-covalently associated with a common β-subunit (CD18). These glycoproteins are members of the integrin supergene family, which also includes the receptors for extracellular matrix glycoproteins such as fibronectin, vitronectin, and laminin (58).

The involvement of the CD11/CD18 antigen complex in neutrophil adherence is further demonstrated by the use of monoclonal antibodies. Monoclonal antibodies directed at individual subunits or combinations of subunits within this complex can inhibit responses that are dependent on neutrophil adherence in vitro (57). Such studies have shown that, in response to chemoattractants, the adhesion active site in neutrophils is primarily contained in the CD11b/CD18 (Mac-1) glycoprotein (57). In vivo, systemic administration of monoclonal antibodies recognising this glycoprotein inhibit neutrophil accumulation at inflammatory sites (59). In addition to a role in adherence, CD11b/CD18 is the CR3 receptor, which mediates the binding and phagocytosis of iC3b-coated particles (60). CR3 also expresses a binding site for bacterial endotoxins (LPS) (60). Although

TABLE I. Adhesive Glycoproteins on Neutrophils and Vascular Endothelial Cells

Endothelial cells	Neutrophils
ELAM-1	LFA-1 (CD11a/CD18)
GMP-140 (CD62)	Mac-1 (CD11b/CD18, CR3)
ICAM-1 (CD54)	p150,95 (CD11c/CD18,CR4)
ICAM-2	MEL-14 antigen/Leu-8

the CR3 binding sites for iC3b and LPS are distinct, they appear to be functionally related in the process of bacterial phagocytosis. CD11c/CD18, like CD11b/CD18, appears to have iC3b-binding activity and it has thus been designated as CR4 (61).

Neutrophils exposed to an inflammatory stimulus exhibit enhanced adhesiveness and increased surface expression of CD11b/CD18, mobilised from intracellular stores (57). Because of this association, it has been suggested that the increase in expression of this molecule may play an important role in the mechanism of enhanced neutrophil adhesiveness in vivo. However, recent in vitro evidence has dissociated up-regulation of CD11b/CD18 from neutrophil adhesiveness (62–64). Furthermore, there is in vivo evidence suggesting that neutrophil accumulation in response to chemoattractants does not require an increase in the surface expression of CD18-containing molecules (65). It is possible that neutrophil accumulation in vivo induced by the local generation of mediators such as C5a may be dependent on a qualitative, rather than a quantitative, change in neutrophil surface expression of glycoproteins in the CD11/CD18 antigen complex. This qualitative change may be in the form of clustering or a conformational change in these molecules.

In addition to the CD11/CD18 antigen complex, the role of other leukocyte cell surface glycoproteins in neutrophil–endothelial cell interactions is being investigated. One such molecule is the murine lymphocyte homing receptor, defined by monoclonal antibody MEL-14. Besides lymphocytes, MEL-14 antigen is also expressed on neutrophils and is involved in the interaction of neutrophils with endothelial cells in vitro (66). In mice, systemically administered MEL-14 antibody inhibits neutrophil migration into subcutaneously implanted sponges. Interestingly, there is a rapid down-regulation (shedding) of MEL-14 antigen in association with neutrophil extravasation in vivo and neutrophil activation in vitro (66). It has been suggested that this process could provide a rapid de-adhesion mechanism necessary for the neutrophil to proceed from binding to the endothelium to migrating through the venular wall or for release of the neutrophil from the endothelium after diapedesis (66). Hence, MEL-14 antigen or its human leukocyte equivalent, Leu-8 (67), may mediate the adherence of neutrophils to venular endothelial cells under basal conditions.

In addition to neutrophils, endothelial cells also express cell surface adhesive glycoproteins that may contribute to the pattern and kinetics of neutrophil migration into inflammatory sites. In vitro, endothelial cells can be rendered adhesive for neutrophils when stimulated with bacterial endotoxins, IL-1 or TNF. These stimuli increase the endothelial cell surface expression of a glycoprotein designated intercellular adhesion molecule-1 (ICAM-1 or CD54) (57) and induce the expression of endothelial leukocyte adhesion molecule-1 (ELAM-1) (68). ICAM-1 is a cell surface glycoprotein originally defined by a monoclonal antibody that inhibits phorbol ester-stimulated lymphocyte aggregation (57). ICAM-1 is expressed by both hematopoietic and nonhematopoietic cells, basally expressed on some tissues and induced on others after stimulation. By contrast, ELAM-1 is only detectable on activated endothelium. Antibody-blocking experiments have implicated both ICAM-1 and ELAM-1 in the adhesion of neutrophils to endothelial cells (68–70). The adherence of neutrophils to IL-1-stimulated endothelial cells is at least partly dependent on the cell surface expression of ELAM-1 and ICAM-1. With respect to ICAM-1, this interaction is CD18 dependent and seems to involve CD11a/CD18 (LFA-1) (69, 70). The neutrophil–endothelial cell interaction triggered by chemotactic stimulation of neutrophils is dependent on an interaction between CD11b/CD18 (Mac-1) on the neutrophil and basally expressed ICAM-1 on endothelial cells (69,70). By contrast, the ligand on neutrophils for ELAM-1 is not believed to be a member of the CD11/CD18 antigen complex and remains uncharacterised (68). In vivo, ELAM-1 and ICAM-1 expression have been detected at inflammatory skin sites (71). Furthermore, a monoclonal antibody recognising ICAM-1 inhibits neutrophil accumulation into PMA-induced inflamed rabbit lungs (72).

The relative importance and contribution of the neutrophil and endothelial cell adhesive glycoproteins in neutrophil migration in vivo are still undetermined. The rapid onset and the transient nature of neutrophil adherence induced by chemotactic factors in vitro suggest a role for neutrophil adhesive glycoproteins in neutrophil accumulation during acute inflammation. Basally expressed ICAM-1 on the endothelium may also be involved in this process. Another endothelial cell surface molecule that may prove an important mediator of neutrophil influx during an acute inflammatory response is the rapidly inducible (< 5 mins) granule membrane protein-140 (GMP-140, CD62) (73). However, the functional role of this molecule, which has certain structural similarities to ELAM-1 and MEL-14 antigen (74), is not clear. The time course of induction of ELAM-1 (maximum at 4–6 hr) and its high turnover rates are also consistent with the transient nature of neutrophil accumulation during acute inflammation, whereas the prolonged expression of induced ICAM-1 (maintained > 48 hr) suggests a role in chronic inflammatory processes (74).

NEUTROPHIL EMIGRATION AND INCREASED MICROVASCULAR PERMEABILITY

In response to an inflammatory stimulus, neutrophil adhere to microvascular endothelial cells, migrate through the vessel wall, and enter the surrounding tissue. This process is intimately associated with increased microvascular permeability to plasma proteins. This section discusses the mechanism of neutrophil emigration through the vessel wall and the role of the neutrophil in increased microvascular permeability.

Neutrophil Emigration Through the Vessel Wall

The passage of neutrophils through the endothelial barrier involves the penetration of a pseudopodium into the junctions between adjacent endothelial cells, rapidly followed by the rest of the neutrophil (49). The neutrophil then becomes sandwiched between endothelial cells and the basement membrane with the interendothelial cell junctions apparently closing. As the extravasating neutrophil reaches the basement membrane, the continued emigration of the cell is delayed until the tough matrix barrier is penetrated. Although the mechanisms involved in neutrophil extravasation are largely unknown, an interesting possibility is a role for specific neutrophil receptors for laminin. Laminin, a glycoprotein ubiquitous to all basement membranes, has also been reported to be chemotactic for neutrophils (75). Neutrophils may penetrate the basement membrane by using laminin as a stimulus and an attachment factor. The migration of the neutrophil through the vessel wall and across the basement membrane may involve the digestion of barrier extracellular matrix proteins. The neutrophil contains a variety of granular proteolytic enzymes that can be exocytosed on stimulation (49). It has been suggested that the neutrophil-induced loss of basement membrane integrity associated with neutrophil diapedesis in vitro is transient and that basement membrane defects are repaired by the overlying endothelium via a process that is dependent on protein synthesis (76). This is in agreement with early reports showing that microscopic examinations of vessel walls exposed to neutrophil traffic in vivo fail to identify defects or alterations in basement membrane structure (77).

Once outside the vessel wall, the neutrophil can move under the influence of a concentration gradient toward the site of generation of the chemoattractant. At the focus of the inflammatory response, the neutrophil is capable of exhibiting various cellular responses such as phagocytosis of particles, release of proteolytic granular enzymes, and generation of toxic oxygen metabolites, all of which ultimately result in the killing and removal of the infecting agent.

Neutrophil–Endothelial Cell Interaction and Microvascular Leakage

Mediators that increase microvascular permeability can be divided into two categories, depending on whether their effects are dependent on neutrophils (7). Histamine, bradykinin, and PAF appear to enhance microvascular permeability by a direct action on venular endothelium. However, the permeability increasing activity of chemoattractant mediators such as C5a, FMLP, and LTB_4 is dependent on their ability to induce neutrophil accumulation. Thus, depletion of circulating neutrophils inhibits inflammatory edema responses induced by C5a, FMLP, and LTB_4 but has no effect on responses to histamine, bradykinin, and PAF (7). These observations can explain the neutrophil dependence of edema formation in various inflammatory conditions, such as the Arthus reaction (78,79). These findings suggest a causal relationship between the stimulated interaction of neutrophils with venular endothelial cells and increased microvascular permeability. Although the mechanisms involved in this process are not yet fully understood, it is plausible that a neutrophil-derived chemical factor mediates the neutrophil-dependent edema formation. Neutrophils can release products capable of altering endothelial function (49). These products include granular enzymes, toxic oxygen metabolites, and biologically active lipid mediators. Although stimulated neutrophils generate PAF, PAF is not involved in edema formation induced by C5a, FMLP, or LTB_4 in rabbit skin (34).

SUMMARY

Neutrophil accumulation in vivo is a vital component of host defence against foreign organisms. This complex process is initiated by the generation of extravascular chemical signals that induce the adherence of neutrophils to venular endothelial cells. Neutrophil–endothelial cell interactions can involve the active participation of both cell types. The adherence component of this interaction is mediated by certain cell surface glycoproteins expressed on neutrophils and endothelial cells. The passage of the neutrophil from the vascular compartment to the inflamed tissue involves the migration of the neutrophil through interendothelial cell junctions and the penetration of the basement membrane. Despite much research, many aspects of neutrophil–endothelial cell interaction in vivo, which also mediates increased microvascular permeability, are not yet fully understood. A better understanding of these in vivo events involving neutrophils and other leukocyte types will be of considerable value in the development of therapeutic strategies for inflammatory disorders.

REFERENCES

1. Ward PA, Lepow IH, Newman LJ. Bacterial factors chemotactic for polymorphonuclear leukocytes. Am J Pathol 1968;52:725–736.
2. Keller H, Sorkin E. Studies on chemotaxis V. On the chemotactic effect of bacteria. Int Arch Allergy Appl Immunol 1967;31:505–517.
3. Schiffmann E, Showell HJ, Corcoran BA, Ward PA, Smith E, Becker EL. The isolation and partial characterization of neutrophil chemotactic factors from Escherichia coli. J Immunol 1975;114:1831–1837.
4. Schiffmann E, Corcoran BA, Wahl SA. N-formylmethionylpeptides as chemoattractants for leukocytes. Proc Natl Acad Sci USA 1975;72:1059–1062.
5. Marasco WA, Phan SH, Krutzsch H, Showell HJ, Feltner DE, Nairn R, Becker EL, Ward PA. Purification and identification of formyl-methionyl-leucyl-phenylalanine as the major peptide neutrophil chemotactic factor produced by Escherichia coli. J Biol Chem 1984;259:5430–5435.
6. Snyderman R, Pike MC. Chemoattractant receptors on phagocytic cells. Annu Rev Immunol 1984;2:257–281.

7. Wedmore CV, Williams TJ. Control of vascular permeability by polymorphonuclear leukocytes in inflammation. Nature (Lond) 1981;289:646–650.
8. Colditz IG, Movat HZ. Kinetics of neutrophil accumulation in acute inflammatory lesions induced by chemotaxins and chemotaxinogens. J Immunol 1984; 133:2169–2173.
9. Cybulsky MI, Colditz IG, Movat HZ. The role of interleukin-1 in neutrophil leukocyte emigration induced by endotoxin. Am J Pathol 1986;124:367–372.
10. Pohlman TH, Stanness KA, Beatty PG, Ochs HD, Harlan JM. An endothelial cell surface factor(s) induced in vitro by lipopolysaccharide, interleukin 1 and tumor necrosis factor-α increases neutrophil adherence by a CDw18-dependent mechanism. J Immunol 1986;136:4548–4553.
11. Baggiolini M, Walz A, Kunkel SL. Neutrophil-activating peptide-1/interleukin 8, a novel cytokine that activates neutrophils. J Clin Invest 1989;84:1045–1049.
12. Guthrie LA, McPhaid LC, Henson PM, Johnston RB. Priming of neutrophils for enhanced release of oxygen metabolites by bacterial lipopolysaccharide. Evidence for increased activity of superoxide-producing enzyme. J Exp Med 1984; 160:1656–1671.
13. Jose PJ. Complement-derived peptide mediators of inflammation. Br Med Bull 1987;43:336–349.
14. Hugli TE. Structure and function of the anaphylatoxins. Springer Semin Immunopathol 1984;7:193–219.
15. Chenoweth DE, Hugli TE. Demonstration of specific C5a receptor on intact human polymorphonuclear leukocytes. Proc Natl Acad Sci USA 1978;75:3943–3947.
16. Perez HD, Kelly E, Chenoweth D, Elfman F. Identification of the C5a des Arg cochemotaxin. Homology with vitamin D-binding protein (Group-specific component globulin). J Clin Invest 1988;82:360–363.
17. Williams TJ, Jose PJ. Mediation of increased vascular permeability after complement activation: Histamine-independent action of rabbit C5a. J Exp Med 1981;153:136–153.
18. Jose PJ, Forrest MJ, Williams TJ. Detection of the complement fragment C5a in inflammatory exudates from the rabbit peritoneal cavity using radioimmunassay. J Exp Med 1983;158:2177–2182.
19. Forrest MJ, Jose PJ, Williams TJ. Kinetics of the generation and action of chemical mediators in zymosan-induced inflammation of the rabbit peritoneal cavity. Br J Pharmacol 1986;89:719–730.
20. Movat HZ, Rettl C, Burrowes CE, Johnston MG. The in vivo effect of leukotriene B4 on polymorphonuclear leukocytes and the microcirculation. Comparison with activated complement (C5a des Arg) and enhancement by prostaglandin E2. Am J Pathol 1984;115:233–245.
21. Rampart M, Williams TJ. Evidence that neutrophil accumulation induced by interleukin-1 requires both local protein biosynthesis and neutrophil CD18 antigen expression in vivo. Br J Pharmacol 1988;94:1143–1148.
22. Jose PJ, Moss IK, Maini RN, Williams TJ. Measurement of the chemotactic complement fragment C5a in rheumatoid synovial fluids by radioimmunoassay: role of C5a in the acute inflammatory phase. Ann Rheum Dis 1990; in press.
23. Samuelsson B. Leukotrienes: Mediators of immediate hypersensitivity reactions and inflammation. Science 1983;220:568–575.

24. Brain SD, Williams TJ. Prostaglandins, leukotrienes, related compounds and their inhibitors. In: Shuster S, Greaves M, eds. Handbook of Experimental Pharmacology. Vol. 87. Springer-Verlag: Berlin, Heidelberg, 1989;347–366.
25. Rampart M, Williams TJ. Polymorphonuclear leukocyte-dependent plasma leakage in the rabbit skin is enhanced or inhibited by prostacyclin, depending on the route of administration. Am J Pathol 1986;124:66–73.
26. Walsh CE, Waite BM, Thomas MJ, DeChatelet LR. Release and metabolism of arachidonic acid in human neutrophils. J Biol Chem 1981;256:7228–7234.
27. Payan DG, Goldman DW, Goetzl EJ. Biochemical and cellular characteristics of the regulation of human leukocyte function by lipoxygenase products of arachidonic acid. In: Chakrin LW, Bailey DM, eds. The Leukotrienes Chemistry and Biology. Orlando, Florida: Academic Press, 1984;231–245.
28. Camp RDR, Mallet AI, Woolard PM, Brain SD, Black AK, Greaves MW. The identification of hydroxy fatty acids in psoriatic skin. Prostaglandins 1983;26: 431–448.
29. Mullane KM, Read N, Salmon JA, Moncada S. Role of leukocytes in acute myocardial infarction in anesthetized dogs: Relationship to myocardial salvage by anti-inflammatory drugs. J Pharmacol Exp Ther 1984;228:510–522.
30. Zimmerman GA, McIntyre TM. Neutrophil adherence to human endothelium in vitro occurs by CDw18 (Mo-1,Mac-1/LFA-1/GP150,95) glycoprotein-dependent and -independent mechanisms. J Clin Invest 1988;81:531–537.
31. Hanahan DJ. Platelet-activating factor: A biologically active phosphoglyceride. Annu Rev Biochem 1986;55:483–509.
32. Lynch JM, Henson PM. The intracellular retention of newly synthesized platelet-activating factor. J Immunol 1986;137:2653–2661.
33. Humphrey DM, Hanahan DJ, Pinckard RN. Induction of leukocytic infiltrates in rabbit skin by acetyl glyceryl ether phosphorylcholine. Lab Invest 1982;47: 227–234.
34. Hellewell PG, Williams TJ. Antagonism of PAF-induced oedema formation in rabbit skin: A comparison of different antagonists. Br J Pharmacol 1989;97:171–180.
35. Balkwill FR, Burke F. The cytokine network. Immunol Today 1989;10:299–303.
36. Dinarello CA. Biology of interleukin 1. FASEB J 1988;2:108–115.
37. Pober JS. Cytokine-mediated activation of vascular endothelium. Am J Pathol 1988;133:426–433.
38. Movat HZ. Tumor necrosis factor and interleukin-1: Role in acute inflammation and microvascular injury. J Lab Clin Med 1987;110:668–681.
39. Wang JM, Bersani L, Mantovani A. Tumor necrosis factor is chemotactic for monocytes and polymorphonuclear leukocytes. J Immunol 1987;138:1469–1474.
40. Shalaby MR, Palladino MA, Hirabayashi SE, Eessalu TE, Lewis GD, Shepard HM, Aggarwal BB. Receptor binding and activation of polymorphonuclear neutrophils by tumor necrosis factor-alpha. J Leukocyte Biol 1987;41:196–204.
41. Mrowietz U, Schroder J-M, Christophers E. Recombinant human tumor necrosis factor α lacks chemotactic activity for human peripheral blood neutrophils and monocytes. Biochem Biophys Res Commun 1988;153:1223–1228.
42. Rampart M, De Smet W, Fiers W, Herman AG. Inflammatory properties of recombinant tumor necrosis factor in rabbit skin in vivo. J Exp Med 1989;169: 2227–2232.

43. Metcalf D. The molecular biology and functions of the granulocyte–macrophage colony-stimulating factors. Blood 1986;67:257–267.
44. Weisbart RH, Golde DW, Clark SC, Wong GG, Gasson JC. Human granulocyte–macrophage colony-stimulating factor is a neutrophil activator. Nature (Lond) 1985;314:361–363.
45. DiPersio JF, Billing P, Williams R, Gasson JC. Human granulocyte-macrophage colony-stimulating factor and other cytokines prime human neutrophils for enhanced arachidonic acid release and leukotriene B_4 synthesis. J Immunol 1988;140:4315–4322.
46. Watson ML, Lewis GP, Westwick J. Increased vascular permeability and polymorphonuclear leukocyte accumulation in vitro in response to recombinant cytokines and supernatant from interleukin 1-treated human synovial cell cultures. Br J Exp Pathol 1989;70:93–101.
47. Cunha FQ, Ferreira SH. The release of a neutrophil chemotactic factor from peritoneal macrophages by endotoxin: Inhibition by glucocorticoids. Eur J Pharmacol 1986;129:65–76.
48. Issekutz AC, Megyeri P, Issekutz TB. Role for macrophage products in endotoxin-induced polymorphonuclear leukocyte accumulation during inflammation. Lab Invest 1987;56:49–59.
49. Harlan JM. Leukocyte–endothelial interactions. Blood 1985;65:513–525.
50. Hoover RL, Karnofsky MJ, Austen KF, Corey EJ, Lewis RA. Leukotriene B_4 action on endothelium mediates augmented neutrophil/endothelial adhesion. Proc Natl Acad Sci USA 1984;81:2191–2193.
51. Tonnesen MG, Smedley LA, Henson PM. Neutrophil-endothelial cell interactions. Modulation of neutrophil adhesiveness induced by complement fragments C5a and C5a des arg and formyl-methionyl-leucyl-phenylalanine in vitro. J Clin Invest 1984;74:1581–1592.
52. Nourshargh S, Edwards AJ, Williams TJ. Effect of pertussis toxin on neutrophil accumulation in vivo and neutrophil surface CD18 expression in vitro. Br J Pharmacol 1989;96:40P.
53. Nagai K, Katori M. Possible changes in the leukocyte membrane as a mechanism of leukocyte adhesion to the venular walls induced by leukotriene B_4 and fMLP in the microvasculature of the hamster cheek pouch. Int J Microcirc 1988;7:305–314.
54. Colditz IG, Movat HZ. Desensitization of acute inflammatory lesions to chemotaxins and endotoxin. J Immunol 1984;133:2163–2168.
55. Williams TJ, Jose PJ, Forrest MJ, Wedmore CV, Clough GF. Interactions between neutrophils and microvascular endothelial cells leading to cell emigration and plasma protein leakage. In: Meiselman HJ, Lichtman MA, LaCelle PL, eds. White Cell Mechanics: Basic Science and Clinical Aspects. New York: Alan R. Liss, Inc., 1984;195–208.
56. Rotrosen D, Malech HL, Gallin JI. Formyl peptide leukocyte chemoattractant uptake and release by cultured human umbilical vein endothelial cells. J Immunol 1987;139:3034–3040.
57. Kishimoto TK, Larson RS, Corbi AL, Dustin ML, Staunton DE, Springer TA. The leukocyte integrins. Ad Immunol 1989;46:149–182.
58. Hynes RO. Integrins: A family of cell surface receptors. Cell 1987;48:549–554.
59. Rosen H, Gordon S. Current status review: Adhesion molecules and myelomonocytic cell–endothelial interactions. Br J Exp Pathol 1989;70:385–394.

60. Wright SD, Levin SM, Jong MTC, Chad Z, Kabbash LG. CR3 (CD11b/CD18) expresses one binding site for Arg-Gly-Asp-containing peptides and a second site for bacterial lipopolysaccharide. J Exp Med 1989;169:175–183.
61. Myones BL, Dalzell JG, Hogg N, Ross GD. Neutrophil and monocyte cell surface p150,95 has iC3b-receptor (CR_4) activity resembling CR_3. J Clin Invest 1988;82: 640–651.
62. Buyon JP, Abramson SB, Philips MR, Slade SG, Ross GD, Weissmann G, Winchester RJ. Dissociation between increased surface expression of Gp165/95 and homotypic neutrophil aggregation. J Immunol 1988;140:3156–3160.
63. Philips MR, Buyon JP, Winchester R, Weissmann G, Abramson SB. Up-regulation of the iC3b receptor (CR3) is neither necessary nor sufficient to promote neutrophil aggregation. J Clin Invest 1988;82:495–501.
64. Vedder NB, Harlan JM. Increased surface expression of CD11b/CD18 (Mac-1) is not required for stimulated neutrophil adherence to cultured endothelium. J Clin Invest 1988;81:676–682.
65. Nourshargh S, Rampart M, Hellewell PG, Jose PJ, Harlan JM, Edwards AJ, Williams TJ. Accumulation of [111] In-neutrophils in rabbit skin in allergic and non-allergic inflammatory reactions in vivo: Inhibition by neutrophil pretreatment in vitro with a monoclonal antibody recognising the CD18 antigen. J Immunol 1989;142:3193–3198.
66. Kishimoto TK, Jutila MA, Berg EL, Butcher EC. Neutrophil Mac-1 and MEL-14 adhesion proteins inversely regulated by chemotactic factors. Science 1989; 245:1238–1241.
67. Camerini D, James SP, Stamenkovic I, Seed B. Leu-8/TQ1 is the human equivalent of the Mel-14 lymph node homing receptor. Nature (Lond) 1989;342:78–82.
68. Luscinskas FW, Brock AF, Arnaout MA, Gimbrone MA. Endothelial-leukocyte adhesion molecule-1-dependent and leukocyte (CD11/CD18)-dependent mechanisms contribute to polymorphonuclear leukocyte adhesion to cytokine-activated human vascular endothelium. J Immunol 1989;142:2257–2263.
69. Smith CW, Rothlein R, Hughes BJ, Mariscalco MM, Rudloff HE, Schmalstieg FC, Anderson DC. Recognition of an endothelial determinant for CD18-dependent human neutrophil adherence and transendothelial migration. J Clin Invest 1988;82:1746–1756.
70. Smith CW, Marlin SD, Rothlein R, Toman C, Anderson DC. Co-operative interactions of LFA-1 and Mac-1 with intercellular adhesion molecule-1 in facilitating adherence and transendothelial migration of human neutrophils in vitro. J Clin Invest 1989;83:2008–2017.
71. Munro JM, Pober JS, Cotran RS. Tumor necrosis factor and interferon-gamma induce distinct patterns of endothelial activation and associated leukocyte accumulation in skin of papio anubis. Am J Pathol 1989;135:121–133.
72. Barton RW, Rothlein R, Ksiazer J, Kennedy C. The effect of anti-intercellular adhesion molecule-1 on phorbol-ester-induced rabbit lung inflammation. J Immunol 1989;143:1278–1282.
73. Johnston GI, Cook RG, McEver RP. Cloning of GMP-140, a granule membrane protein of platelets and endothelium: Sequence similarity to proteins involved in cell adhesion and inflammation. Cell 1989;56:1033–1044.
74. Bevilacqua MP, Stengelin S, Gimbrone MA, Seed B. Endothelial leukocyte adhesion molecule 1: an inducible receptor for neutrophils related to complement regulatory proteins and lectins. Science 1989;243:1160–1164.

75. Terranova VP, DiFlorio R, Hujanen ES, Lyall RM, Liotta LA, Thorgeirsson U, Siegal GP, Schiffmann E. Laminin promotes rabbit neutrophil motility and attachment. J Clin Invest 1986;77:1180–1186.
76. Huber AR, Weiss SJ. Disruption of the subendothelial basement membrane during neutrophil diapedesis in an in vitro construct of a blood vessel wall. J Clin Invest 1989;83:1122–1136.
77. Hurley JV. An electron microscopic study of leukocyte emigration and vascular permeability in rat skin. Aust J Exp Biol Med Sci 1963;41:171–186.
78. Stetson CA. Similarities in the mechanisms determining the Arthus and Schwartzman phenomena. J Exp Med 1951;94:347–358.
79. Humphrey JH. The mechanism of Arthus reactions. I. The role of polymorphonuclear leucocytes and other factors in reversed passive Arthur reactions in rabbits. Br J Exp Pathol 1955;36:268–289.

The Endothelium: An Introduction to Current Research, pages 187–208

16
Neutrophils and the Pulmonary Microvasculature

C. HASLETT AND J.B. WARREN

Departments of Medicine (Respiratory Division) (C.H.) and Clinical Pharmacology (J.B.W.), Royal Postgraduate Medical School, London W12 ONN, England

INTRODUCTION

The complex interplay among the microvasculature, mediators, and leucocytes that constitutes inflammation has evolved as an essential host response to infection and trauma. That this response is effective can be judged by the high proportion of patients who, by virtue of a massive local cellular infiltration of mostly neutrophil granulocytes, survived lobar pneumococcal pneumonia during the pre-antibiotic era. The neutrophil is the archetypal acute inflammatory cell whose importance is highlighted by the high morbidity and mortality of diseases characterized by neutrophil malfunction or neutropenia. It is the first cell to migrate from the microvasculature to the scene of perturbation, where it rapidly kills organisms such as the *S. pneumoniae*. Furthermore, it appears that some of the subsequent events at the evolving inflammatory site, such as the formation of oedema (1) and monocyte migration (2) may depend on the initial neutrophil infiltration.

The reliability and effectiveness of inflammation as a host-defense mechanism depends on the diversity of its component parts. The monocyte can thus perform many of the inflammatory functions of the neutrophil, although its response is generally slower. However, the neutrophil remains the most rapidly responsive nucleated inflammatory cell and contains the most powerful internal reactive oxygen generating system. Within the vast range of inflammatory mediators, there are many examples of such redundancy but, as with a spider web, the loss of a few strands does not necessarily influence overall effectiveness. This diversity of the inflammatory response clearly contributes to its effectiveness, yet it also complicates the prospect of pharmacological intervention.

In recent years, it has become apparent that inflammation, paradoxically employing mechanisms identical to those used in host defense, is involved in many of the inflammatory diseases that afflict modern Western society. The neutrophil has been implicated in most of these diseases (3); this cell contains many substances having the potential to cause tissue damage (Table I). Many of these potentially histotoxic contents are likely to have evolved in order to aid the rapid transit of the neutrophil through tissues and its effective destruction of bacteria. It is generally considered that a balance exists between the potential for inflammatory tissue injury (e.g., proteases) and tissue protective systems (e.g., antiproteases) to restore normal function rapidly with minimal disruption. In some circumstances, however, this balance can be tipped towards excessive injury and the development of persistent inflammation. Under such circumstances, proteases derived from the neutrophil may play a part in chronic inflammation not only by injuring tissue directly, but also by cleaving matrix proteins into chemotactic fragments (4), which in turn attract more inflammatory cells to the site. Why inflammation under certain circumstances should be beneficial with minimal tissue injury and, under other circumstances, causes excess injury, is a major challenge in trying to understand common pulmonary diseases such as chronic bronchitis and emphysema, adult respiratory distress syndrome (ARDS), neonatal respiratory distress syndrome, the lung vasculitides, and the chronic lung scarring diseases such as pneumoconiosis and fibrosing alve-

TABLE I. Substances That Have the Potential to Cause Tissue Damage

Potentially histotoxic neutrophil products	Potentially pro-inflammatory mediators
Oxidants and radicals	
Superoxide anion	Platelet activating factor (PAF)
Hydrogen peroxide	Thromboxane B_2 (Tx B_2)
Hydroxyl radical	Leukotriene B_4 (LTB$_4$)
Hypochlorous acid	Plasminogen activator
Chloramines	5-HETE
Nitric oxide (NO)	
Proteolytic enzymes	
Elastase	
Gelatinase	
Collagenase	
Cathepsins	
Lysozyme	
Neuraminidase	
Heparanase	
Others	
Cationic proteins	

olitis. In some of these disorders, for example, in ARDS and pulmonary vasculitis, there is evidence that the disease begins in the pulmonary microvessels, whereas in others the persistent accumulation of inflammatory cells in the lung parenchyma is associated with permanent architectural disruption and scarring. In the former, neutrophil interaction with the pulmonary endothelium obviously plays a key role. In the latter, this interaction is also important in that neutrophil migration into the lung parenchyma is in part controlled by the endothelium. Widespread disruption of the delicate microcirculation of the lung by inflammatory oedema, cellular proliferation, or scarring has profound effects, causing rapidly progressive respiratory failure, often fatal, as well as an increased susceptibility to pulmonary infection.

The lung normally contains about three times the number of neutrophils that are present in the rest of the circulation. A significant number of these (the marginated pool) are in dynamic equilibrium with the circulating pool and can be released by exercise or adrenaline. The retention of leucocytes by the lung may have evolved as an important defense against the inevitable exposure to inhaled microorganisms and toxins or it may function as a rapid release pool in stress or injury. However, this concentration of potentially destructive cells in the lung may help explain why the lung is at particular risk from injury triggered by systemic or distant insults in ARDS. Although the existence of this close association between the lung microvasculature and circulating neutrophil was suspected during the 1930s (5), the mechanisms of this interaction are only just beginning to unfold.

The marginated pool can be further expanded by the addition of sequestered neutrophils in conditions such as endotoxemia without necessarily causing overt lung injury (6). Thus, the presence per se of neutrophils does not equate with injury. The circumstances leading to neutrophil-mediated pulmonary vascular injury, such as in ARDS and models of acute lung injury, have recently come under closer scrutiny. Injury appears to depend on a combination of factors including the degree and dynamics of neutrophil–endothelial contact, the state of priming/activation of the neutrophil and the type of toxic agent released. Much of this information has come from in vitro experiments because the human pulmonary microvasculature is virtually inaccessible in life. However, advances in external imaging and cell labelling techniques, together with the use of invasive techniques in experimental animals, are shedding more light on cellular events in situ (6–8).

The remainder of this chapter discusses the possible mechanisms of neutrophil sequestration, neutrophil migration, endothelial injury in the pulmonary microcirculation, mediators, and the possibilities for pharmacological intervention. Finally, using ARDS as an example, the question of how future therapy might manipulate some of these events in order to combat inflammatory lung disease is addressed.

NEUTROPHIL SEQUESTRATION IN THE PULMONARY MICROVASCULATURE

To understand the mechanisms whereby neutrophils adhere to, and migrate through, the pulmonary vascular wall in inflammation, it is first necessary to elucidate the mechanisms leading to the formation of the pulmonary marginated neutrophil pool.

The Physiological Pulmonary Marginated Neutrophil Pool

For a review of the original studies that recognized and subsequently investigated the mechanisms underlying its existence, see Worthen et al. (9). This pool is considered to be in dynamic equilibrium with the circulating pool, so that neutrophils may be released in response to hemodynamic changes (e.g., exercise), stress, or adrenaline (10–12) or retained in response to histamine, endotoxin, or hemodialysis (6,13,14). The existence of the marginated pool has been known for more than 50 years, yet its size, its exact site, and the mechanisms of neutrophil sequestration within the pulmonary microcirculation are still being actively investigated.

Since the work of the Clarks (15) and many others, it has been clear that, in vascular beds other than the lung, neutrophils sequester and roll along the post capillary venules. Work by Staub et al. (16) and others (17) suggested that the pulmonary capillaries, rather than the venules, might be the site of neutrophil sequestration within the lung, as confirmed by recent detailed morphometric analysis (18). Furthermore, direct microscopic observation of fluorescent-labelled neutrophils passing through a vital experimental lung window preparation (7) showed that they are temporarily delayed in the pulmonary capillaries. In this experiment, not all neutrophils were delayed, some passed directly through, whereas others were sequestered for up to 20 min. In addition, the profile of different neutrophil sequestration times was similar when first-pass neutrophils were compared with those recirculating later. This observation implies that factors in the local vascular environment have a major influence on the capillary transit times of individual neutrophils.

The widely held assumption that the lung contains nearly all the physiologically releaseable marginated pool has recently been questioned. Studies using peripheral blood neutrophils labelled by techniques that do not appear to affect their function (6,19) indicate that the spleen, and to a lesser extent the liver, may also be physiological sites of sequestration. Recent work in man confirms that the spleen makes a major contribution to the exercise-induced release of neutrophils into the circulation (20). Although the final proportion remains to be established, the lung nonetheless provides an important component of the marginated pool, a factor that may be important in the susceptibility of the lung to injury, as in ARDS triggered by sepsis or distant trauma.

Neutrophil retention within the pulmonary physiological marginated pool is not necessarily determined by neutrophil–endothelial adherence alone. The physical characteristics of neutrophils within the pulmonary microvasculature may well prove more important than the complex cell–cell adhesive forces outlined in Chapter 15. This concept is supported by the observation that leukocyte adherence deficiency (LAD) patients, who have defective neutrophil surface adhesive molecules, still have a marginated pool of neutrophils releasable by exercise. The mean diameter of pulmonary capillaries is 7 μm, some being only 5 μm in diameter (21), whereas the mean neutrophil diameter is 7 μm (22). Most neutrophils will therefore squeeze through the capillaries with an ease proportional to their deformability (which in turn depends on their poorly understood viscoelastic properties) and the pressure gradient.

The impeding forces of physical resistance to deformation and neutrophil–endothelial adhesion must be overcome by the hemodynamic pressure gradient. The low pressure of the pulmonary vascular bed is a major determinant of neutrophil margination, as witnessed by the marked demarginating effects of increased blood flow (11). From the clear observation that reductions in blood flow are directly associated with increased sequestration, it can be predicted that, in the upright position, the difference in blood flow between the apices and bases of the lungs would cause a gradient of neutrophil transit times with greater retention in the apices. This may contribute to the pattern of tissue destruction in conditions such as emphysema. Thus, the dynamics of the pulmonary marginated pool will mainly be determined by hemodynamic forces and the rheological properties of neutrophils. Nonetheless, a low activity of cell–cell adhesion caused by normal background levels of local mediator release cannot be excluded, and adhesive mechanisms are undoubtedly more important in inflammation, where adhesion is a prerequisite of neutrophil migration through the vascular endothelium.

The mechanisms outlined above involved in the physiological sequestration of neutrophils in the pulmonary microcirculation permit some prediction of how this system may be altered in diseases characterized by neutrophil-mediated endothelial injury. It is predictable that minor changes in the rheological properties of neutrophils could have profound effects on the size and dynamics of the pool of neutrophils sequestered in the lung. It is also logical to assume that any process that increases the sequestration of neutrophils would increase the degree and duration of contact with the endothelium. These effects would be magnified not only by the recruitment of neutrophils from the circulating pool but also by any reduction in blood flow caused by inflammatory edema.

Neutrophil Migration Through the Endothelial Barrier

To reach the extravascular space, neutrophils squeeze through endothelial cell junctions, a process termed *diapedesis*. This process was first demonstrated by electron microscopy (23) and does not itself necessarily cause endothelial injury, either ultrastructurally (23,24) or functionally (25). In vitro, neutrophils preferentially adhere to endothelial cells, as compared with smooth muscle cells, fibroblasts, or culture plates, yet much of the "adhesive" interaction between neutrophils and endothelial monolayers in culture represents spontaneous migrations of neutrophils beneath the endothelial monolayer. This in vitro model is useful, as it can be amplified by the addition of chemotactic factors and other inflammatory mediators (26) and may represent a valuable experimental analogy of the process of capillary transmigration in vivo. Neutrophil migration through the endothelial barrier is not only one of the primary cellular events in acute inflammation but is also a key point at which activated cells could cause excessive lung injury. The mechanisms of cellular transmigration are largely unknown, but neither neutrophil proteases nor reactive oxygen intermediates (ROI) are required. Recent studies suggest that the endothelial cell itself contributes to the control of transmigration and even penetration of the endothelial cell basement membrane (27). Other work suggests that prolonging neutrophil contact or alterations of the contact surface could initiate processes favouring endothelial injury (28,29).

Neutrophil–Endothelial Interaction in Inflammation and Microvascular Injury

Metchnikoff and Cohnheim interpreted their classical studies of the early cellular stages of inflammation differently, yet both were correct. Cohnheim believed that alterations in the microvessel were of primary importance, whereas Metchnikoff favoured the local release of leucocyte chemotactic agents. It is now clear that both neutrophil- and endothelial-dependent mechanisms lead to neutrophil sequestration in pulmonary microvessels. Two types of adhesion can be distinguished; the rounded neutrophil rolls along the endothelial surface with transient stops, whereas the flattened neutrophil is bound more avidly (15). In pathological states such as ARDS or the Arthus reaction, the mechanism of the latter type of adhesion is likely to be of profound importance to the subsequent processes that lead to a microenvironment favouring endothelial injury. Since it is difficult to injure endothelial cells in vitro without neutrophil adherence, adhesion may lead to the formation of a protected intercellular microenvironment that favours cell injury. The concept of a microenvironment created by tightly adhesive neutrophils and favouring injury is strengthened by the observation that neutrophil mediated matrix degradation still occurs in the presence of antiproteases (30).

Within the inflammatory pulmonary microenvironment, the expression of adhesive molecules by either cell may then play an important role. Any changes in the ability of the neutrophil to squeeze through the pulmonary capillaries would profoundly influence the size of the sequestered neutrophil pool, the degree and duration of neutrophil–endothelial cell contact, and thus the chances of injury. Although the relative importance of each mechanism is not yet determined, it is likely that they all contribute to the excessive and prolonged sequestration of neutrophils in lung injury (Fig. 1).

The considerable advances in our understanding of the role of the endothelium in the clotting system and in platelet adhesion have not yet been applied to neutrophil–endothelial cell adhesion. Whether vessel wall shear stress and the local production of prostacyclin, prostaglandin E_2 (PGE_2), thromboxane, nitric oxide, and tissue plasminogen activator are important to neutrophil adhesion remains largely unknown.

NEUTROPHIL SURFACE ADHERENCE MECHANISMS

Studies of neutrophils and endothelial cells in vitro show greatly enhanced adherence within one minute of the addition of chemotactic factors and mediators such as platelet activating factor (26,31). The recent interest in the CD11–CD18 glycoprotein complex was initially stimulated by the observation that in patients who are CD11–CD18 deficient (LAD syndrome), neutrophils do not appear in skin ulcers. Furthermore, it was shown that monoclonal antibodies to this surface glycoprotein complex inhibit the adhesion of stimulated neutrophils to endothelial monolayers (32,33). The antibody to the common CD18 component of this group of integrins, MoAb 60.3, was recently shown to prevent neutrophil migration to inflamed skin in vivo (34). However, this important adhesive complex may not represent the whole neutrophil adhesive/migration mechanism in all organs. For example, MoAb 60.3 inhibits shock-induced injury to the gut, but not the lung (35), and similarly blocks *Streptococcus*-induced neutrophil migration in the skin but not in the lung (36). In addition, in patients with the LAD syndrome who died from pulmonary complications, neutrophils have been detected in the lung at necroscopy (Harlan J: personal communication). These results will be difficult to put into perspective until organ differences, different responses to stimuli, and ways of distinguishing migration from vascular sequestration are established. Nevertheless, they leave us with the intriguing possibility that neutrophils may employ different adhesive/migratory mechanisms in different organs, depending on the stimulus.

ENDOTHELIAL SURFACE ADHERENCE MECHANISMS

After treatment with cytokines such as interleukin 1 (IL-1), endothelial cells in vitro express adhesion molecules such as ELAM-1 at a rate similar to the kinetics of neutrophil accumulation following the injection of cyto-

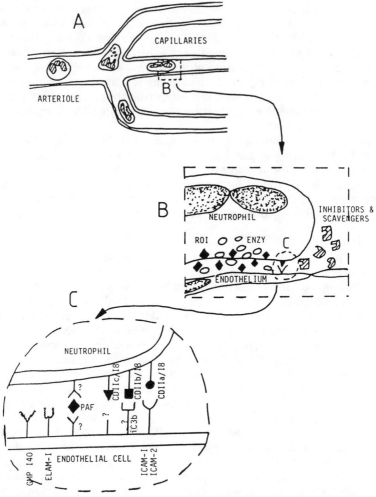

Fig. 1. Progressively magnified view of the mechanisms involved in neutrophil–endothelial cell interactions within the pulmonary microvasculature. **A:** Sequestration is predisposed by the narrow lumen of the pulmonary capillaries compared with the diameter of the neutrophil. Retention is enhanced by the low pressure of the pulmonary vascular bed, and this is increased further when neutrophils become less deformable upon activation. **B:** The close cell–cell contact creates a microenvironment that permits a high concentration of enzymes (ENZY) and other toxic products favouring endothelial injury. Reactive oxygen intermediates (ROI) may be toxic directly or by inactivating enzyme inhibitors. **C:** Specific adhesion molecules occur on the surface of the neutrophil (the CD11/CD18 complex) and on the surface of stimulated endothelial cells (GMP-140, ELAM-1, ICAM-1, and ICAM-2), which may further promote cell–cell adhesion.

kines in skin in vivo. The structures of ELAM-1 (37) and the intercellular adhesion molecules ICAM-1, ICAM-2 (38), and GMP-140 have been elucidated. The exact relationship between neutrophil CD11/CD18 expression and endothelial determinants is uncertain, although ICAM-1 and 2 are ligands for CD11a/CD18. The expression of different adhesion molecules may show stimulus specificity; certainly there are differences in temporal expression. Stimulated neutrophils rapidly express CD11/CD18; stimulated endothelial cells express GMP-140 within a few minutes, ELAM-1 is maximal at approximately 4 hr, ICAM-1 is maximal at 24 hr, and HLA-DR class II antigens are expressed after 3–4 days. Thus, rapid neutrophil sequestration seen early in microvascular injury (6) is more likely to be the result of altered neutrophil properties, whereas later (1–4 hr) amplification of neutrophil sequestration may be more influenced by endothelial surface adhesiveness. However, the rapid endothelial changes associated with platelet activating factor production (39) or complement receptor-mediated processes (40) may also contribute to early neutrophil sequestration in pulmonary microvessels.

ALTERATIONS IN NEUTROPHIL DEFORMABILITY

Changes in the rheological properties of primed and activated neutrophils may be primary or secondary factors in pulmonary microvascular neutrophil sequestration. Worthen et al. (41) showed that neutrophils stimulated by chemotactic factors were retained abnormally by 5-μm polycarbonate filters by a CD11/CD18-independent mechanism. The retention appeared to be caused by decreased cell deformability associated with a rearrangement of intracellular actin. In addition, LPS, a longer-acting mediator, has been shown to cause more prolonged reduction in neutrophil deformability (42). Although pure conjecture, it is possible that alterations in pulmonary capillary endothelial deformability could also contribute to enhanced neutrophil sequestration in inflammatory injury.

However, excessive neutrophil sequestration in pulmonary capillaries per se is not necessarily associated with injury. For example, it has been shown experimentally that a marked increase in neutrophil sequestration can be induced in vivo by the injection of bacterial LPS, which has mainly neutrophil priming effects, without causing capillary injury detectable by electron microscopy or capillary leak (6). Thus tight, persistent adhesions between sequestered neutrophils and endothelial cells are necessary to permit the creation of an intracellular microenvironment favouring injury and the time available for it to occur, but adhesion alone is not sufficient, and the secretory state of adherent neutrophils is the likely essential further factor in the injury equation.

NEUTROPHIL PRIMING AND ACTIVATION

Neutrophils do not secrete injurious agents in their basal state. However, their secretory state can be rapidly amplified by stimuli working through a priming mechanism that does not require protein synthesis. Inflammatory mediators differ in their effects on neutrophils. Some, such as C5a, are good secretagogues, whereas others, such as LPS or PAF alone, are relatively ineffective stimulants of neutrophil secretion. However, even at very low concentrations, these latter two agents may have profound effects on neutrophil responses by a priming mechanism (Fig. 2). It was found that pretreatment of neutrophils with trace amounts of LPS greatly enhanced the release of superoxide in response to secretagogues such as formyl-methionyl–leucyl-phenylalanine (FMLP) (43). Indeed, in some cases there was no detectable FMLP-stimulated superoxide release unless the cells had been previously primed. Similar LPS-priming effects were subsequently demonstrated for stimulated neutrophil lysosomal enzyme release (44). These results suggested that both priming and activation of neutrophils were important; this led to the hypothesis that the combination of both a priming agent (LPS) and an activating agent (C5a), but neither agent alone, would cause neutrophil-dependent pulmonary microvascular injury in vivo (45), an observation subsequently confirmed in vitro (46). These findings suggest that it may be more fruitful to study how different types of relevant mediators interact, rather than search for a final common stimulant of neutrophil-mediated endothelial injury. They also indicate that an understanding of the mechanisms of neutrophil priming will help unravel the pathogenesis of neutrophil-mediated tissue injury.

A variety of biologically relevant agents can effectively prime neutrophils (47). These include bacterial products such as LPS and products of other inflammatory cells such as macrophages and platelets. It appears that some mediators, such as TNF and PAF, are more effective primers than activators.

The intracellular mechanisms of priming are poorly understood. In the LPS system, priming enhances FMLP-stimulated superoxide release independent of FMLP receptor number or affinity (43). A reduced lag time and faster rate of superoxide generation could have resulted from increased NADPH oxidase catalytic activity or from a modification of the signal transduction process. The multiple neutrophil functions modulated by priming agents pari passu with the enhanced stimulated superoxide release suggest that the mechanism of priming occurs early in the signal transduction pathway. Indeed, recent data suggest that modulation of an intracellular calcium-dependent step in signal transduction is of primary importance (48), but how its effects are mediated is unclear.

A variety of neutrophil functions other than stimulated superoxide release and granule enzyme secretion are also modulated by exposure to priming agents. For example, trace concentrations of LPS cause neutrophils to sequester abnormally in pulmonary microvessels in vivo (6); in vitro effects include change of shape, reduced chemotactic response, and increased adhesion. These observations may relate to the recently de-

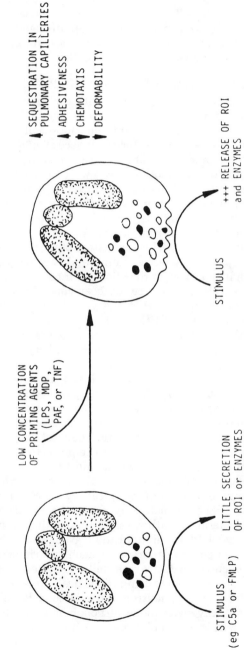

Fig. 2. Stimulation of neutrophils in their normal state with several agents, such as complement fragments (e.g., C5a), causes little release of toxic contents unless they are initially primed with even trace amounts of products, such as bacterial lipopolysaccharide (LPS), which produces the additional effects shown. FMLP, N-formyl-methionyl-leucyl-phenylalanine; MDP, muramyl dipeptide; ROI, reactive oxygen intermediates.

scribed finding of LPS-induced reduced actin polymerisation and reduced deformability of neutrophils (42). How these changes relate to priming, hence enhanced stimulated secretion, is uncertain, although increasing and prolonging sequestration in pulmonary capillaries will create conditions favouring injury by primed and activated cells.

POTENTIALLY INJURIOUS NEUTROPHIL PRODUCTS

There is a long list of neutrophil products with the capacity to injure tissues, some of the more important of which are shown in Table I. Many of these will only be secreted in small amounts, but these could still be toxic to endothelial cells if presented on the external surface of adherent neutrophils. Alternatively, these products might be toxic if disintegration of the neutrophil in the vicinity of the endothelial cell were to lead to high local concentrations. There is little evidence that the latter mechanism is important in the microvessels; in fact, it is remarkable that the inflammatory cell membrane seems to survive within the very microenvironment in which the target cell membrane is destroyed; there are many such examples shown by electron microscopy (49). The elucidation of mechanisms underlying this intriguing, apparently selective, vulnerability is likely to provide some interesting insights into cytoprotection at inflamed sites. Mechanisms of neutrophil secretion have recently been carefully and fully reviewed (49). It has been suggested that the generation of chlorinated oxidants, via the action of the NADPH oxidase and the myeloperoxidase systems, may destroy the antiproteinase enzymes in some species (50). This would substantially increase the half-life, hence the toxicity, of the proteolytic enzymes.

It is difficult to pinpoint which of the many histotoxic agents are relevant to inflammatory tissue injury. During the past decade, ROI have received much attention as primary agents of likely central importance. While their intracellular role in killing microorganisms is undisputed (51), their contribution to tissue injury is uncertain. The most toxic of the ROI are so reactive and unstable that even within the protected intercellular microenvironment, they are likely to be rapidly inactivated. Furthermore, many studies of neutrophil-mediated endothelial injury in vitro have employed neutrophil stimuli of uncertain biological relevance, such as phorbol myristate acetate (PMA), which may drive the neutrophil more selectively down ROI-generating pathways. Moreover, the interpretation of in vivo experiments using ROI inhibitors and scavengers has been problematical; some of the compounds generated in such experiments, such as lipid peroxidation products could derive from cell injury mediated by other primary mechanisms. In experiments using "biologically relevant" neutrophil stimuli, such as C5a and LPS, neutrophil-mediated endothelial injury was not inhibited by ROI scavengers alone, although injury could be inhibited by AAPVCK, a specific neutrophil elastase inhibitor (46). Interestingly, in the same series of experiments, there was a further additive inhibitory effect when catalase and superoxide dismutase were included with AAPVCK, suggesting an obscure collaborative effect of ROI in neutrophil elastase-mediated endothelial injury. Recently, potential indirect effects of ROI in the mediation of tissue injury, such as through the inactivation of antiproteinases, have been extensively reviewed (50).

As with ROI, there are difficulties in evaluating the individual pathogenetic roles of other neutrophil products such as proteinases and cationic proteins (52). Nevertheless, neutrophil elastase is emerging as a prime candidate in the etiology of inflammatory tissue injury. Instillation of neutrophil elastase into the lung causes architectural changes typical of pulmonary emphysema and the observation that α_1-antiprotease deficiency is associated with the development of severe emphysema (53) has supported the proteinase/antiproteinase theory of its etiology. More recently, neutrophil elastase has been found in the lung washings of patients with ARDS (54). This enzymatic activity was first isolated by Janoff and Zeligs in 1968 (55). It is highly cationic and capable of degrading a variety of substrates, including elastin, fibronectin, and proteoglycans. It is certainly toxic to endothelial cells in vitro, but whether this toxicity is enzymatic or cationic is uncertain. Other proteinases such as cathepsin G (also highly cationic) may have roles in vivo. Finally, the neutrophil contains a variety of nonenzymatic cationic proteins that have long been known to be capable of increasing vascular permeability (56) but that have received scant attention of late.

POTENTIAL PHARMACOLOGICAL INTERVENTION

The ability to modulate the destructive interactions between neutrophils and endothelial cells would clearly be a great advantage in therapy of inflammatory diseases. ARDS is an example in which new therapeutic approaches could be based on an increased knowledge of the cell biology of its pathogenesis (Fig. 3), but further analysis of such possibilities also highlights some of the potential problems we are likely to encounter in the treatment of inflammatory diseases.

ARDS is a catastrophic form of acute lung injury, often occurring in young people, which, despite the use of mechanical ventilation, still has a mortality rate of 50–70%. Although there is a wide range of triggering stimuli, the histology of the injured lung is uniform, suggesting common pathogenetic processes. Early in the disease there is evidence of acute injury, with endothelial and epithelial destruction leading to pulmonary edema and markedly reduced gas exchange (57). This early phase is associated with the accumulation of large numbers of inflammatory cells, predominantly neutrophils, and evidence of release of their products (58,-59). Common causes of ARDS include septicaemia and more distant triggers such as multiple trauma and burns. This led to early speculation that

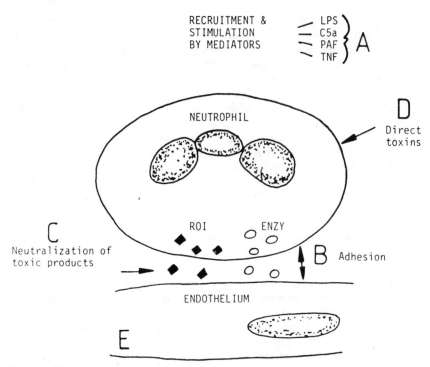

Fig. 3. Schematic representation of the possible methods of pharmacological intervention in the destructive interaction between neutrophils and endothelial cells in ARDS. A, the antagonism of mediators of neutrophil recruitment and stimulation; B, supression of sequestration by inhibiting cell adhesion; C, inhibition of the release of toxic agents from the neutrophil; D, the destruction of neutrophils or of their overall function; and E, cytoprotection of the endothelial cell.

the disease is, at least in part, humorally mediated. That there was often a latent period of 24–48 hr between initial insult and full-blown injury implied that early intervention might abort the later stages of injury. Of those patients who recover, most regain useful lung function.

Current treatment consists of mechanical ventilation with adequate oxygenation and treatment of the provoking condition and its complications. These supportive measures have not improved the appalling mortality rate over the past three decades. Therapy with high doses of corticosteroids, after initial enthusiasm, has been abandoned. Corticosteroids do not improve outcome in controlled clinical trials (60) and may even be detrimental in cases involving sepsis, even though they suppress the production of many inflammatory cytokines. The histological changes are usually advanced beyond endothelial and epithelial injury once the patient is mechanically ventilated, when a complex picture develops of continuing injury, attempts at repair (e.g., type II epithelial cell proliferation) and the interstitial deposition of scar tissue matrix proteins. Many of those who die develop a rapidly progressive form of lung scarring or succumb to secondary gram-negative bacterial infection. Thus attention is focused on early intervention.

There is no established specific pharmacological therapy for ARDS and it is remarkably difficult to alter the course of this condition once it becomes established. The initial injury or insult triggers the release of mediators which cause the abnormal sequestration of neutrophils and other inflammatory cells in the pulmonary microvessels. The outcome of this potentially lethal situation is likely to depend on the degree and type of secretion of injurious agents into the microenvironment between cells. This leads to further amplification caused by the accumulation of more primed and triggered cells. The subsequent endothelial and epithelial injury permits the leak of exudate into the interstitium and alveoli, leading to fibroblast activation and matrix deposition. This process, depicted in Figure 3, suggests a number of possible therapeutic approaches.

A number of mediators may be generated at an early stage as a result of septicaemia, shock, or multiple injury. One such mediator is C5a, which alone can cause lung injury (61), but this has only been shown using large quantities in rats. High concentrations of C5a have been detected in man in ARDS, where its levels do not predict outcome (62), but it can also be similarly detected during hemodialysis, during which ARDS rarely occurs. Although not of primary importance in ARDS, C5a may act in concert with other agents. Gram-negative bacterial endotoxin, or its active constituent lipopolysaccharide (LPS), has also been strongly implicated and can cause neutrophil dependent acute lung injury in sheep (63). The plasma level of endotoxin is a better predictor of outcome in ARDS than C5a (Parsons PE: personal communication). LPS can release tumor necrosis factor (TNF), which, like PAF, has a predominantly priming effect on neutrophils at low concentrations. A combination of LPS as a priming agent and C5a as an activator of neutrophils, but neither agent alone, caused neutrophil-dependent lung injury in rabbits (45). However, the initial development of ARDS seems to involve an interaction between many mediators. The clinical use of specific inhibitors of mediators such as LPS, C5a, TNF, and PAF is likely to be limited, since these mediators are probably released too early to offer any hope of intervention at the triggering stage. Nevertheless, they are also implicated in the later amplification and recruitment phases. It is still impossible to judge which are the critical strands in the web of the inflammatory response, although LPS and TNF are gaining increasing prominence.

Another therapeutic approach might be to reduce the sequestration of neutrophils in the pulmonary microvessels. Adhesive proteins are likely to be important, but it is difficult to assess the relative contribution of other factors such as neutrophil stiffness to the development of ARDS. Again, the initiation of abnormal sequestration is likely to occur too quickly for therapeutic intervention, although amplification and recruitment could be inhibited. Even if it were certain which are the primary adhesive molecules in lung injury, successful inhibition of neutrophil–endothelial adherence might severely inhibit the host defense to infection.

Agents that inhibit the secretion of toxic neutrophil products are too toxic and nonspecific to make this approach viable. The development of inhibitors of products such as neutrophil elastase will be "catalysed" by increasing evidence for their direct involvement in disease. Other toxic neutrophil products may assume prominence in the future, but they are also likely to play essential roles in host defense, such as cell migration and bacterial killing. This central paradox of beneficial inflammation versus destructive inflammation is likely to prove a stumbling block repeatedly.

The approach of immobilizing or killing neutrophils with cytotoxic antibodies can probably be dismissed on the grounds that it would cause further immunosuppression in patients who already have an increased susceptibility to infection. Finally, although there is a large body of evidence that the neutrophil and its products play are important in the pathogenesis of ARDS, an ARDS-like disease can occur in patients with peripheral blood neutropenia (64). This may either represent a different disease, or it may be yet another example of redundancy within the inflammatory response. Under these conditions, it is likely that the monocyte plays a similar role to that normally taken by the neutrophil since it possesses comparable potential toxicity even though it is less responsive. The involvement of monocytes, platelets, lymphocytes, and their interactions with neutrophils in the early development of ARDS needs considerable further study.

If it is not possible to minimize tissue damage by interfering with neutrophil function without causing immunosuppression, it may be possible to try the alternative approach of pharmacological protection of endothelial and epithelial cells. The phenomenon of cytoprotection by prostaglandins was first described in gastrointestinal cells, and it has been suggested that it also occurs in many other tissues. There is no convincing evidence that prostaglandins cytoprotect endothelial cells against injury, but several studies have examined exogenous prostaglandins and the pharmacological manipulation of endogenous arachidonic acid metabolites.

Of the many arachidonic acid metabolites that have been implicated as of potential importance (e.g., the thromboxanes, prostacyclin, PGE_2, and $PGF_{2\alpha}$), none plays a key role in ARDS, although inhibitors of cyclo-oxygenase or thromboxane synthestase reduce pulmonary hypertension and injury in some animal models (65,66). One metabolite of particular interest is leukotriene B_4 (LTB_4). It is a potent neutrophil chemotactic agent whose main source may be stimulated alveolar macrophages. LTB_4 not only causes neutrophil chemotaxis and infiltration in the skin but also plays a key role in myocardial reperfusion injury (67). The compound BW755c markedly antagonises the effect of LTB_4 and substantially limits neutrophil-mediated myocardial damage caused by reperfusion injury in animal models. BW755c is nonspecific in that it also inhibits lipoxygenase and cyclo-oxygenase and has a small effect on phospholipase. Further work on BW755c has been curtailed by its liver toxicity and because there is unfortunately no safer alternative.

A small clinical trial of ibuprofen in ARDS has recently given encouraging results (Brigham K: personal communication). This drug not only inhibits cyclo-oxygenase but also has some effect on lipoxygenase, but its exact anti-inflammatory mechanism is unknown (68). If one of the main mechanisms of neutrophil sequestration is reduced neutrophil deformability, drugs that improve the rheological properties of cells may reduce pulmonary microvascular sequestration. Claims that such drugs improve tissue perfusion in peripheral vascular disease have not been substantiated. Nonetheless, it has been proposed that this is one mechanism by which a methylxanthine derivative, pentoxyfylline, improves leukocyte filterability. It has also been claimed that incubating isolated neutrophils with pentoxyfylline decreases neutrophil adherence, decreases superoxide production, decreases granule release and increases directed migration (69). Whether this will improve clinical outcome is yet to be determined.

Specific measures to prevent neutrophil–endothelial adhesion are sparse. The infusion of PGE_1 inhibits neutrophil adhesion and injury (70), although clinical trials of efficacy are still not available. Another approach is to antagonize the detrimental effects of released mediators. Two prime targets are TNF and interleukin 1 (Il-1), both of which promote neutrophil adhesion and are directly toxic to the endothelium. They can also trigger the release of superoxide, the discharge of neutrophil granules (71) and can promote the release of neutrophil chemotactic activity from endothelial cells (72). PAF is another mediator that is released from many inflammatory cell types besides the neutrophil in both allergic and toxic reactions. PAF is capable of causing pulmonary hypertension (although in low doses it is a vasodilator, partly through the release of EDRF) and an increase in endothelial permeability, although any role in ARDS is speculative. Clinical trials using antagonists to TNF and Il-1 would help put their importance into perspective, but it may be that the diversity of the inflammatory response makes the antagonism of a single mediator an untenable approach.

The overall prospect for pharmacological intervention may seem poor, but the above analysis does indicate the need to identify accurately the exact mechanisms of neutrophil-mediated endothelial injury and distinguish them from those used in host defense. If this is not the case, it may prove possible to identify a time window when the neutrophil temporarily does more harm than good, and it is of overall benefit to antagonize its destructive potential. For such trials, it is important to develop better markers of early ARDS in patients at high risk of developing ARDS.

SUMMARY

The neutrophil is an essential part of our host defense yet it also has enormous destructive potential. Neutrophil–endothelial interaction is crucial to the early stages of inflammation and it is likely that, in beneficial inflammation, mechanisms have evolved to minimize tissue injury. The loss of any one of a number of fine controls could lead to excessive injury and a destructive spiral. Once established, this chain of events is difficult to halt without seriously compromising host defense. A better understanding of the molecular mechanisms of neutrophil–endothelial interaction is likely to provide rational therapy for inflammatory diseases of the lung and elsewhere.

REFERENCES

1. Wedmore CV, Williams TJ. Control of vascular permeability by polymorphonuclear leukocytes in inflammation. Nature (Lond) 1981;289:646–650.
2. Doherty DE, Downey GP, Worthen GS, Haslett C, Henson PM. Monocyte retention and migration in pulmonary inflammation. Lab Invest 1988;59:200–213.
3. Malech HD, Gallin JI. Neutrophils in human diseases. N Engl J Med 1988;37: 687–694.
4. Vartio T, Seppa H, Vaheri A. Susceptibility of soluble and matrix fibronectin to degradation by tissue proteinases, mast cell chymase and cathepsin G. J Biol Chem 1981;256:471–477.
5. Vejlens G. The distribution of leukocytes in the vascular system. Acta Pathol Microbiol Immunol Scand [A] 1938;33(suppl):11–33.
6. Haslett C, Worthen GS, Giclas PA, Morrison DC, Henson JE, Henson PM. The pulmonary vascular sequestration of neutrophils in endotoxaemia is initiated by an effect of endotoxin on the neutrophil in the rabbit. Am Rev Respir Dis 1987;136:9–18.
7. Lien DC, Wagner WW, Capen RL, Haslett C, Hanson WL, Hofmeister SE, Henson PM, Worthen GS. Physiological neutrophil sequestration in the lung: Visual evidence for localization in capillaries. J Appl Physiol 1987;62:1236–1243.
8. MacNee W, Wiggs B, Belzberg AS, Hogg JC. The effect of cigarette smoking on neutrophil kinetics in human lungs. N Engl J Med 1989;321:924–928.
9. Worthen GS, Lien DC, Tonnesen MG, Henson PM. Interactions of endothelium with other cell types and blood components. In: Ryan US, ed. Pulmonary Endothelium in Health and Disease. New York: Marcel Dekker, 1987.
10. Athens JW, Haab OP, Raab So, et al. Leukokinetic studies. IV. The total blood, circulating and marginal granulocyte pools and the granulocyte turnover rate in normal subjects. J Clin Invest 1961;40:989–995.

11. Muir AL, Cruz M, Martin BA, Thommasen H, Beizberg A, Hogg JC. Leukocyte kinetics in the human lung: Role of exercise and catecholamines. J Appl Physiol 1984;57:711–719.

12. Doerschuk CM, Allard MF, Lee S, Brumwell ML, Hogg JC. Effect of epinephrine on neutrophil kinetics in rabbit lungs. J Appl Physiol 1989;65:401–407.

13. Bierman HR, Byron RL, Kelley H, Cordes F, White LP, Littleman A. The influence of intra-arterial administration of histamine upon the circulating leukocytes of man. Blood 1953;8:315–203.

14. Craddock PR, Fehr J, Brigham KL, Kronenberg RS, Jacob HS. Complement and leukocyte-mediated pulmonary dysfunction in hemodialysis. N Engl J Med 1977;296:769–774.

15. Clark ER, Clark EL. Observations on changes in blood vascular endothelium in the living animal. Am J Anat 1935;57:385–438.

16. Staub NE, Schultz EL, Albertine KH. Leukocytes and pulmonary microvascular injury. Ann NY Acad Sci 1982;38:332–343.

17. Perlo S, Jalowayski AA, Durand CM, West JB. Distribution of red and white blood cells in alveolar walls. J Appl Physiol 1975;38:117–124.

18. Doerschuk CM, Allard MF, Martin BA, MacKenzie A, Autor AP, Hogg JC. Marginated pool of neutrophil in rabbit lungs. J Appl Physiol 1987;65:1806–1815.

19. Saverymuttu SH, Peters AM, Danpure HJ, Reavy HJ, Osman S, Lavender JP. Lung transit of ^{111} Indium-labelled granulocytes. Relationship to labelling techniques. Scand J Haematol 1983;30:151–160.

20. Peters AM, Stuttle AWJ, Allsop P, Gwillam ME, Hall GM, Arnot RN, Lavender JP. Response of the splenic platelet and neutrophil pool to vigorous exercise. (submitted).

21. Weibel ER. Morphometry of the human lung. New York: Academic, 1963.

22. Wintrobe M, Lee G, Boggs D, Bithell T, Foerster J, Athens J, Leukens J (eds). Granulocytes—Neutrophils, eosinophils and basophils. In: Clinical Haematology. 8th Ed. Philadelphia, Lea & Febiger, 1981;192.

23. Marchesi VT, Florey HW. Electron micrographic observations on the emigration of leukocytes. Q J Exp Physiol 1960;45:343–348.

24. Hurley JV. An electron microscopic study of leukocyte emigration and vascular permeability in rat skin. Aust J Exp Biol Med Sci 1963;41:171–179.

25. Worthen GS, Gumbay RS, Larsen GL, Henson PM. Prostaglandin E_2 enhances platelet-activating factor-induced neutrophil migration but not vascular permeability. Am Rev Respir Dis 1983;127:57–62.

26. Tonnesen MG, Smedley LA, Henson PM. Neutrophil–endothelial cell interactions. Modulation of neutrophil adhesiveness induced by complement fragments C5a and C5a des arg and formyl-methionyl-leucyl-phenylalanine in vitro. J Clin Invest 1984;74:1581–1592.

27. Huber AR, Weiss SJ. Disruption of the subendothelial basement membrane during neutrophil diapedesis in an in vitro construct of the blood vessel wall. J Clin Invest 1989;83:1122–1136.

28. Nathan CF. Neutrophil activation on biological surfaces—Massive secretion of hydrogen peroxide in response to products of macrophages and lymphocytes. J Clin Invest 1987;80:1550–1560.

29. Parsons PE, Suguhara K, Cott GR, Mason RJ, Henson PM. The effect of neutrophil migration and prolonged neutrophil contact on epithelial permeability. Am J Pathol 1987;129:302–312.
30. Campbell EJ, Campbell MA. Pericellular proteolysis by neutrophils in the presence of proteinase inhibitors: Effects of substrate opsonization. J Cell Biol 1988; 106:667–676.
31. Zimmerman GA, McIntyre TM, Prescott SM. Thrombin stimulates neutrophil adherence by an endothelial cell-dependent mechanism: Characterization of the response and relationship to platelet-activating synthesis. Ann NY Acad Sci 1986;485:349–367.
32. Ross GD. Complement and complement receptors. Curr Opin Immunol 1989;2: 50–62.
33. Kishimoto TK, Larson RS, Corbi AL, Dustin ML, Staunton DE, Springer TA. The leukocyte integrins. Adv Immunol 1989;46:149–182.
34. Nourshargh S, Rampart M, Hellewell PG, Jose PJ, Harlan JM, Edwards AJ, Williams TJ. Accumulation of ^{111}In-neutrophils in rabbit skin in allergic and non-allergic inflammatory reactions in vivo. J Immunol 1989;142:3193–3198.
35. Vedder NB, Winn RK, Rice CL, Chi EY, Arfors A-E, Harlan JM. A monoclonal antibody to the adherence-promoting glycoprotein, CD18, reduces organ injury and improves survival from hemorrhagic shock and resusitation in rabbits. J Clin Invest 1988;81:939–944.
36. Doerschuk CM, Winn RK, Harlan JM. Role of CD11/CD18 in neutrophil (PMN) emigration in response to endotoxin induced pneumonia in rabbits. FASEB J 1989;3:A1281.
37. Bevilacqua MP, Stengelin S, Gimbrone MA, Seed B. Endothelial leukocyte adhesion molecule 1: An inducible receptor for neutrophils related to complement regulatory proteins and lectins. Science 1989;243:1160–1164.
38. Staunton DE, Dustin MI, Springer TA. Functional cloning of ICAM-2, a cell adhesion ligand for LFA-1 homologous to ICAM-1. Nature (Lond) 1989;339:61–64.
39. McIntyre TM, Zimmerman GA, Prescott SM. Leukotrienes C_4 and D_4 Leukotrienes C_4 and D_4 stimulate human endothelial cells to synthesize platelet-activating factor and bind neutrophils. Proc Natl Acad Sci USA 1986;83:2204–2208.
40. Marks RM, Todd RF, Ward PA. Rapid induction of neutrophil–endothelial adhesions by endothelial complement fixation. Nature (Lond) 1989;339:314–317.
41. Worthen GS, Schwab B, Elson EL, Downey GP. Mechanics of stimulated neutrophils: Cell stiffening induces retention in capillaries. Science 1989;245:183–185.
42. Erzurum SC, Downey GP, Worthen GS. Bacterial lipopolysaccharide mediates microfilament-dependent retention of neutrophils in model capillaries. Am Rev Respir Dis 1985;139:A298.
43. Guthrie LA, McPhail LC, Henson PM, Johnston RB. The priming of neutrophils for enhanced release of oxygen metabolites by bacterial lipopolysaccharide. J Exp Med 1984;160:1656–1671.
44. Haslett C, Guthrie LA, Kopaniak MM, Johnston RB, Henson PM. Modulation of multiple neutrophil functions by preparative methods or trace concentrations of lipopolysaccharide. Am J Pathol 1985;119:101–110.

45. Worthen GS, Haslett C, Rees AJ, Gumbay RS, Henson JE, Henson PM. Neutrophil-mediated pulmonary vascular injury: Synergistic effects of trace amounts of lipopolysaccharide and neutrophil stimuli on vascular permeability and neutrophil sequestration in the lung. Am Rev Respir Dis 1987;136:19–28.
46. Smedly LA, Tonnesen MG, Sandhaus RA, Haslett C, Guthrie LA, Johnston RB, Henson PM, Worthen GS. Neutrophil-mediated injury to endothelial cells: Enhancement by endotoxin and essential role of neutrophil elastase. J Clin Invest 1986;77:1233–1243.
47. Haslett C, Savill JS, Meagher L. The neutrophil. Curr Opin Immunol 1989;2:10–18.
48. Forehand JR, Pabst MJ, Philips WA, Johnston RB. Lipopolysaccharide priming of human neutrophils for an enhanced respiratory burst—Role of intracellular free calcium. J Clin Invest 1989;83:74–83.
49. Henson PM, Henson JE, Fittschen C, Kimani G, Bratton DL, Riches DWH. Phagocytic cells: Degranulation and secretion. In: Gallin JI, Goldstein IM, Synderman R, eds. Inflammation: Basic Principles and Clinical correlates. New York: Raven Press, 1988;363–390.
50. Weiss SJ. Tissue destruction by neutrophils. N Engl J Med 1989;320:365–376.
51. Klebanoff SJ. Phagocytic cells: Products of oxygen metobolism In: Gallin JI, Goldstein IM, Synderman R, eds. New York: Raven Press, 1988;391–444.
52. Gleisner JM. Lysosomal factors in inflammation. In: Glynn LE, Houck JC, Weissman G, eds. Handbook of Inflammation. Vol. 1. Amsterdam: Elsevier, 1979.
53. Eriksson S. Studies in alpha-1-antitrypsin deficiency. Acta Med Scand 1965;432(suppl):1–85.
54. Lee CT, Fein AM, Lippman M, Holtzman H, Kimbel P, Weinbaum G. Elastolytic activity in pulmonary lavage fluid from patients with adult respiratory-distress syndrome. N Engl J Med 1981;304:192–196.
55. Janoff A, Zeligs JD. Vascular injury and lysis of basement membrane in vitro by neutral protease of human leukocytes. Science 1968;161:702–704.
56. Ranadive NS, Cochrane CG. Basic proteins in rat neutrophils that increase vascular permeability. Clin Exp Immunol 1970;6:905–911.
57. Stevens JH, Raffin TA. Adult respiratory distress syndrome. I. Aetiology and mechanisms. Postgrad Med J 1984;60:505–513.
58. Rinaldo JE, Rodgers R. Adult respiratory distress syndrome: Changing concepts of lung injury. N Engl J Med 1982;396:900–909.
59. Weiland JE, Davies WB, Holter JF, Mohammed JR, Dorinsky PM, Gadek JE. Lung neutrophils in the adult respiratory distress syndrome: Clinical and pathophysiological significance. Am Rev Respir Dis 1986;133:218–215.
60. Bernard GR, Luce JM, Sprung CL, et al. High dose corticosteroids in patients with the adult respiratory distress syndrome. N Engl J Med 1987;317:1565–1570.
61. Till GO, Johnson KJ, Kunkel R. Intravascular activation of complement and acute lung injury. J Clin Invest 1982;69:1126–1135.
62. Duchateau J, Haas M, Schreyen H, Radoux L, Sprangers I, Noel FX, Braun M, Lamy M. Complement activation in patients at risk of developing the adult respiratory distress syndrome. Am Rev Respir Dis 1984;130:1058–1064.
63. Meyrick B, Brigham KL. Acute effects of E Coli endotoxin in the pulmonary microcirculation of anaesthetized sheep. Lab Invest 1983;48:458–470.

64. Braude S, Apperley J, Krausz T, Goldman JM, Royston D. Adult respiratory distress syndrome after allogenic bone marrow transplantation: Evidence for a neutrophil independent mechanism. Lancet 1985;1:1239–1242.
65. Begley CJ, Ogletree JL, Meyrick BO, Brigham KL. Modification of pulmonary responses to endotoxemia in awake sheep by steroidal and nonsteroidal anti-inflammatory agents. Am Rev Respir Dis 1984;130:1140–1146.
66. Frolich J, Ogeltree M, Brigham KL. Gram negative endotoxemia in sheep: pulmonary hypertension correlated to pulmonary thromboxane synthesis. Adv Prostaglandin Thromb Res 1980;7:745.
67. Mullane KM, Read N, Salmon JA, Moncada S. Role of leukocytes in acute myocardial infarction in anesthetized dogs: Relationship to myocardial salvage by anti-inflammatory drugs. J Pharmacol Exp Ther 1984;228:510–522.
68. Rampart M, Williams TJ. Suppresion of inflammatory oedema by ibuprofen involving a mechanism independent of cyclo-oxygenase inhibition. Biochem Pharmacol 1986;35:581–586.
69. Mandell GL. ARDS, neutrophils, and pentoxifylline. Am Rev Respir Dis 1988; 138:1103–1105.
70. Chopra J, Webster RO. PGE1 inhibits neutrophil adherence and neutrophil-mediated injury to cultured endothelial cells. Am Rev Respir Dis 1988;138:915–920.
71. Tracey KJ, Lowry SF, Cerami A. Cachetin/TNF-α in septic shock and septic adult respiratory distress syndrome Am Rev Respir Dis 1988;138:1377–1379.
72. Strieter RM, Kunkel SL, Showell HJ, Remick DG, Phan SH, Ward PA, Marks RM. Endothelial cell gene expression of a neutrophil chemotactic factor by TNF-α, LPS, and IL-1β. Science 1989;243:1467–1469.

The Endothelium: An Introduction to Current Research, pages 209–227
© 1990 Wiley-Liss, Inc.

17

Vasculitis and Endothelium

H.L.C. BEYNON, G.H. NEILD, C.D. PUSEY, AND M.J. WALPORT
Rheumatology Unit (H.L.C.B., M.J.W.) and Renal Unit (C.D.P.),
Department of Medicine, Royal Postgraduate Medical School,
Hammersmith Hospital, London W12 ONN, and Renal Unit, St.
Philip's Hospital, London WC2A 2EX (G.H.N.), England

INTRODUCTION

Systemic vasculitis or angiitis may be defined as an inflammatory disorder of blood vessels that usually results in necrosis of the vessel wall with subsequent vascular occlusion. There are a group of diseases, such as Wegener's granulomatosis and polyarteritis nodosa, in which vasculitis appears to represent the primary pathology, but vasculitis may also develop as part of a spectrum of inflammatory pathology affecting many tissues, for example, in systemic lupus erythematosus (SLE) and rheumatoid arthritis.

Attempts to classify the vasculitides have included such criteria as vessel size, histological changes of the vessel wall, and underlying pathogenesis. Zeek (1) in 1952 classified vasculitic diseases into five groups based on vessel wall size: (i) periarteritis nodosa, (ii) hypersensitivity angiitis, (iii) allergic granulomatous arteritis, (iv) rheumatic arteritis, and (v) temporal arteritis. This has formed the prototype for subsequent attempts at classification (2,3). The clinical features of the individual vasculitides are not described here; the reader is referred to the review by Conn and Hunder (4).

There can be no definitive classification of vasculitis as long as the etiology and pathogenesis remain unknown, which is the case for the majority of vasculitic illnesses. Even when vasculitis has been associated with a specific infection, hepatitis B virus (HBV), the clinical features and pathology may be diverse, ranging from polyarteritis nodosa to localised vasculitic lesions affecting skin and kidneys (5).

Nevertheless, preliminary attempts at the classification have been useful in the definition of groups of patients with apparently similar manifestations of disease, and of great clinical importance, in predicting prognosis and response to treatment. For example, rapidly progressive glomerulone-

TABLE I. Classification of Primary Systemic Vasculitis

Vessel size	Granulomata present	Granulomata absent
Large	Giant cell arteritis	Takayasu's arteritis
Medium	Churg–Strauss syndrome	Polyarteritis nodosa
Small	Wegener's granulomatosis	Microscopic polyarteritis
		Schönlein-Henoch purpura
		Hypersensitivity vasculitic

phritis and lung haemorrhage associated with Wegener's granulomatosis and microscopic polyarteritis respond well to early aggressive immunosuppressive therapy, including plasma exchange (6). The recent discovery of autoantibodies to the cytoplasm of normal human neutrophils, which show high sensitivity and specificity for Wegener's granulomatosis and microscopic polyarteritis (7,8), has provided some validation for empirical clinical schemes of classification, although the role of these autoantibodies in disease causation is uncertain (Table I).

The original view that endothelial cells were damaged as passive targets of inflammation has been radically altered by a recent appreciation that they may play an active role in the pathogenesis of many of the vasculitic illnesses. Endothelial cell activation, in response to stimulation by cytokines, may promote inflammation and allow endothelial cells to influence the immune response [reviewed by Cotran and Pober (9,10)]. Such changes include (i) procoagulant activity, mediated by increased synthesis of tissue factor and plasminogen activator inhibitor, and decreased thrombomodulin synthesis (11); (ii) stimulated adhesion of leucocytes, promoted by increased expression of endothelial adhesion molecules such as ICAM-1 (12) and ELAM-1 (13); (iii) upregulation of expression of class I and II HLA molecules, allowing endothelial cells to act as antigen presenting cells (14–19), and as targets for cytotoxic T lymphocytes; (iv) cytokine production, particularly membrane-bound interleukin 1 (IL-1) (20); and (v) changes in cell morphology (21) that may promote increased vascular permeability. The following have been suggested as causative mediators of vasculitis: (i) immune complexes, (ii) antiendothelial cell antibodies, (iii) cytotoxic lymphocytes, and (iv) viruses; each in turn is considered.

VASCULITIS MEDIATED BY IMMUNE COMPLEXES

The formation of immune complexes of antibodies with foreign antigens is a central part of adaptive immunity. The mononuclear phagocytic system is an efficient scavenger of such immune complexes. However, under certain circumstances, immune complexes apparently escape this system and deposit in other tissues causing inflammation (22,23). The association of serum sickness with systemic necrotising vasculitis in man was first described in 1937 by Clark and Kaplan (24). Animal models of serum sickness developed during the 1940s and 1950s [reviewed by Cochrane and Koffler (25)] have formed the experimental basis of our current understanding of vasculitis mediated by immune complexes, although the relevance of these models to the natural occurrence of vasculitis in humans remains uncertain.

ANIMAL MODELS
Acute Serum Sickness

Rabbits injected with bovine serum albumin developed circulating immune complexes at the time of immune elimination of the antigen, with subsequent deposition in arteries and glomeruli (25). Electron micrographs implied that immune complexes and colloidal carbon (a tracer macromolecule) entered between endothelial cells (26). It was proposed that the increased vascular permeability followed from antigen interaction with immunoglobulin E (IgE)-coated basophils, which led to the release of platelet-activating factor (PAF), with subsequent release of vasoactive amines from platelets (27,28), platelet depletion was associated with diminished immune complex deposition (28). There was also evidence of recruitment of neutrophils by complement following deposition of immune complexes, which could be abrogated by depletion of complement using cobra venom factor (29). Evidence for the pathogenic role of neutrophils in this model of necrotising vasculitis came from observations that depletion of polymorphonuclear cells prevented the development of vasculitis (30).

Arthus Reaction

Injection of antigen into the skin of sensitised animals was followed by a vasculitis mediated by the local formation of immune complexes. Immune complexes formed in the walls of blood vessels were rapidly removed by neutrophils with 90% disappearance in 24–48 hr (31). Subsequent experiments in vitro showed that neutrophils, activated by immune complexes in vessel walls, released proteases that digested proteins such as fibronectin (32) and generated a respiratory burst with formation of hydrogen peroxide and superoxide anion (33), causing endothelial cell detachment and lysis with vessel wall damage and occlusion.

VASCULITIS MEDIATED BY IMMUNE COMPLEXES IN HUMANS
Systemic Lupus Erythematosus

Systemic lupus erythematosus (SLE) is often considered the prototype of a disease mediated by immune complexes. Complement activity in sera from patients with SLE is reduced, is related to disease activity (34–36), and improves with treatment. Complement deposition has also been identified in inflamed tissues (37–39).

Many tests to identify soluble immune complexes in serum and plasma have been devised and sera from patients with lupus almost invariably provide a test bed for such assays (40). Possibly the most reliable assays for immune complexes are those that detect combinations of neoantigens of complement proteins and immunoglobulins, such as the conglutinin assay (41,42) and more recent assays using monoclonal antibodies to neoantigens expressed in C3b, iC3b, and C3dg (43). All these assays produce positive results in sera from patients with SLE, which in general correlate with disease activity.

The occurrence of immune complexes containing DNA and anti-dsDNA in lupus plasma is controversial. Tan et al. (44) identified DNA and anti-dsDNA in sera and plasma, and DNA and anti-dsDNA have been identified as constituents of cryoglobulins in lupus patients (45,46). Harbeck et al. (47) reported an increase in the levels of measurable anti-dsDNA antibodies after treating lupus plasma with DNAase. This latter observation, is difficult to reconcile with the more recent report that anti-dsDNA antibodies may protect short stretches of complexed DNA from digestion with DNAase (48). Others have failed to detect DNA/anti-dsDNA immune complexes in lupus sera (49). Difficulty in the demonstration of such immune complexes in the circulation may either reflect their very rapid transit time, which has been demonstrated experimentally in mice (50), or alternatively such immune complexes may form in situ. The overall conclusion that can be drawn from a large number of studies is that small amounts of circulating immune complexes, of largely unknown composition, may be found in patients with SLE.

The probable role of anti-DNA antibodies in causing disease has recently been reviewed (51). DNA and anti-DNA antibodies were found in renal tissue (52,53) and in skin (54,55). Anti-DNA antibodies could be eluted from renal tissue (53) and were concentrated compared with their levels in serum (52). Most workers found correlations between the levels in sera of anti-dsDNA antibodies and disease activity, in both cross-sectional and longitudinal studies, although almost everyone identified some patients with very high levels of anti-dsDNA and apparently inactive disease and vice versa (56–59).

It remains unclear how anti-dsDNA antibodies localise to tissues and several possibilities have been considered (i) that complexes comprising anti-dsDNA/DNA are deposited from plasma; (ii) that dsDNA is deposited in tissues and immune complexes form in situ (60); and (iii) that anti-dsDNA antibodies bind to other cross-reacting antigens in tissues such as lupus-associated membrane protein, LAMP (61,62), or proteoglycan heparan sulfate, which is a normal constituent of glomerular basement membrane (63).

Vasculitis Associated With Hepatitis B Infection

Cases of polyarteritis nodosa associated with chronic carriage of hepatitis B antigen were first described in 1970 by Gocke and colleagues (64).

Subsequently Levo et al. (65) reported a strong association between carriage of hepatitis B surface antigen and mixed cryoglobulinaemia, a finding that has not been confirmed by others (66). Hepatitis B infection has also been associated with cutaneous vasculitis (5) and membranous glomerulonephritis; the latter association is reportedly common in Japan and France but is rare in Britain and North America (67). Circulating immune complexes from patients with vasculitis in association with chronic carriage of HBV have been shown to contain viral antigen, and vasculitis is accompanied by low complement levels, cryoglobulins, and deposits of immunoglobulin and complement in affected vessel walls (67). Why so few of the world's 200 million carriers of HBV develop vasculitis or glomerulonephritis, and the explanation for the geographical variation remains unknown.

Essential Mixed Cryoglobulinaemia

Cryoglobulins are immunoglobulins that precipitate in the cold and dissolve on rewarming. Three types of circulating cryoglobulin may be identified. Type I cryoglobulins are monoclonal immunoglobulins (e.g., myeloma, Waldenstrom's macroglobulinaemia). Types II and III are mixed cryoglobulins; type II cryoprecipitate is typically a combination of monoclonal IgM rheumatoid factor and polyclonal IgG, whereas type III cryoprecipitates usually contain polyclonal IgM, IgG, and C3. The disease, mixed essential cryoglobulinaemia, is associated with type II cryoglobulins and is a vasculitic illness characterised by arthralgia and rash, and may be complicated by diffuse proliferative or mesangiocapillary glomerulonephritis, and by neuropathy (68). Immunoglobulins (of the type in the precipitate) and complement have been demonstrated in glomeruli and vasculitic lesions in association with low serum levels of complement (68, 69).

Drugs and Vasculitis

Many drugs have been implicated in the development of vasculitis, including sulfonamides (70), penicillin (71), and streptokinase (72); in some cases, immune complexes and cryoglobulins containing the drug and specific antibodies have been demonstrated in sera from patients with vasculitis (72).

In most cases of vasculitis presumed to be mediated by immune complexes, however, the responsible antigen is not identified, and there is only indirect evidence in the form of low serum complement levels, cryoglobulins, and rheumatoid factors to support this form of pathogenesis. Histologically, there may be evidence only of complement and fibrin deposition in vessel walls, although this may relate to the age of the biopsy material, as illustrated by the Arthus reaction (31).

THE ROLE OF ENDOTHELIUM IN IMMUNE COMPLEX VASCULITIS

The above scheme of disease mediated by immune complexes disease portrays the endothelial cell in a passive role, damaged by the products of neutrophils and platelets thereby permitting deposition of immune complexes. However, there is some evidence that endothelial cells express complement and Fc receptors and hence may have the capacity to bind immune complexes directly. Some authors have detected Fc receptors on unstimulated endothelial cells (73–76), although these findings have not confirmed by others (77–79).

Receptors for C1q on endothelial cells were first demonstrated by Linder and colleagues (80), and this observation has subsequently been confirmed (74,77,81). Daha and co-workers (77) demonstrated that endothelial C1q receptors bound the collagenous part of C1q and that binding was saturable. Cultured endothelial cells bound heat aggregated immunoglobulin and thyroglobulin/anti-thyroglobulin immune complexes only after pre-incubation with C1q, evidence against the presence of Fc receptors on unstimulated endothelial cells. The physiological significance of endothelial surface C1q receptors is questionable; intact C1 cannot bind to C1q receptors (82) and, although C1 inhibitor rapidly dissociates C1r and C1s from activated C1 (83), immune complexes bearing C1q have not been shown to exist in the circulation. If C1q receptors on endothelial cells were able to bind circulating immune complexes this would serve to localise immune complexes to endothelial cells. Alternatively, such receptors might augment the binding of immune complexes binding to endothelium by other mechanisms, for example DNA/anti-DNA immune complexes attached to basement membrane (60) in the vicinity of endothelium.

Herpes viruses possess genes for Fc and complement receptors that may be expressed on the surface of infected cells. Herpes simplex virus 1 (HSV-1) infection of cultured human umbilical endothelial cells is followed by expression of Fc and C3b receptors within 4 hr (78). Likewise, herpes simplex virus 2 (HSV-2), cytomegalovirus, and herpes zoster virus (HSV) have been shown to induce Fc receptors on endothelial cells (79,84,85). The Fc receptor of HSV-1 appears to be glycoprotein E (86), and the C3b receptor is glycoprotein C (87). Expression of these receptors is thought to be a mechanism for the protection of infected cells from destruction by specific antibody and complement. However, such receptors might also serve to localise immune complexes to infected endothelium and cause injury.

VASCULITIS MEDIATED BY CIRCULATING AUTOANTIBODIES

There have been many studies suggesting a role for antibodies directed against endothelium in the aetiology of vasculitis. Some of these studies require critical appraisal, as there are important methodological difficulties in the identification of true anti-endothelial cell antibodies. In particular, endothelium is bathed in vivo in plasma containing antibodies. It should therefore be very difficult to detect anti-endothelial antibodies of high binding constant, unless these are present in gross antibody excess. Many of the assays for anti-endothelial antibodies have measured binding to endothelial cells fixed in microtitre plates. These assays may measure binding of immunoglobulins of relatively low binding constant, which may be of little pathophysiological significance.

Kawasaki Syndrome

Kawasaki syndrome is characterized by a diffuse panvasculitis, with endothelial necrosis, immunoglobulin deposition, and a mononuclear infiltrate of small and medium-sized blood vessels (88). Sera from patients with acute Kawasaki syndrome were shown to enhance endothelial cell proliferation in vitro significantly, although no molecule to explain this activity was characterised (89). The acute phase of illness is marked by a reduction in the number of circulating CD8+ lymphocytes, an increase in the numbers of CD4+ cells and up to 1,000-fold increase in the number of B cells secreting immunoglobulins (90,91). Studies in acute Kawasaki syndrome have demonstrated two types of antibodies that bound endothelium (92,93). IgM from patients with acute Kawasaki syndrome induced complement-dependent lysis of human umbilical and saphenous vein endothelial cells after pretreatment with γ-interferon (IFN-2) but had no effect on resting endothelial cells, or on dermal fibroblasts or vein smooth muscle cells even after stimulation with IFN-γ (92). The anti-endothelial cell antibodies were only absorbed out by endothelial cells which had been activated by IFNγ, discounting the possibility that they were directed against class I MHC molecules. In a separate series of experiments, Leung et al. (93) showed that IgM and IgG from patients with acute Kawasaki syndrome were able to lyse, specifically and in a complement-dependent manner, endothelial cells that had been pretreated with interleukin 1 (IL-1) and tumour necrosis factor (TNF) for 4 hr. These cytokines have previously been shown to induce expression of ELAM-1 on endothelial cells (13). Convalescent sera and controls were negative.

The antigens induced by IL-1 and TNF appeared distinct from those induced by γ-interferon in several ways: (i) *time course:* antigens induced by IL-1 and TNF appeared by 4–6 hr and disappeared by 24 hr even in continued presence of the mediator, whereas IFN-γ required 72 hr to induce its effect; (ii) *antibody class:* antibodies induced by IFN-γ-stimulated endothelium were exclusively of the IgM class; and (iii) *differential cross-absorption of antibodies:* only IFN-γ-treated cells were able to absorb out antibodies directed against interferon-treated endothelial cells and, conversely, only IL-1- and TNF-treated cells were able to absorb out antibodies against IL-1- and TNF-stimulated cells (92,93).

The pathogenic role of these antibodies in vivo is unknown. It is possible that Kawasaki syndrome has a viral aetiology; one study has found evidence of retrovirus-associated reverse transcriptase in peripheral blood monocytes from patients with Kawasaki syndrome (94). A viral infection of this nature could cause cytokine stimulation of vascular endothelium leading to the induction of new antigens, which in turn stimulate the production of at least two different types of pathogenic anti-endothelial cell antibodies. This hypothesis is highly speculative.

Systemic Lupus Erythematosus

Anti-endothelial cell antibodies were found in sera from patients with active disease (95), which bound saturably via the $F(ab)_2$ domain to endothelial cells, deposit complement on endothelial surfaces, induce prostacyclin release, cause platelets to adhere, and disrupt the endothelial monolayer. Others (96,97) have shown circulating anti-endothelial cell antibodies in a variety of connective tissue diseases, including SLE and rheumatoid arthritis, but these antibodies have not been shown to be in any way pathogenic. It is possible that anti-endothelial cell antibodies require cofactors to induce vascular damage. The addition of peripheral blood mononuclear cells was shown to induce endothelial cell cytotoxicity in combination with anti-endothelial cell antibodies from some patients with active SLE (98). Cytokine stimulation of endothelium may be necessary for mediation of the pathogenic affects of anti-endothelial cell antibodies (as discussed above); there is evidence for increased cytokine production in SLE (99). One study (100) identified antibodies in sera from patients with SLE that reacted with cultured endothelial cells and increases production of procoagulant tissue factor, which could promote vascular thrombosis. Defective release of tissue plasminogen activator has been found in patients with systemic or cutaneous vasculitis (101).

Wegener's Granulomatosis and Microscopic Polyarteritis

Wegener's granulomatosis and microscopic polyarteritis form part of the spectrum of primary systemic vasculitis. Both affect principally small blood vessels and lead to focal necrotising glomerulonephritis. The pathological changes are similar in both conditions, with a leucocytoclastic vasculitis and fibrinoid necrosis of small muscular arteries, although the presence of granulomata is a feature only of Wegener's granulomatosis. The clinical syndromes are also similar, although destructive lesions of the upper and lower respiratory tracts are peculiar to Wegener's granulomatosis (102). The pathogenesis of these disorders remains obscure, although they have been found to respond well to immunosuppressive therapy (103). Therapeutic plasma exchange was introduced at a time when it was believed that immune complexes were important in pathogenesis, although there was little evidence to support this notion. However, the apparent benefit from plasma exchange supports a role for humoral factors. It was therefore of great interest when autoantibodies to the cytoplasm of neutrophils and monocytes (ANCA) were described in association with Wegener's granulomatosis (7), and subsequently also in microscopic polyarteritis (8). Subsequent studies have confirmed that ANCA are a highly specific and sensitive test for active Wegener's granulomatosis and microscopic polyarteritis (104). Two different patterns of cytoplasmic staining of neutrophils have been observed: a diffuse cytoplasmic pattern (C-ANCA), and a perinuclear pattern (P-ANCA). It is becoming clear that the cytoplasmic pattern is more closely associated with Wegener's granulomatosis, whereas perinuclear staining is found in patients with microscopic polyarteritis, as well as in some cases of idiopathic rapidly progressive glomerulonephritis and other forms of vasculitis (105). The target antigen(s) may be different in each type. There is now reasonable evidence that myeloperoxidase is the target of P-ANCA, and a 29-kD serine protease is the target of C-ANCA (106).

The role of ANCA in the pathogenesis of vasculitis has not been established, although it has been suggested that they may lead to activation of neutrophils, hence vascular damage. Indirect evidence that these antibodies are relevant to disease is provided by observations of a relationship of positive tests for ANCA with relapses in disease activity during follow-up evaluation of patients with Wegener's granulomatosis and microscopic polyarteritis (107). Perhaps more interesting are recent findings that antibodies from patients with Wegener's granulomatosis and microscopic polyarteritis bind to glomerular endothelial (and epithelial) cells in culture (108), and that circulating anti-endothelial cell antibodies can be detected in ANCA-positive patients using an enzyme-linked immunosorbent assay (ELISA) with fixed endothelial cells (Savage COS: personal communication). However, cross-absorption studies suggest that anti-endothelial cell activity is separate to anti-neutrophil activity, and more work is required in this area. In particular, it will be important to determine whether the activation state of endothelium (hence the presence of inducible adhesion molecules) influences the binding of antibodies and whether sera from patients have cytotoxic effects on endothelial cells.

Other Vasculitic Illnesses

Antibodies reactive with vascular endothelium have also been reported in other diseases associated with vasculitis (Table II). In hairy cell leukaemia, cross-reacting antibodies between hairy cells and endothelial cells may in part be responsible for the vasculitis associated with the leukaemia (109).

Anti-endothelial cell antibodies directed against non-HLA molecules on graft endothelium have been detected in a proportion of recipients of renal allografts, who developed either accelerated or chronic graft rejection. Anti-endothelial cell antibodies have been detected in eluates from these

TABLE II. Classification of Vasculitic Illnesses in Which
Vasculitis Is Only a Part of the Pathology

Primary "autoimmune" diseases
  Systemic lupus erythematosus (SLE)
  Rheumatoid arthritis
  Polymyositis/dermatomyositis
  Scleroderma
  Behçet's disease

Malignancy
  Carcinoma
  Lymphoma
  Hairy cell leukaemia

Mixed essential cryoglobulinaemia

Infection
  Infective endocarditis
  Hepatitis B
  Syphilis
  Kawasaki syndrome (infectious etiology not established beyond doubt)

grafts, suggesting that antibodies reactive with the endothelium from the transplanted kidney may take part in graft rejection (110,111). Leung et al. (112) identified IgG and IgM complement-fixing antibodies that lysed human umbilical vein endothelial cells in sera from children with acute haemolytic-uraemic syndrome. Interestingly, pretreatment of the endothelial cells with IFN-γ resulted in loss of this lytic activity, raising the possibility that in this disease IFN-γ induces the specific loss, or alteration in structure, of molecules present on resting endothelial cells.

Anti-endothelial Cell Antibodies: Cause or Effect of Vasculitis?

The question as to whether anti-endothelial cell antibodies are a cause or consequence of vascular damage has not been answered. That such antibodies are only detected with low frequency in sera from patients with diabetes and atherosclerosis argues against them developing as a general consequence of vascular damage (96).

If pathogenic anti-endothelial cell antibodies are present in patients with SLE (95), a question that needs to be resolved is: What determines binding of such antibodies in vivo? In a flare of SLE, not all organs are involved at the same time. An explanation for the restriction of diseases to particular vessels could be variation in the type and density of surface endothelial cell antigens from organ to organ. There is some evidence in support of this hypothesis. The monoclonal antibody, OKM5, showed differential binding to endothelial cells present in different parts of the kidney; the antibody was reactive with renal medullary endothelial cells but not glomerular or cortical small vessel endothelium (113).

Vasculitis Mediated by Other Humoral Factors

There have been reports that sera from patients with rheumatoid arthritis, SLE, systemic sclerosis, and systemic necrotising vasculitis can mediate endothelial cytotoxicity by antibody-independent mechanisms (99,114). The nature of these mediators is unknown. Blake and colleagues (115) proposed that oxidised low-density lipoprotein (LDL) may be such a factor but found that levels in stored sera were much higher than in fresh sera, casting doubt on the physiological significance of these observations.

CELL-MEDIATED IMMUNE MECHANISM OF VASCULITIS

Vasculitis marked by a perivascular lymphocytic infiltration and by absence of neutrophils is found in certain types of cutaneous (116) and systemic vasculitis (117). Endothelial cells are capable of accessory function in presenting antigen to lymphocytes. Splenic lymphocytes from BALB/c mice could be activated by co-culturing in vitro with an endothelial mouse cell line ME-2 (118). These lymphocytes, when injected into synegeneic mice, induced vasculitic lesions. It was proposed that splenic lymphocytes were activated by endothelial antigens on the ME-2 cells and cross-reactive antigens were present on BALB/c endothelial cells.

Moyer and Reinisch (119) attempted to elucidate the pathogenesis of cell-mediated vascular damage by constructing a model in vitro using vascular smooth muscle cells and splenocytes from lupus-prone MRL/1pr mice. Vascular smooth muscle cells were able to recruit and activate splenocytes, culminating in cytotoxicity of the vascular smooth muscle cells. They proposed that vascular smooth muscle cells might play an active role in promoting lymphocyte influx in vivo. Subsequently, Hart and colleagues (120), using BALB/c mice, sensitised lymphocytes in vitro to syngeneic smooth muscle cells, and on transfer to syngeneic recipients were able to induce in vivo microvessel vasculitis that was granulomatous in nature in 20% of cases.

Evidence is scanty of vascular damage mediated by cells in humans. Increased lymphocyte-mediated toxicity to human endothelial cells has been reported in a small number of patients with giant cell arteritis and Takayasu's arteritis (121). The occurrence of granulomata containing lymphocytes and epithelioid cells in Wegener's granulomatosis and Churg–Strauss vasculitis (122) implies that cell-mediated immunity is a part of the immunopathology. Further evidence to support such a mechanism is provided by the finding of a predominance of CD4+ lymphocytes in periglomerular and interstitial infiltrates in renal biopsies from patients with active Wegener's granulomatosis (123). In these diseases, Fauci (3) proposed that sensitised lymphocytes react with antigen and release lymphokines that result in monocyte accumulation and transformation into macrophages. Release of lysosomal enzymes leads to vessel wall damage and transformation of macrophages into epithelioid cells and multinucleate giant cells forming granulomata.

VASCULITIS INDUCED BY VIRUSES

Viruses are known to induce vasculitis in at least two ways. The first is mediated by the host immune response to persisting viral antigens, usually in the form of circulating immune complexes, Aleutian disease of the mink (124), and hepatitis B-associated vasculitis (discussed above) are examples of this type of pathology. The second mechanism of induction of vasculitis follows from direct replication of viruses in vascular endothelial cells. Equine viral arteritis is the prime example (124), but it is likely that the arteritis that occasionally complicates herpes zoster ophthalmicus is due to direct invasion by the zoster virus (125). It is also probable that some viruses induce vascular injury by triggering a cellular immune response to their presence in and around blood vessels (126), and the viral induction of Fc and complement receptors on endothelial cells has been discussed above.

MARKERS OF VASCULITIC ACTIVITY

Nonspecific markers that have been used to monitor vasculitic activity include C-reactive protein, erythrocyte sedimentation rate (ESR), serum alkaline phosphatase, neutrophilia, and thrombocytosis. Factor VIII-related antigen (von Willebrand factor), which is synthesised and stored in endothelial cells, has been studied as a marker of vasculitic activity. Although levels are nonspecifically elevated in noninflammatory peripheral vascular disease, diabetes, and surgical trauma, levels are elevated in systemic necrotising vasculitis and large vessel vasculitis, and there are data showing that levels reflect disease activity (127,128).

CONCLUSION

The etiology and pathogenetic mechanisms of the various forms of systemic vasculitis have been reviewed. Animal models of vasculitis mediated by immune complexes and lymphocytes have been helpful, although their relevance to human disease remains uncertain. Recent advances in endothelial cell biology suggest an active role for endothelium in mediating inflammation. In the future, the development of monoclonal antibodies to cytokines and/or cytokine-induced endothelial cell antigens may provide a method of abrogating endothelial and vascular damage. Although there is considerable evidence for the role of autoimmunity in many forms of vasculitis in man, we remain far from an accurate understanding of the etiology and pathogenesis of most cases of vasculitis.

REFERENCES

1. Zeek PM. Periarteritis nodosa: A critical review. Am J Clin Pathol 1952;22:777–790.

2. Lie JT. Classification and immunodiagnosis of vasculitis: A new solution or promises unfilled? J Rheumatol 1988;15(5):728–731.
3. Fauci AS. The spectrum of vasculitis. Clinical, pathologic, immunologic, and therapeutic considerations. Ann Intern Med 1978;89:660–676.
4. Conn DL, Hunder GC. Vasculitis and Related Disorders. In: Kelley WN, Harris ED, Ruddy S, Sledge CB, eds. Textbook of Rheumatology. Philadelphia: WB Saunders, 1989;1167–1193.
5. Sergent JS. Extrahepatic manifestations of hepatitis B infection. Bull Rheum Dis 1983;33:37–42.
6. Hind CRK, Pareskevakou H, Lockwood CM, Evans DJ, Peters DK, Rees AJ. Prognosis after immunosupression of patients with crescenteric nephritis requiring dialysis. Lancet 1983;1:263–265.
7. Van der Woude FJ, Raasmussen N, Lobatto S, Wiik A, Permin H, Van Es LA, Van der Giessen M, Van der Hem GK, The TH. Autoantibodies against neutrophils and monocytes: Tool for diagnosis and marker of disease activity in Wegener's granulomatosis. Lancet 1985;1:425–429.
8. Savage COS, Winearls CG, Jones S, Marshall PD, Lockwood CM. Prospective study of radioimmunoassay for antibodies against neutrophil cytoplasm in diagnosis of systemic vasculitis. Lancet 1987;1:1389–1393.
9. Cotran RS, Pober JS. Endothelial activation: Its role in inflammatory and immune Reactions. In: Simionescue N, Simionescue M, eds. Endothelial Cell Biology. New York: Plenum Press, 1988;335–344.
10. Pober JS. Cytokine-mediated activation of vascular endothelium. Am J Pathol 1989;133:426–433.
11. Stern DM, Handley DA, Nawroth PP. Endothelium and the regulation of coagulation. In: Simionescue N, Simionescue M, eds. Endothelial Cell Biology. New York: Plenum Press, 1988;275–308.
12. Pober JS, Lapierre LA, Stolpen AH, et al. Activation of cultured human endothelium cells by recombinant lymphotoxin: Comparisons with tumour necrosis factor and interleukin-1 species. J Immunol 1987;138:3319–3324.
13. Bevilaqua MO, Pober JS, Mendrick DL, Cotran RS, Gimbrone MA Jr. Identification of an inducible endothelial leucocyte adhesion molecule ELAM1. Proc Natl Acad Sci USA 1987;84:9238–9242.
14. Hirshberg H, Bergh OJ, Thorsby E. Antigen-presenting properties of human vascular endothelial cells. J Exp Med 1980;152:249s–255s.
15. Ashida ER, Johnson AR, Lipsky PE. Human endothelial cell–lymphocyte interaction. Endothelial cells function as accessory cells necessary for mitogen-induced human T lymphocyte activation in vitro. J Clin Invest 1981;67:1490–1499.
16. Pober JS, Gimbrone MA Jr. Expression of 1a like antigens by human vascular endothelial cells is inducible in vitro: Demonstration by monoclonal antibody binding and immunoprecipitation. Proc Natl Acad Sci USA 1982;79:6641–6648.
17. Moreas JR, Stansty P. A new antigen system expressed in human endothelial cells. J Clin Invest 1977;66:449–454.
18. Gibofsky A, Jaffe EA, Fotino M, Becker CG. The identification of HLA antigens on fresh and cultured human endothelial cells. J Immunol 1975;115:730–733.
19. Teitel JM, Shore A, Mc Barron J, Schiavone A. Enhanced T cell activation due to combined stimulation by both endothelial cells and monocytes. Scand J Immunol 1989;29:165–173.

20. Kurt Jones EA, Fiers W, Pober JS. Membrane bound Il-1 induction on human endothelial cells and dermal fibroblasts. J Immunol 1987;139:2317–2324.
21. Stolpen AH, Guinan EC, Fiers W, Pober JS. Recombinant tumour necrosis factor and immune interferon act singly and in combination to reorganise human vascular endothelial morphology. Am J Pathol 1986;123:16–24.
22. Kimberly RP. Immune complexes in the rheumatic diseases. Rheum Dis Clin North Am 1987;13:583–596.
23. Schifferli JA, Ng YC, Peters DK. The role of complement and its receptors in the elimination of immune complexes. N Engl J Med 1986;315:488–492.
24. Clark E, Kaplan BJ. Endocardial, arterial and other mesenchymal alterations associated with serum sickness disease in man. Arch Pathol 1937;24:458.
25. Cochrane CG, Koffler D. Immune complex disease in experimental animals and man. Adv Immunol 1973;16:185.
26. Cochrane CG. Studies on localisation of antigen–antibody complexes and other macromolecules in vessels. J Exp Med 1963;142:242.
27. Majno G, Shea SM, Leventhal M. Endothelial contraction induced by histamine type mediators. J Cell Biol 1969;42:647–473.
28. Cochrane CG. Mechanisms involved in deposition of immune complexes in tissues. J Exp Med 1971;134:75–89.
29. Ward PA, Cochrane CG, Muller Eberhard HJ. The role of serum complement in chemotaxis of leucocytes in vitro. J Exp Med 1965;122:327–346.
30. Kniker W, Cochrane CG. Pathogenic factors in vascular lesions of experimental serum sickness. J Exp Med 1965;122:83–98.
31. Cochrane CG, Weigle WO, Dixon FJ. The role of polymorphonuclear leucocytes in the initiation and cessation of the Arthus reaction. J Exp Med 1959; 110:481.
32. Harlan J, Killen P, Harker LA, Striker GE, Wright DG. Neutrophil mediated endothelial injury: In vitro mechanism of cell detachment. J Clin Invest 1981; 68:1394–1403.
33. Sachs T, Moldow CF, Craddock PR, Bowers TK, Jacob HS. Oxygen radicals mediate endothelial cell damage by complement-stimulated granulocytes. J Clin Invest 1978;61:1161–1167.
34. Townes AS, Stewart CR, Osler AG. Immunologic studies of systemic lupus erythematosus. Bull Johns Hopkins Med J 1963;112:202–219.
35. Schur PH, Sandson J. Immunologic factors and clinical activity in systemic lupus erythematosus. N Engl J Med 1968;278:533–538.
36. Lloyd W, Schur PH. Immune complexes, complement and antiDNA in exacerbations of systemic lupus erythematosus. Medicine (Baltimore) 1981;60:208–217.
37. Lachman PJ, Muller Eberhard HJ, Kunkel HG, Paronetto F. The localisation of in vivo bound complement in tissue sections. J Exp Med 1962;115:63–82.
38. Tann EM, Kunkel HG. An immunofluorescent study of skin lesions in systemic lupus erythematosus. Arthritis Rheum 1966;9:37–46.
39. Biesecker G, Katz S, Koffler D. Renal localisation of the membrane attack complex in systemic lupus erythematosus nephritis. J Exp Med 1981;154:1779–1794.
40. Theofilopoulos AN, Dixon FJ. The biology and detection of immune complexes. Adv Immunol 1979;28:89–220.

41. Casali P, Bossus A, Carpentier MA, Lambert PH. Solid phase enzyme immunoassay or radioimmunoassay for the detection of immune complexes based on their recognition by conglutinin, conglutinin binding test. Clin Exp Immunol 1977;29:342–354.
42. Eisenberg RA, Theofilopoulus AN, Dixon FJ. Use of bovine conglutinin for the assay of immune complexes. J Immunol 1977;118:1428–1434.
43. Aguadu MT, Lambris JD, Tsokos GC, et al. Monoclonal antibodies against complement 3 neoantigens for detection of immune complexes and complement activation. J Clin Invest 1985;76:1418–1426.
44. Tan EM, Schur PH, Carr RI, Kunkel HG. Deoxyribonucleic acid (DNA) and antibodies to DNA in serum of patients with systemic lupus erythematosus. J Clin Invest 1966;45:1732.
45. Davis JS, Godfrey SM, Winfield JB. Direct evidence for circulating DNA/anti-DNA complexes in systemic lupus erythematosus. Arthritis Rheum 1978;21:17–22.
46. Adu D, Dobson J, William DG. Effects of soluble aggregates of IgG on the binding, uptake and degradation of the C1q subcomponent by adherent guinea pig macrophages. Clin Exp Immunol 1981;43:605.
47. Harbeck RJ, Bardana EJ, Kohler PF, Carr RI. DNA-anti-DNA complexes; their detection in systemic lupus erythematosus sera. J Clin Invest 1973;52:789–795.
48. Burdick G, Emlen W. Effect of antibody excess on the size and stoichemistry and DNAase resistance of DNA-antiDNA immune complexes. J Immunol 1985;135:2593–2597.
49. Izui S, Lambert PH, Miescher PA, Hay FC, Nineham J, Roitt IM. Routine assay for detection of immune complexes of known immunoglobulin class using solid phase C1q. Clin Exp Immunol 1977;30:384–392.
50. Emlen W, Mannick M. Clearance of circulating DNA-antiDNA immune complexes. J Exp Med 1982;155:1210–1215.
51. Fournie GJ. Circulating DNA and lupus nephritis. Kidney Int 1988;33:487–497.
52. Koffler D, Shur PH, Kunkel HG. Immunological studies concerning the nephritis of systemic lupus erythematosus. J Exp Med 1967;126:607–624.
53. Krishnan C, Kaplan MH. Immunopathologic studies of systemic lupus erythematosus. Antinuclear reaction of gammaglobulin eluted from homogenates and isolated glomeruli of kidneys from patients with systemic lupus erythematosus nephritis. J Clin Invest 1967;46:569–579.
54. Tan EM, Kunkel HG. An immunofluorescent study of skin lesions in systemic lupus erythematosus. Arthritis Rheum 1966;9:37–46.
55. Landry M, Mitchell W. Systemic lupus erythematosus; studies of the antibodies bound to the skin. J Clin Invest 1973;52:1871–1880.
56. Schur PH, Sandson J. Immunologic factors and clinical activity in systemic lupus erythematosus. N Engl J Med 1968;278:533–538.
57. Pincus T, Schur PH, Rose JA, Decker JL, Talal N. Measurement of serum DNA binding activity in systemic lupus erythematosus. N Engl J Med 1969;281:702–705.
58. Bardana EJ, Harbeck RJ, Hoffman AA, Pirofksy B, Carr R. The prognostic and therapeutic implications of DNA–antiDNA complexes in systemic lupus erythematosus. Am J Med 1975;59:515–522.

59. Cameron JS, Lessof MH, Ogg CS, Williams BD, Williams DG. Disease activity in nephritis of systemic lupus erythematosus in relation to serum complement concentration. Clin Exp Immunol 1976;25:418–427.

60. Izui S, Lambert PH, Miescher PA. In vitro demonstration of a particular affinity of glomerular basement membrane and collagen for DNA. J Exp Med 1976;144: 428–443.

61. Jacob L, Lety MA, Louvard D, Back JF. Binding of a monoclonal anti-DNA autoantibody to identical protein(s) present on the surface of several human cell types involved in lupus pathology. J Clin Invest 1985;75:315–317.

62. Jacob L, Lety MA, Choquette D, et al. Presence of antibodies against a cell surface protein, cross reactive with DNA, in systemic lupus erythematosus, a marker of disease activity. Proc Natl Acad Sci USA 1987;84:2956–2959.

63. Faaber P, Capel PJA, Rijke GSM, Vierwinden G, Van De Putte LBA, Koene RAP. Cross reactivity of anti-DNA antibodies with proteoglycan. Clin Exp Immunol 1984;55:502–508.

64. Gocke DJ, Hsu K, Morgan C. Bombardier S, Lochshiu M, Christian CL. Association between polyarteritis and Australian antigen. Lancet 1970;2:1149–1153.

65. Levo Y, Gorevic PD, Kassab IIJ, Zucker-Franklin D, Franklin EC. Association between hepatitis B virus and essential mixed cryoglobulinaemia. N Engl J Med 1977;296:1501–1504.

66. Popp JW, Dienstag JL, Wands JR, Block KJ. Essential mixed cryoglobulinaemia without evidence for hepatitis B infection. Ann Intern Med 1980;92:379–383.

67. Shusterman M, London WT. Hepatitis B and immune complex disease. N Engl J Med 1984;310:43–45.

68. Ponticelli C, D'Amico G. Essential mixed cryoglobulinaemia. In: Schrier RW, Gottshalk CW, eds. Diseases of the Kidney. Boston: Little, Brown, 1988;2377.

69. Cream JJ. Immunofluorescent studies of the skin in cryoglobulinaemic vasculitis. Br J Dermatol 1971;84:48.

70. Rose GA, Spencer H. Polyarteritis nodosa. Q J Med 1957;26:43.

71. Waugh D. Myocarditis, arteritis and focal hepatic, splenic and renal granulomas apparently due to penicillin sensitivity. Am J Pathol 1952;28:437.

72. Davies KAA, Mathieson P, Winearls CG, Rees AJ, Walport MJ. Serum sickness and acute renal failure after Streptokinase therapy for myocardial infarction. Clin Exp Immunol 1990;80:83–88.

73. Lyss AP, Finko R, Knight K, Bina M, Reeber M, Cines DB. Interaction of IgG with human endothelial cells. Clin Res 1989;30:323A.

74. Andrews BS, Shadford M, Cunningham P, Davis 1V JS. Demonstration of a C1q receptor on the surface of human endothelial cells. J Immunol 1981;127:1075–1080.

75. Johnson PM, Trenchev P, Faulk WP. Immunological studies of human placentae. Binding of complexed immunoglobulin by stromal endothelial cells. Clin Exp Immunol 1975;22:133.

76. Matre R. Similarities of Fc gamma receptors on trophoblast and placental endothelial cells. Scand J Immunol 1977;6:953–958.

77. Daha MR, Miltenburg AMM, Hiemstra PS, Klar-Mohamad N, Van Es LA, Van Hinsbergh VWM. The complement subcomponent C1q mediates binding of

immune complexes and aggregates to endothelial cells in vitro. Eur J Immunol 1988;18:783–787.

78. Cines DB, Lyss AP, Bina M, Corkey R, Kefalides NA, Friedman HM. Fc and C3 receptors induced by herpes simplex virus on cultured endothelial cells. J Clin Invest 1982;69:123–128.

79. Ryan US, Schultz DR, Ryan JW. Fc and C3b receptors on pulmonary endothelial cells: Induction by injury. Science 1981;214:557–558.

80. Linder E. Binding of C1q and complement activation by vascular endothelium. J Immunol 1981;126:648–657.

81. Zhang SC, Schultz DR, Ryan US. Receptor mediated binding of C1q on pulmonary endothelium cells. Tissue Cell 1986;18:13–18.

82. Veerhuis R, Van Es LA, Daha MR. Effects of soluble aggregates of IgG on the binding, uptake and degradation of the C1q subcomponent by adherent guinea pig macrophages. Eur J Immunol 1985;15:881–887.

83. Ziccardi RJ, Cooper NR. Active disassembly of the first complement component C1 by C1 inactivator. J Immunol 1979;123:788–792.

84. Para MF, Goldstein L, Speak PG. Similarities and differences in the Fc binding glycoprotein of Herpes simplex virus types 1 and 2 and tentative mapping of the viral genome for this glycoprotein. J Virol 1982;41:137–144.

85. Smiley ML, Hoxie JA, Friedman H. Herpes simplex virous type 1 infection of endothelial, epithelial, and fibroblast cells induces a receptor for C3bi. J Immunol 1985;134:2673–2678.

86. Baucke RB, Spear PG. Membrane proteins specified by herpes simplex virus on cultured human endothelial cells. J Virol 1979;32:779.

87. Friedman HM, Cohen GH, Eisenberg C, Seidel CA, Cines DB. Glycoprotein C of herpes simplex virus 1 acts as a receptor for the C3b complement component on infected cells. Nature (Lond) 1884;309:633.

88. Yaragihara R, Todd JK. Acute febrile mucocutaneous lymph node syndrome. Am J Dis Child 1980;134:603–614.

89. Hashimoto Y, Yoshinoya S, Aikawa T, Mitamura T, Miyoshi Y, Murariaka M, Miyamotot T, Yamase Y, Kawasaki Y. Enhanced endothelial cell proliferation in acute Kawasaki disease (mucocutaneous lymph node disease). Pediatr Res 1986;20:943–946.

90. Leung DYM, Siegel RL, Grady S, Krensky A, Meade A, Reinherz EL, Geha A. Immunoregulatory abnormalities in mucocutaneous lymph node syndrome. Clin Immunol Immunopathol 1982;23:100–112.

91. Leung DYM, Chu ET, Wood M, Grady S, Meade R, Geha RS. Immunoregulatory T cell abnormalities in mucocutaneous lymph node syndrome. J Immunol 1983;130:2002–2004.

92. Leung DYM, Collins T, Lapierre LA, Geha RS, Pober JS. Immunoglobulin M antibodies present in the acute phase of Kawasaki syndrome lyse cultured vascular endothelial cells stimulated by gamma interferon. J Clin Invest 1986; 77:1428–1435.

93. Leung DYM, Geha RS, Newburger JW, Burns JW, Fiers W, Lapiere IA, Pober JS. Two monokines Interleukin 1 and Tumour necrosis factor, render cultured vascular endothelial cells susceptible to lysis by antibodies circulating during acute Kawasaki syndrome. J Exp Med 1986;164:1958–1972.

94. Burns JC, Geha RS, Schneeberger EE, Newburger JW, Rosen FS, Glezen LS, Huang AS. Polymerase activity in lymphocyte culture supernatants from patients with acute Kawasaki disease. Nature (Lond) 1986;323:814–815.

95. Cines DB, Lyss AP, Reeber M, Bina M, DeHoratius RJ. Presence of complement fixing antiendothelial cell antibodies in systemic lupus erythematosus. J Clin Invest 1984;73:611–625.

96. Rosenbaum J, Pottinger BE, Woo P, Black CM, Loizous S, Byron MA, Pearson JD. Measurement and characterisation of circulating antiendothelial cell IgG in connective tissue diseases. Clin Exp Immunol 1988;72:450–456.

97. Shingu M, Hurd ER. Sera from patients with systemic lupus erythematosus reactive with human endothelial cells. J Rheumatol 1981;8:581–586.

98. Penning CA, French MAH, Rowell NR, Hughes P. Antibody dependent cellular toxicity of human vascular endothelium in systemic lupus erythematosus. J Clin Lab Immunol 1985;17:125–130.

99. Ramirez F, Williams RC, Sibbitt WL, Searles RP. Immunoglobulin from systemic lupus erythematosus serum induces interferon release by normal mononuclear cells. Arthritis Rheum 1986;29:326–336.

100. Tannenbaum SH, Finsko R, Cines DB. Antibody and immune complexes induce tissue factor production by human endothelial cells. J Immunol 1986; 137:1532–1537.

101. Jordan JM, Allen NB, Pizzo SV. Defective release of tissue plasminogen activator in systemic and cutaneous vasculitis. Am J Med 1987;82:397–400.

102. Fauci AS, Haynes BF, Kanz P, Wolff SM. Wegener's granulomatosis: Prospective clinical and therapeutic experience with 85 patients for 21 years. Ann Intern Med 1983;98:76–85.

103. Pusey CD, Lockwood CM. Plasma exchange for glomerular disease. In: Robinson RR, ed. Nephrology. New York: Springer-Verlag, 1984;1474–1485.

104. Savage COS, Winearls CG, Evans DJ, Rees AJ, Lockwood CM. Microscopic polyarteritis, presentation, pathology and prognosis. Q J Med 1985;56:467–484.

105. Pusey CD, Lockwood CM. Autoimmunity in rapidly progressive glomerulonephritis. Kidney Int 1989;35:929–937.

106. Falk RJ, Jennette JC. Anti-neutrophil cytoplasmic antibodies with specificity for myeloperoxidase in patients with systemic vasculitis and idiopathic necrotising and crescentic nephritis. N Engl J Med 1988;318:1651–1657.

107. Molle B, Specks U, Ludeman J, Rohrback MS, DeRenee RA, Gross WL. ANCA their immunodiagnostic value in Wegener's granulomatosis. Ann Intern Med 1989;111:28–40.

108. Abbott F, Jones S, Lockwood CM, Rees AJ. Autoantibodies to glomerular antigens in patients with Wegener's granulomatosis. Nephrol Dial Transplant 1989;4:1–8.

109. Posnett DN, Marboe CC, Knowles D M, Jaffe EA, Kunkel HG. A membrane antigen selectively present on hairy cell leukaemia cells, endothelial cells and epidermal basal cells. J Immunol 1984;132:2700–2702.

110. Cerilli J, Brasile L. Endothelial cell autoantigens. Transplant Proc 1980; 12(3/1):37–42.

111. Paul LC, Carpenter CB. Antibodies against renal vein endothelial alloantigens. Transplant Proc 1980;12(3/1):42–45.

112. Leung DYM, Havens PL, Moake JL, Kim M, Pober JS. Lytic anti-endothelial cell antibodies in haemolytic uraemic syndrome. Lancet 1988;2:183–186.
113. Knowles DM, Tolidjian B, Marboe C, D'Agati V, Grimes M, Chess I. Monoclonal antibodies OKM1 and OKM5 possess distinctive tissue distributions including differential reactivity with vascular endothelium. J Immunol 1984; 132:2170–2173.
114. Drenk F, Mensing H, Serbin A, Deicher H. Studies on endothelial cell cytotoxic activity in sera of patients with progressive systemic sclerosis, Raynaud's syndrome, rheumatoid arthritis and systemic lupus erythematosus. Rheum Int 1985;5:259–263.
115. Blake DR, Winyard P, Scott DGI, Brailsford S, Blann A, Lunec J. Endothelial cell cytotoxicity in inflammatory vascular diseases: the possible role of oxidised lipoprotein. Ann Rheum Dis 1985;44:176–182.
116. Soter NA. Clinical presentations and mechanisms of necrotising angiitis of the skin. J Invest Dermatol 1976;67:354–359.
117. Epstein WL. Granulomatous hypersensitivity. Prog Allergy 1967;11:36–88.
118. Hart MN, Sadewasser KL, Cancilla PA, Debault LE. Experimental autoimmune type of vasculitis resulting from activation of mouse lymphocytes to cultured endothelium. Lab Invest 1983;48:419–427.
119. Moyer CF, Reinisch CL. The role of vascular smooth muscle cells in experimental autoimmune vasculitis. Am J Pathol 1984;117:380–390.
120. Hart MN, Tassell SK, Sadewasser KL, Schelper RL, Moore SA. Autoimmune vasculitis resulting from in vitro immunization of lymphocytes to smooth muscle cells. Am J Pathol 1985;119:448–455.
121. Scott DGI, Blake DR, Blann A, et al. The role of lymphocytes and serum factors in vasculitic diseases. Ann Rheum Dis 1989;43:116.
122. McClusky RT, Fienberg R. Vasculitis in primary vasculitides, granulomatoses, and connective tissue diseases. Hum Pathol 1983;14:305–315.
123. Wilmink JM, Meyer CJLM, Surachno J, Ten Veen KH, Balk TG, Schellekens PTA. Clinical and immunological follow up of patients with severe renal disease in Wegener's granulomatosis. Am J Nephrol 1985;5:21–29.
124. Henson JB, Crawford TB. The pathogenesis of virus induced arterial disease— Aleutian disease and equine viral arteritis. Ad Cardiol 1974;13:183–191.
125. Reyes MG, Fresco R, Chokroverty S, Salud EQ. Virus like particles in granulomatous angiitis of the central nervous system. Neurology (NY) 1976;26:797–799.
126. Sergent JS. Vasculitidies associated with viral infections. Clin Rheum Dis 1980;6:339–349.
127. Woolf AF, Wakerley G, Wallington TB, Scott DGI, Dieppe PA. Factor V111 related antigen in the assessment of vasculitis. Ann Rheum Dis 1987;46:441–447.
128. Nusinow SR, Federeci AD, Zimmerman TS, Curd JG. Increased von Willebrand factor antigen in the plasma of patients with vasculitis. Arthritis Rheum 1984;27:1405–1410.

The Endothelium: An Introduction to Current Research, pages 229–252
© 1990 Wiley-Liss, Inc.

18
Dynamic Interactions Between Lymphocytes and Vascular Endothelial Cells

ANN AGER
Immunology Group, Department of Cell and Structural Biology,
University of Manchester, Manchester M13 9PT, England

INTRODUCTION

Lymphocytes gain access to tissues directly from the blood. In so doing, the first hurdle or barrier that lymphocytes must cross is the monolayer of endothelial cells that lines all blood vessels. The distribution of lymphocytes within the body is markedly nonrandom both inside and outside lymphoid tissues. This could reflect either selective entry or specific retention of lymphocytes following random entry or indeed a combination of both. There is now a substantial body of experimental evidence that supports the selective entry of lymphocytes into tissues from the blood following molecular recognition between lymphocytes and vascular endothelial cells (EC). The process of extravasation can be divided into at least three separate stages: adhesion to the luminal surface of EC, migration of lymphocytes from the luminal to abluminal surface of EC, and detachment from EC for subsequent entry into tissues. The selection of lymphocytes could occur either at the initial adhesion step or during the subsequent migration stage.

Recent experimental evidence has identified three separate families of molecule on the lymphocyte surface that mediate adhesion to specialised postcapillary or high endothelial venules (HEV) in lymph nodes. Because of their ability to direct lymphocytes into lymph nodes (LN), these adhesion molecules have been called lymph node homing receptors (LNHR). The products of two of these three gene families are known not to be restricted to lymphocytes but are, in fact, widely distributed on all leucocytes. Since lymphocyte extravasation into all tissues, including LN, is regulated independently of other leucocytes there must be a crucial *second signal,* which mediates the selective migration of lymphocytes across vascular endothelia. This may be an as yet undiscovered adhesion molecule that is selectively expressed by lymphocytes. Alternatively, the selection of lymphocytes may occur during the process of translocation from the luminal to abluminal surface of EC. Thus lymphocyte migration would be regulated independently of adhesion to EC. An obvious prediction of this proposal is that migration would not necessarily be an automatic consequence of adhesion to the luminal surface of EC. Although lymphocytes and neutrophils may use similar molecules to adhere to EC, they would each respond to different stimuli in order to migrate out of blood vessels.

This chapter briefly reviews the distinct patterns of lymphocyte distribution around the body in order to outline the considerable heterogeneity in lymphocyte-EC interactions that underlies the specific migration of lymphocyte subsets. There are several excellent reviews of this subject, and the reader is referred to these for further information. This is followed by descriptions of two experimental animal models in which the adhesion of lymphocytes to EC in vivo is regulated independent of migration. Finally, an in vitro model is described that we have developed for the study of lymphocyte migration into LN using HEV endothelium cultured from rat LN. We have found that lymphocytes adhere to the exposed surfaces of these high endothelial cells (HEC) in a nonrandom manner. A random subpopulation of bound lymphocytes migrated between adjacent HEC to a position underneath the HEC layer. We are currently trying to determine the stimuli used by lymphocytes to migrate in this in vitro assay. It is hoped that this approach may contribute to our understanding of the mechanisms underlying the selective extravasation of lymphocytes in vivo.

DISTRIBUTION OF LYMPHOCYTES WITHIN THE BODY

Lymphocytes are a heterogeneous cell population that can be subdivided according to several different criteria, such as phenotype (T- vs. B-cells), function (T-helper vs. T-cytotoxic cells), and activation state (naive vs. memory cells). In the absence of recent antigenic stimulation, all lymphocytes are small, nondividing cells. Following antigen encounter, those lymphocytes that bear clonally distributed receptors for antigen are activated to the large cell, or lymphoblast state. After clonal expansion, these cells will differentiate into either memory cells or effector cells, such as immunoglobulin-secreting plasma cells and cytotoxic T-cells, which are ultimately involved in antigen elimination.

The distribution of lymphocytes within the body is markedly nonrandom, and it is possible to subdivide lymphocytes according to their tissue distribution. In normal individuals, the majority of all nondividing lymphocytes ($\sim 80\%$) are found in the so-called secondary lymphoid organs, the spleen and lymph nodes. A property of these cells that is unique amongst other leucocytes is that they are nomadic; they have recently migrated from the blood and, within a few hours, they will return to the blood to be distributed once again to lymphoid tissues. This process occurs constitutively in the absence of antigen and it is called lymphocyte recirculation. The continual traffic of lymphocytes through lymphoid organs optimises the chances of encounter between the low numbers of antigen specific lymphocytes in the body and antigen which is processed for presentation to lymphocytes in lymphoid tissues. In addition, it allows the distribution of cellular products of the immune response, such as memory cells and effector cells, throughout the entire immune system (1). The traffic of recirculating lymphocytes through LN in different regions of the body is not entirely random. The most marked asymmetry is seen between peripheral lymph nodes, such as the brachial and axillary lymph nodes (LN), and lymphoid tissues associated with mucosal surfaces, such as the Peyer's patches in the gut wall (2). This asymmetry is not simply restricted to the major lymphocyte subsets. There are populations of both T- and B-lymphocytes that preferentially migrate to either peripheral LN or gut associated lymphoid tissues (GALT). For example, IgA secreting plasma cells are preferentially found in Peyer's patches, and IgG secreting plasma cells are found in peripheral LN. These observations form the basis of a secretory immune system which functions in the mucosa independently of the peripheral immune system (3).

Lymphoblasts show a markedly different pattern of tissue distribution from non-dividing cells. Adoptive transfer studies of blasts in S-phase of the cell cycle show that, although they will migrate to lymphoid tissues, lymphoblasts show a predilection for nonlymphoid tissues such as the lung, liver, intestine, and skin. In general, lymphoblasts do not recirculate through lymphoid tissues as do the majority of nondividing lymphocytes. Lymphoblasts provide a particularly striking example of cells that return or home to their site of generation. Peripheral LN blasts preferentially colonise the skin and peripheral LN, whereas gut derived blasts preferentially colonise the gut and its' associated LN (4). Thus lymphoblasts are a likely source of those nondividing lymphocytes that demonstrate tissue specific homing. Lymphoblasts are known to contain precursors of effector cells, since blasts that colonise the gut wall differentiate into IgA secreting plasma cells (3). There is now substantial evidence to support the view that tissue-specific migration is restricted to those lymphocytes that have already responded to antigen, i.e., memory and effector cells (5).

Adoptive transfer studies of nondividing lymphocytes to normal recipients have shown that lymphocytes will localise in nonlymphoid tissues in significant but lower numbers than those entering lymphoid tissues on a weight basis; these tissues are those with extensive mucosal surfaces that are potential sites of antigen entry such as the lungs, liver, intestine, and skin. Lymphocytes collected from afferent lymphatics draining a skin site in the sheep have a substantially different phenotype and function from those recirculating through lymphoid tissues (6). Whether this is true for lymphocytes that enter other nonlymphoid organs remains to be determined. In addition, it cannot be concluded from this experimental animal model that lymphocyte entry into nonlymphoid tissues is a constitutive process entirely independent of antigen, since these animals were not maintained in a germ free environment.

There are other subpopulations of lymphocytes that demonstrate distinct patterns of tissue distribution. The intraepithelial lymphocyte is found in the mucosal lining of the gut (7) and in mice cells bearing the $\gamma\delta$ T-cell receptor (TCR) are found in the gut mucosa (8) as well as in the skin (9). Neither of these lymphocyte populations fits into the category of the majority of B-cells and T-cells (bearing the $\alpha\beta$ TCR), which have the capacity to recirculate through lymphoid tissues; thus, these lymphocytes may function in an entirely different manner. For example, they may be effector cells that are unable to undergo further clonal expansion and differentiation into memory cells. They would therefore not need to recirculate through lymphoid tissues and would be distributed at sites of potential antigen penetration such as the skin and mucosal surfaces.

The level of lymphocyte migration into nonlymphoid tissues is dramatically increased during inflammation. The entry of different lymphocyte subsets appears to be tightly regulated and is exquisitely dependent on the nature of the inflammatory response [for review, see Parrot and Wilkinson (10)]. For example, increased numbers of lymphoblasts will enter sites of inflammation in the skin irrespective of whether the inflammatory stimulus is immune or nonimmune. If the inflammatory stimulus elicits a local cell-mediated immune response, blast cell entry is followed by the entry of nondividing lymphocytes such as in delayed type hypersensitivity lesions to recall antigens and in organ allografts undergoing rejection. The relationship between these infiltrating lymphocytes and lymphocytes that recirculate through lymphoid tissues remains to be determined. However, blood vessels with the characteristic morphology of HEV have been reported at sites of chronic inflammation, which suggests that recirculating cells may enter these nonlymphoid sites. In so doing, they may use *recognition molecules,* which are related to those used for LN entry (11). A crucial step in the chronicity of inflammation may be the ability of EC to respond to local environmental stimuli in order to recruit recirculating lymphocytes from the blood. It will therefore be important to determine the signals required for the induction and maintenance of HEV phenotype and function in blood vessels outside of lymph nodes (see Chapter 21).

MOLECULAR RECOGNITION BETWEEN LYMPHOCYTES AND ENDOTHELIAL CELLS

The interaction between lymphocytes and high endothelial venule (HEV) endothelium that controls entry into LN has been studied extensively, and more is known about lymphocyte–endothelial interactions in LN than in any other organ. The adhesion of lymphocytes to HEV has been studied in vitro using the frozen section assay in which lymphocytes selectively adhere to the cross-sectional areas of HEV in sectioned LN at low temperatures. This assay provided the first demonstration that the extent of lymphocyte migration into LN could be explained by the large numbers of lymphocytes that adhere to these specialised blood vessels rather than to other blood vessels. The nonrandom distribution of lymphocytes between peripheral LN and GALT seen in vivo is demonstrable in vitro using the frozen section assay. A crucial observation was that lymphomas preferentially bind to HEV in either peripheral LN or Peyer's patches strictly according to their tissue specific migration pathways in vivo. It was therefore proposed that separate sets of recognition molecules mediate lymphocyte migration into either peripheral LN or GALT (2).

Using the frozen section assay, three separate families of molecule on the lymphocyte surface have now been shown to mediate tissue specific adhesion to HEV in either peripheral LN or Peyer's patches. Because of their ability to direct the migration or homing of lymphocytes, they have been called lymph node homing receptors (LNHR). Other molecules on the lymphocyte surface have been shown to mediate adhesion in the frozen section assay, although they operate in a nontissue specific manner, such as LFA-1; they are thus thought to function as accessory molecules (12,13). A natural prediction from these observations is that HEV express ligands for LNHR in a tissue specific manner. Recently, several HEV-specific antigens have been identified that are expressed either in peripheral LN or in GALT, some of which mediate adhesion in the frozen section assay. Because of their ability to direct the homing of lymphocytes to specific lymphoid organs they have been called vascular addressins. The identities and distribution of LNHR and vascular addressins have been reviewed recently in several articles (14,15) and are not discussed in detail here. The gene for a molecule with significant homology to the mouse peripheral LNHR defined by MEL-14 has recently been cloned and sequenced from a human cDNA library (16). It appears to be the pan-leucocyte antigen Leu8 (17).

The distribution of vascular addressins described thus far is specific for HEV under basal conditions. However, LNHR are expressed on leucocytes other than lymphocytes and thus at first sight this proposed receptor–ligand interaction does not explain the selective extravasation of lymphocytes into LN. For example the MEL-14 antigen is expressed by neutrophils, although it is somewhat larger at 100 kd instead of the 90-kd form found on lymphocytes (18). In fact, Lewinsohn et al. have shown that neutrophils adhere to HEV in the frozen section assay via cell surface MEL-14 antigen (18). However, neutrophils do not constitutively migrate across HEV in vivo. The CD44 molecule is expressed by all haemopoietic cells, although post-translational modification gives rise to multiple forms of this molecule (19). If there are lymphocyte specific forms of these molecules, recognition between a homing receptor on the lymphocyte surface and its ligand, a vascular addressin, selectively expressed by HEV could explain the selective extravasation of lymphocytes into LN. It can be envisaged that coupling of a LNHR to the lymphocyte cytoskeleton following ligand engagement could result in stimulated lymphocyte motility. Apart from presenting a vascular addressin, HEV would function as a passive partner in the extravasation of lymphocytes. If there are no distinct forms of LNHR on lymphocytes, alternative recognition events will have to be considered to explain the selective entry of lymphocytes into LN. One possibility is that the adhesion of lymphocytes to EC should be considered independent of the subsequent migration of lymphocytes. It then becomes possible to propose a lymphocyte specific migration stimulus emanating either from the vascular endothelium directly or from it's immediate environment. Although there is no direct evidence to support this proposal, there is substantial indirect evidence to implicate either the EC and/or it's microenvironment in lymphocyte extravasation.

As described in Chapter 17, HEV are lined with a type of activated endothelium. These high endothelial cells (HEC) are an extremely heterogeneous population of cells. Systematic studies of HEV in sections of LN have shown that there are preferred or "hot" spots of lymphocyte extravasation within the HEV network (20). It is possible that vascular addressins are expressed at higher levels in these areas. Alternatively, HEC may secrete higher levels of a lymphocyte migration stimulus that directs the movement of lymphocytes, i.e., a chemotactic or haptotactic factor. A possible role for secreted HEC products in lymphocyte extravasation is supported by the observation that the orientation of Golgi apparatus within HEC is preferentially directed towards migrating lymphocytes (21). In addition, HEC constitutively secrete a sulphated glycoconjugate, probably a glycolipid, at the luminal surface. This metabolic pathway is not readily identifiable in non-HEV or "flat" EC and thus has been proposed to function during lymphocyte extravasation (22). More recently the identification of IL-8 as a chemotactic factor for lymphocytes and its production by cytokine-activated EC introduces a further possible candidate for the proposed lymphocyte migration stimulus. However, IL-8 also has powerful effects on neutrophil migration both in vivo and in vitro and thus may not demonstrate absolute specificity for lymphocytes, although there is evidence to support this (23).

There are two experimental animal models that demonstrate clearly that lymphocyte migration is not an automatic consequence of adhesion to the luminal surface of HEV in vivo. The dynamic interactions between fluorescently labelled lymphocytes and HEV in Peyer's patches of the mouse have been recorded by time-lapse video microscopy. In this study, Bjerknes et al. (24) found that following adhesion to the luminal surface of HEV lymphocytes either detached or they migrated across the blood vessel wall. A careful statistical analysis demonstrated that some lymphocytes underwent multiple attachments in series and the greater the number of attachments the greater the chances of extravasation. However, following detachment, some lymphocytes were carried away from the node via the blood. Thus, there are multiple types of lymphocyte adhesion to HEC, and migration is not an automatic consequence of all types of adhesive events. Presumably the adhesive interaction has to be of sufficient affinity to either engage the lymphocyte cytoskeleton directly or to hold the lymphocyte long enough in order to receive a "second signal" that allows the lymphocyte to proceed to the migration stage.

The second model involves the permanent ligation of afferent lymphatics that drain cells and fluid into a LN from the surrounding tissues. This operation has dramatic effects on the phenotype and function of HEV, which have been described in detail in Chapter 21. Briefly, over a 6-week period following deafferentisation, HEC lose their cuboidal morphology and adopt the morphology of "flat" EC lining non-HEV blood vessels (21). There is a dramatic reduction in the level of lymphocyte extravasation from these blood vessels, which falls to 2% of control levels 6 weeks after deafferentisation (25). Hendricks *et al.* have measured the adhesion of lymphocytes to HEV in deafferentisated LN using the frozen section assay and found that there is a time-dependent reduction in lymphocyte adhesion. However, 6 weeks after operation lymphocyte adhesion was still significant at 25% of control levels (26). At this time, lymphocyte migration into these operated LN was reduced to 2% of control levels in vivo (25). Thus, although lymphocytes bound reasonably well to HEV in vitro, they did not migrate across the vessel wall in vivo. A possible explanation for these results is that the proposed lymphocyte migration stimulus is either missing or too low in deafferentisated LN to support the actual extravasation of lymphocytes. The source of such a stimulus could either be HEC directly or the LN microenvironment immediately surrounding HEV.

AN IN VITRO MODEL OF LYMPHOCYTE EXTRAVASATION INTO LYMPH NODES

The precise role of HEV endothelium in lymphocyte extravasation is poorly understood, since these cells are not viable in the frozen section assay. In order to study the contribution of the vascular endothelium to lymphocyte extravasation, we have chosen an in vitro model using cultured vascular endothelial cells. In particular, we have established lines of HEV endothelium from rat lymph nodes for this work [see Ager (27) and Chapter 21]. The interaction between lymphocytes and flat endothelial cells cultured from nonlymphoid tissues, such as umbilical vein, have been studied by other groups. Where appropriate these results will be contrasted and compared with those we have obtained using cultured high endothelial cells (HEC).

We have found that recirculating lymphocytes adhered to the exposed surfaces of cultured HEC in a nonrandom manner. Following adhesion a random subpopulation of lymphocytes actively migrated between adjacent HEC to a position underneath the endothelial layer. Cultured HEC bound recirculating lymphocytes at 50-fold higher levels than flat, non-HEV EC and at 15-fold higher levels than nonendothelial cells. The directional movement of lymphocytes only occurred in cultures of HEC. It is proposed that cultured HEC provides a new in vitro model of lymphocyte migration into LN from the blood. It should be possible to study the regulation of vascular addressin expression by HEC and the directional migration of lymphocytes in this in vitro model.

Interactions Between Recirculating Lymphocytes and Cultured High Endothelial Cells

These results have been described in detail (28). Briefly, recirculating lymphocytes were collected from the thoracic ducts of rats and plated on top of monolayer cultures of HEC in 8-well chamber slides for 60 min at 37°C. After removal of nonaherent lymphocytes by vigorous washing, all remaining lymphocytes were bound to cultured HEC. Lymphocytes were not attached to uncovered areas of the glass slide. Phase-contrast microscope analysis of HEC-adherent lymphocytes revealed two populations of cells. The first population (type I) was phase-light and round and the second population (type II) was phase dark (Fig. 1A). The morphology of type I cells was identical to that of lymphocytes in suspension. Type I and type II lymphocytes were readily distinguished from one another by light microscope analysis of fixed and stained preparations. Type I lymphocytes had an average diameter of 4 μm. Staining with toluidine blue did not reveal any intracellular detail, rather, type I lymphocytes were stained a uniform blue. Type II lymphocytes were large, flat cells with an average diameter of 7 μm. The nucleus and a rim of cytoplasm were clearly visible in type II cells after toluidine blue staining. Because of the marked differences in morphology between type I and type II cells it was possible that type II lymphocytes had flattened on to the exposed surfaces of HEC. Alternatively, they could be between HEC and the tissue culture dish where a flattened morphology was adopted due to lack of space.

The question of whether type II lymphocytes were on top of or below HEC was answered definitively using scanning electron microscopy. All cells bound to the exposed surface of HEC were spherical, type I lymphocytes. These cells had an average diameter of 4 μm and had numerous microvilli distributed over their surfaces (Fig. 1B). Type II lymphocytes were not seen bound to HEC surfaces in scanning electron micrographs. Characteristic crescent shaped defects were seen in HEC cytoplasm. Through these defects type II lymphocytes were clearly visible underneath HEC. In contrast to type I cells, type II lymphocytes were smooth surfaced,

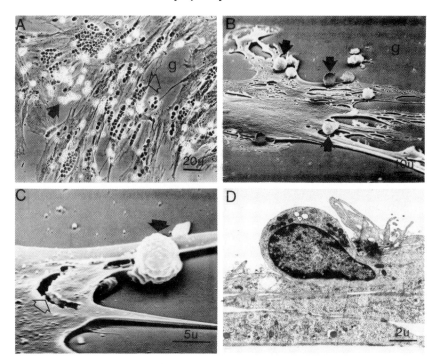

Fig. 1.   Interaction of thoracic duct lymphocytes with cultured high endothelial cells. **A:** Phase-contrast micrograph of TDL bound to HEC. Lymphocytes adhered selectively to HEC and not to serum coated glass (g). Two populations of lymphocytes were seen: type I cells, which are phase-light and round (closed arrow), and type II lymphocytes which are phase-dark (open arrow). Bar: 20 μm. ×500. **B:** Scanning electron micrograph showing numerous type I lymphocytes bound to the exposed surface of HEC (closed arrows). Bar: 10 μm. ×1,000. **C:** Scanning electron micrograph in which a type II, flattened lymphocyte can be seen underneath HEC through a characteristic crescent-shaped defect in HEC cytoplasm (open arrow). A type I lymphocyte bound to the surface of HEC is also visible (closed arrow). Bar: 5 μm. ×400. **D:** Transmission electron micrograph of a lymphocyte migrating across HEC. The lymphocyte has an organelle-free, protruding pseudopod between overlapping layers of HEC cytoplasm. Bar: 2 μm. ×7,950.

presumably following retraction of their microvilli. Type II lymphocytes were flattened between HEC and the culture support up to an average diameter of 7 μm and a maximum thickness of 2 μm (Fig. 1C). Further analysis by electron microscopy showed that lymphocytes partially underneath HEC had an organelle-free, protruding pseudopod which was between overlapping layers of HEC cytoplasm (Fig. 1D). The disappearance of microvilli from the surface of type II lymphocytes and the redistribution of organelles in these cells suggested that the lymphocyte actively migrated in this assay. The transition from type I to type II was confined to those lymphocytes that migrated to a position underneath the HEC monolayer. This will be referred to as lymphocyte migration across cultured HEC. Experiments were designed to identify these two lymphocyte populations in order to determine their relationship.

Differential Adhesion of Lymphocytes to Cultured Vascular Cells

Lymphocyte adhesion to cultured HEC was compared directly with adhesion to non-HEV endothelial cells and to nonendothelial cells. Using fixed and stained preparations type I, spherical lymphocytes were readily distinguished from type II, flattened cells by high-power light microscopy. The number of lymphocytes bound was expressed as a percentage of the lymphocytes plated. For a direct comparison of lymphocyte adhesion to these three cell types, the results were expressed per mg of cultured cell protein to accommodate differences in cell size.

The results in Figure 2A show that lymphocyte adhesion to cultured HEC was 50-fold higher than that to aortic endothelial cells and 15-fold higher than that to aortic adventital fibroblasts. The number of type II, migrated lymphocytes was expressed as a fraction of total bound lymphocytes (types I + II) to give the lymphocyte migration index. After 60 min incubation 25% of HEC-adherent lymphocytes were underneath the endothelial layer. Of the low numbers of lymphocytes bound to aortic endothelial cells, all were type I, spherical cells. Type II, flattened lymphocytes were not found. Similarly, all lymphocytes bound to aortic fibroblasts were of the type I, spherical morphology (Fig. 2B).

Cultured HEC constitutively expressed "adhesion molecules" for recirculating lymphocytes at 50-fold higher levels than either non-HEV endothelial cells or nonendothelial cells in culture. Although cell types other than HEC supported low levels of lymphocyte adhesion, they did not support the migration of lymphocytes from their upper to lower surfaces as found using cultured HEC. The nature of the proposed adhesion molecules expressed by cultured HEC is unknown. Increased adhesion of lymphocytes to HEC could reflect increased expression of vascular addressins. Alternatively, increased adhesion to HEC could reflect the absence of an endogenous inhibitor of lymphocyte adhesion in comparison with other vascular cells. For convenience, I will refer to the expression of adhesion molecules by cultured HEC to account for differential levels of lymphocyte adhesion. However, it should be borne in mind that lymphocyte adhesion in this assay may be controlled by more than one type of molecule.

Effects of Cytokines on Lymphocyte–Endothelial Cell Interactions

Lymphocyte adhesion to non-HEV endothelial cells is stimulated above basal levels following preincubation of EC with a range of inflammatory cytokines. Haskard et al. have reported that T-cell adhesion to human

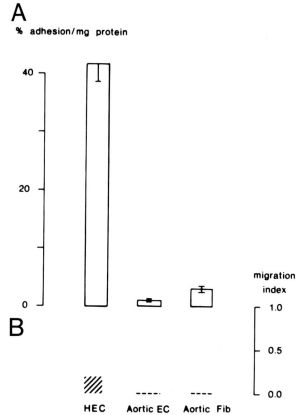

Fig. 2. Interactions of thoracic duct lymphocytes with cultured vascular cells. **A:** The total number of lymphocytes bound (types I and II) per vascular cell was measured by light microscopy and expressed as a percentage of the lymphocyte number plated. Results were expressed per mg of vascular cell protein for direct comparison with HEC. **B:** The number of type II, migrated lymphocytes was expressed as a fraction of total bound cells (types I and II) to give the lymphocyte migration index.

umbilical vein endothelial cells (HUVEC) was maximally elevated by two-fold following a 4-hr incubation of EC with either interleukin 1 (IL-1) or tumour necrosis factor (TNF). Lymphocyte adhesion was also elevated by pretreatment of HUVEC with interferon (IFN)-γ. Effects were detectable within 4 hr, although they were not maximal until 24 hr of treatment. Increased lymphocyte adhesion in this model was dependent on *de novo* synthesis of adhesion molecules by HUVEC. Although their identities are not yet determined, the increased adhesion of T-cells to cytokine-activated HUVEC was not mediated by LFA-1/ICAM1 or 2 interactions as found for lymphocyte adhesion to unstimulated HUVEC (29). These workers propose that cytokine-activated HUVEC provides an in vitro model of vascular endothelium in inflamed nonlymphoid tissues.

In a rat model, Hughes *et al.* have shown that pretreatment of brain capillary EC with either human rTNF or rat rIFN-gamma increased the adhesion of lymphocytes. The effects were detectable within 4 hr of treating EC although the effect of IFN-γ was not maximal until after 24 hr. There was some overlap between the effects of TNF and IFN-γ, since pretreatment with a combination of the two gave less than additive effects. Pretreatment of rat brain capillary EC with either human rIL-1α or β for ≤ 3 days had no effect on lymphocyte adhesion. Adhesion to IFN γ activated EC was reduced to basal levels of adhesion by MRC-OX42, a mouse monoclonal antibody against complement receptor 3. The effect of OX42 on basal lymphocyte adhesion was not reported; thus, it cannot be concluded that the blocking activity of OX42 was restricted to the cytokine inducible component. This conclusion is substantiated by the fact that although OX42 antigen was detected in low amounts on rat brain capillary EC, the level was not affected by IFN-γ treatment (30).

The fact that lymphocyte adhesion to HEC was 50-fold higher than to aortic EC prompted the question whether the elevated adhesion of lymphocytes to HEC was mediated by cytokine action on HEC. Since HEC were isolated from antigen activated LN and primary LN cultures were "contaminated" for up to 10 days with lymph node macrophages (27) the possible presence of macrophage derived cytokines, such as IL-1 and TNF, in HEC cultures must be considered. The fact that there was a differential adhesion of lymphocytes to HEC and aortic EC suggested that adhesion was not simply mediated by endotoxin activation of vascular cells (29), since all cells were maintained in identical stocks of growth media.

Media conditioned for 4–5 days by primary LN cultures ($\geq 70\%$ HEC), subcultured HEC ($\geq 95\%$ purity) and adventitial fibroblasts were collected and screened for either IL-1 or TNF activity. Using an IL-1 dependent subclone of the D10.G4 cell line, media conditioned by primary LN cultures significantly reduced the uptake of ^{3}H-thymidine in comparison with control growth media (RPMI 1640 plus 20% FCS) from 1,500 cpm to 200 cpm. Media conditioned by either subcultured HEC lines or adventitial fibroblasts had no effect on proliferation of D10.G4 cells. Thus IL-1 activity was not detectable in cultures of rat HEC at any stage of culture. TNF activity in conditioned media was assayed by monitoring killing of L929 cells in the presence of actinomycin D. TNF activity was below the threshold of detection at < 20 U/ml in all media tested. Thus TNF activity was not present in either primary LN cultures or subcultures of HEC. IFN-γ activity was not assayed directly. In a separate study, prolonged incubation (≥ 9 days) with 100 U/ml IFN-γ significantly inhibited HEC proliferation (see Chapter 21). The inclusion of a mouse monoclonal antibody to rat IFN-γ had no significant effect on the proliferation of HEC over a period of 9 days, indicating that high levels of IFN-γ activity were not present in cultures of HEC. The lack of readily detectable IL-1, TNF, or IFN-γ in cultures of HEC suggests that the high level of lymphocyte adhesion to HEC we have measured is independent of cytokine activity. Interestingly, the 50-fold higher level of lymphocyte adhesion to HEC over flat EC is much greater than the published increases in lymphocyte adhesion to flat EC after cytokine treatment, which are a maximum of two- to four-fold.

In Chapter 21, it has been proposed that cultured HEC constitutively express the phenotype of cytokine activated, flat or non-HEV endothelial cells in a cytokine independent manner. In order to determine the relationship between HEC and flat EC, we have asked whether HEC demonstrate a cytokine inducible component of lymphocyte adhesion similar to that shown by flat EC. The effects of cytokines on the adhesion of thoracic duct lymphocytes to cultured HEC were studied directly. In these experiments, total lymphocyte adhesion to cultured HEC was quantitated using radiolabelled lymphocytes. This radioassay does not allow type I, surface bound and type II, migrated lymphocytes to be quantitated separately. Briefly, HEC were plated in 24-well cluster plates at subconfluent density and incubated for up to 3 days with either control media (RPMI 1640 plus 5% FCS) or test media. Incubation media were removed and 5×10^6 ^{3}H-leucine labelled lymphocytes in either control (RPMI 1640 plus 1% FCS) or test media were plated per well. After 60 min at 37°C nonadherent cells were removed by vigorous washing and the HEC layer plus adherent lymphocytes were solubilised in 1 M NH_4OH for liquid scintillation counting. A direct comparison with the microscope assay showed that the number of lymphocytes bound was directly proportional to radioactivity associated with the HEC layer. Results were expressed as a percentage of total radioactivity plated. To accommodate possible effects of the various pretreatments on HEC proliferation, the number of HEC was determined at the end of each experiment by electronic particle counting after detachment using trypsin:EDTA. For comparison between experiments, results were expressed as percentage lymphocyte adhesion per 10^5 HEC (number of HEC per well at confluence). There was considerable variation between the absolute level of lymphocyte adhesion to HEC between experiments. The effects of cytokines were therefore expressed relative to untreated HEC to give fold increases in lymphocyte adhesion.

Human recombinant IL-1α up to 17.5 U/ml had no effect on lymphocyte adhesion when included in the assay. Pretreatment of rat HEC with 17.5 U/ml human rIL-1α for 4, 24, or 72 hr were also without effect on lymphocyte adhesion (Fig 3). Pretreatment of HEC with 200 U/ml human rTNF-α significantly stimulated lymphocyte adhesion in a time-dependent manner; however, the effects were small. After pretreatment for 24 hr, adhesion was increased 1.09-fold and after 72 hr adhesion was a little higher at 1.26-fold (Fig. 3). The stimulatory effect of TNF-α was not detectable after 4 hr pretreatment of HEC. TNF-α was also without effect on lymphocyte adhesion when included in the assay. Pretreatment of HEC with 200 U/ml rat rIFN-γ significantly stimulated lymphocyte adhesion, but only after prolonged pretreatment for 72 hr. The level of stimulation was considerably variable between experiments, ranging from 1.1- to 2.0-fold. Pretreatment with IFN-γ for shorter periods was either without effect (≤ 100 U/ml for 4 hr) or significantly reduced lymphocyte adhesion (200 U/ml for 24 hr) in comparison with untreated controls (Fig. 3). The combined effects of TNFα and IFN-γ on HEC were synergistic rather than additive. When HEC were pretreated for 3 days with a mixture of TNF and IFN-γ, both at 200 U/ml, lymphocyte adhesion was increased by an average of 3.29-

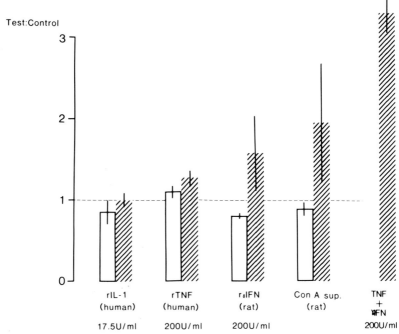

Fig. 3. Effect of cytokine pretreatment of high endothelial cells on the adhesion of thoracic duct lymphocytes. HEC were plated at 3×10^4/15-mm-diameter well and preincubated in triplicate for either 1 (open bars) or 3 (hatched bars) days with cytokines as shown. Preincubation media were removed and the adhesion of ^{3}H-leucine-labelled TDL was measured after 60 min at 37°C. Results were expressed relative to control HEC, which were either pretreated in control media (for effects of IL-1, TNFα and IFN-γ) or in media conditioned by unstimulated LNC (for effects of Con A supernatants). Results are mean $\pm$SD. (4–6).

fold. This was a consistent observation in three separate experiments in which lymphocyte adhesion to pretreated HEC ranged from 2.9- to 3.6-fold higher than to untreated HEC. If the effects of these two cytokines were additive the combination would increase adhesion by 2.1-fold, which is significantly less than the actual increase measured.

To investigate the effects of rat lymphokines other than IFN-γ, HEC were pretreated for 1–3 days with media conditioned by either un-stimulated or mitogen pulsed lymph node cells (LNC), prepared as previously described (see Chapter 21). Lymphocyte adhesion to HEC pretreated with media conditioned by Con A pulsed LNC (Con A LNC media) was compared directly with that to HEC pretreated with media conditioned by unstimulated LNC (LNC media). As shown in Figure 3, the effects of Con A LNC media were similar to those of IFN-γ. Lymphocyte adhesion was stimulated but only after prolonged (3 days) pretreatment of HEC. The level of stimulation varied considerably between experiments from 1.1 to 2.5-fold. Lymphocyte adhesion to HEC was slightly but significantly inhibited after 24-hr incubation in Con A LNC media at 87% of the level of adhesion to HEC incubated in control LNC media. It has already been reported that media conditioned by LNC had a marked inhibitory effect on HEC proliferation; this effect was independent of mitogen activation (Chapter 21). Lymphocyte adhesion to HEC pretreated with LNC media was therefore compared directly with adhesion to untreated HEC in the same experiment. In five separate experiments, pretreatment of HEC with LNC media consistently increased lymphocyte adhesion. The effect was detectable after 24 hr and was consistent at 72 hr at 1.48-fold and 1.67-fold, respectively. For example, in one experiment lymphocyte adhesion to un-treated HEC was 11.3%. It was increased to 23.0% after 3 days preincubation of HEC in LNC media. Adhesion was higher at 31.8% after 3 days incubation in Con A LNC media.

As previously reported for human and rat non-HEV endothelial cells, lymphocyte adhesion to cultured HEC can be upregulated by pretreatment of HEC with various cytokines. However there were marked differences between HEC and flat EC with respect to both time course and magnitude of effects using individual cytokines. Although IL-1 rapidly induced the expression of adhesion molecules on human EC, this cytokine had no efect on rat EC, either brain capillary EC or HEC. The lack of effect of human IL-1 on rat cells did not appear to be due to species specificity of action, although these results should be confirmed with rat IL-1. TNF stimulated lymphocyte adhesion to HEC, but the effects were smaller and later in onset (>24 hr) than were those reported for other types of EC. Thus, lymphocyte adhesion molecules are not rapidly inducible (within 4 hr) on HEC by inflammatory cytokines as is the case for non-HEV endothelium. This may reflect the fact that HEC represents a type of cytokine activated endothelium, as discussed previously, and as such the expression of cytokine inducible lymphocyte adhesion molecules is already maximally upregulated. In this context, it is noteworthy that an early-onset increase in lymphocyte adhesion (detectable by 24 hr) was not stimulated by IFN-γ pretreatment of HEC, as has been shown in flat EC. However, there was a substantial late-onset effect of IFN-γ, which was clearly detectable after 72-hr pretreatment of HEC. Late-onset effects similar to IFN-γ were also demonstrable in supernatants collected from con A pulsed LNC, which have been shown to contain significant amounts of IFN-γ. In the absence of mitogen activation, LNC also secreted nondialysable factors that upregulated the expression of lymphocyte adhesion molecules by HEC. This activity was distinct from that of either IFN-γ, since it's effect was detectable within 24 hr, or TNF, since it's effect was equal after 24 and 72 hr pretreatment.

Effect of Cytokines on Lymphocyte Migration Across Cultured High Endothelial Cells

The interactions of type I, surface bound lymphocytes and type II, migrated lymphocytes with resting and cytokine activated HEC were compared, to determine if they were regulated independently. Cultured HEC were pretreated for 3 days with the following: control media (RPMI 1640 plus 5% FCS); a mixture of TNFα and IFN-γ, both at 200 U/ml; LNC media; Con A LNC media. After removal of incubation media, lymphocyte adhesion was measured after 60 min at 37°C by microscope analysis. In order to determine whether cytokine activation of HEC altered the distribution of lymphocytes above and below the endothelial layer, the adherent cells were separated into type I, surface bound and type II, migrated cells and the migration index calculated as previously described. By directly comparing migration indices it is possible to determine whether type I and type II lymphocytes were equally effected by cytokine activation of HEC.

Quantitation of total lymphocyte adhesion by microscope analysis gave similar results to those obtained using radiolabelled lymphocytes. Lymphocyte adhesion to cultured HEC was increased following pretreatment for 3 days with a TNFα/IFN-γ mixture, LNC media and Con A LNC media, although the effects were greater than those measured previously using the radioassay (Table I). The lymphocyte migration index in untreated HEC was an average of 0.21 + 0.15 (± SD, n = 11). Thus after 60 min incubation, 21% of total bound lymphocytes were underneath the endothelial layer. Of the total cells bound to TNF/IFN-treated HEC, a slightly higher percentage were underneath the endothelial layer after 60 min incubation with a migration index of 0.29 ± 0.14 (±SD, n = 12). Similarly, HEC pretreated with LNC media supported increased lymphocyte migration over untreated HEC. For example, in one experiment, the migration index was increased twofold from 0.19 to 0.40. Con A LNC media pretreatment of HEC also stimulated lymphocyte migration, but to a lesser extent;

TABLE I. Relative Adhesion of Thoracic Duct Lymphocytes to Cytokine-Pretreated High Endothelial Cells [a]

	Fold increase in lymphocyte adhesion	
	Radioassay	Microscope assay
TNF/IFN	3.29 + 0.32 (4)	4.87 + 2.38 (11)
LNC media	1.67 + 0.33 (11)	4.50 + 1.37 (3)
Con A LNC media	2.58 + 1.00 (11)	6.35 + 0.70 (3)

[a]HEC were pretreated for 3 days with the following: control media (RPMI 1640 plus 5% FCS); a TNFα/IFN-γ mixture; LNC media; Con A LNC media. Preincubation media were removed and lymphocyte adhesion was measured as described in the legend to Figure 3. Results were expressed relative to HEC pretreated with control media to give fold increases. Results are means ±SD (4–11).

in the same experiment, the migration index was increased from 0.19 to 0.30. Since lymphocyte adhesion assays were performed in the absence of pretreatment media, these results show that activation of HEC by cytokines increases the absolute level of expression of adhesion molecules. However, activation of HEC by cytokines had a greater effect on the interaction of those lymphocytes that migrate from the upper to lower surfaces in this assay.

In a separate series of experiments (28), phenotypic analyses of adherent lymphocytes using subset specific antibodies has shown that the adhesion of lymphocytes subsets (B-cells vs. CD4+ T-cells vs. CD8+ T-cells) is a nonrandom process. However, the distribution of these lymphocyte subsets above and below the endothelial layer were not significantly different. This suggests that type II, migrated cells are a random subpopulation of total bound cells. Although the signals for migration have not been identified in this assay, the interaction of lymphocytes with cytokine activated HEC clearly show that the proportion of those lymphocytes that migrate underneath the HEC layer can be directly controlled by high endothelial cells.

Differential Adhesion of Lymphocyte Subsets to Cultured High Endothelial Cells

We have already reported that adhesion of lymphocytes to HEC is a nonrandom process. Immunocytochemical analysis of HEC-adherent lymphocytes showed that B-cells were enriched over T-cells and in the adherent T-cell fraction CD8+ cells were enriched over CD4+ cells (28). This nonrandom adhesion of lymphocytes was investigated further by studying the relative adhesion of purified populations of lymphocyte subsets. In these experiments, B-cells, CD4+ T-cells and CD8+ T-cells were purified from thoracic duct lymphocytes by depletion using mouse anti-rat subset specific monoclonal antibodies to label the unwanted subsets (W3/25 for CD4+-cells; OX-8 for CD8+-cells; OX6 and OX12 for B-cells) and immunomagnetic beads coated with goat anti-mouse immunoglobulin to remove antibody coated cells. Isolated subsets were checked for purity using FITC-conjugated mouse anti-rat subset specific monoclonal antibodies and for contamination using FITC-sheep anti-mouse immunoglobulin. Contaminating cells were <5% and purity >95% in the following experiments. Lymphocytes were labelled with ^{3}H-leucine and the adhesion of each lymphocyte subset was compared directly with the adhesion of unseparated cells in individual experiments. The ratio of purified lymphocyte subset adhesion to unseparated lymphocyte adhesion was calculated to permit direct comparisons between individual experiments.

The adhesion of unseparated cells was consistent in three experiments, ranging from 9.0% to 11.3%. When compared directly with adhesion of unseparated cells in the same experiment the results in Table II show that B-cell and CD8+ T-cell adhesion were both greater at 163% and 135%, respectively. The adhesion of CD4+ T-cells was much lower at 14% of unseparated cells. Thus, cultured HEC express adhesion molecules for B-cells and CD8+ T-cells at 11.0-fold and 9.0-fold higher levels, respectively, than those for CD4 + T-cells. The relative adhesion of purified lymphocyte subsets are in good agreement with those previously reported using the microscope assay to analyse HEC-adherent cells using unseparated lymphocyte populations (28). This suggests that the adhesion of each of these three lymphocyte subsets is regulated independently of one another. It is proposed that the adhesion of B-cells, CD4+ T-cells, and CD8+ T-cells is controlled by the expression of subset specific adhesion molecules on the surface of HEC. The low level of CD4+ T-cell adhesion to cultured HEC is somewhat surprising, particularly because the percentage of CD4+ T-cells in cervical LN (from which HEC were cultured) is similar to that in peripheral blood at 37% and 31%, respectively. Since we have already reported the loss of an activated phenotype in HEC, as they

TABLE II. Relative Adhesion of Lymphocyte Subsets to High Endothelial Cells[a]

	% Lymphocyte adhesion		Ratio separated: unseparated
	Unseparated TDL	Separated TDL	
B	10.13	16.54	1.63
CD8+	9.03	12.22	1.35
CD4+	11.26	1.63	0.14

[a]B-cells, CD4+ T-cells and CD8+ T-cells were purified from TDL by depletion of unwanted subsets and the adhesion of purified subsets compared directly with unseparated TDL in the same experiment using ^{3}H-leucine labelled lymphocytes. Results are percentage lymphocyte adhesion/10^5 HEC (mean of three observations, SD ≤10%). The ratio of separated to unseparated cells was calculated.

are held in vitro in the absence of a LN microenvironment (Chapter 21), it is possible that cultured HEC have selectively down-regulated the expression of adhesion molecules for CD4+ T-cells in comparison with those for CD8+ T-cells and B-cells. Cytokine pretreatment of HEC increased the total expression of lymphocyte adhesion molecules. We have therefore investigated whether cytokine pretreatment of HEC had differential effects on the expression of subset-specific adhesion molecules. For these experiments, HEC were pretreated for 3 days with a mixture of TNFα and IFN-γ, both at 200 U/ml, and the cytokines removed before measuring the adhesion of each lymphocyte subset in comparison with unseparated cells as described above.

As shown in Tables III–V and described in Figure 3, unseparated lymphocyte adhesion was increased threefold following pretreatment of HEC with a TNF/IFN mixture. The adhesion of all three lymphocyte subsets was increased but to different extents. For example, in one experiment the adhesion of TDL to cytokine activated HEC was 2.64-fold that to untreated HEC, whereas the adhesion of CD4+ T-cells was greater at 4.52-fold (Table III). In comparison, the increase in CD8+ T-cell adhesion to cytokine activated HEC was less than that of unseparated cells at 2.92-fold and 3.72-fold, respectively (Table IV). Similarly, the increase in B cell adhesion to cytokine activated HEC was less than that of unseparated cells at 2.35-fold and 3.65-fold, respectively (Table V). However, in spite of differential effects on the adhesion of lymphocyte subsets, the relative adhesion of CD4+ T-cells to cytokine activated HEC was still fourfold lower than that of CD8+ T-cells and B-cells (which were now equal at 105% of unseparated cells).

The identities of the proposed adhesion molecules remains to be determined. However, there are several possible explanations for the differential adhesion of lymphocyte subsets to cultured HEC. Either there are separate families of LNHR and vascular addressins that independently

TABLE III. Relative Adhesion of CD4+ T-Cells to Resting and Cytokine-Activated High Endothelial Cells[a]

	% Lymphocyte adhesion		Ratio separated: unseparated
	Unseparated TDL	Separated CD4+ T-cells	
Control	6.89 ± 0.44	1.00 ± 0.12	0.14
TNF/IFN	18.19 ± 0.88	4.52 ± 0.29	0.25
Fold increase	2.64	4.52	

[a]HEC were pretreated for 3 days with either control media or a TNFα/IFN-γ mixture before measuring the adhesion of unseparated TDL and CD4+ T-cells. Results are percentage lymphocyte adhesion ±SD (3). The ratio of separated to unseparated cells and fold increases in the adhesion of either unseparated or separated TDL after cytokine pretreatment are presented.

TABLE IV. Relative Adhesion of CD8+ T-Cells to Resting and Cytokine–Activated High Endothelial Cells[a]

	% Lymphocyte adhesion		Ratio separated: unseparated
	Unseparated TDL	Separated CD8+ T-cells	
Control	5.58 + 0.07	7.55 + 0.54	1.35
TNF/IFN	20.75 + 0.01	22.05 + 0.67	1.06
Fold increase	3.72	2.92	

[a]Unseparated TDL and CD8+ T-cell adhesion were measured as described in the legend to Table III.

TABLE V. Relative Adhesion of B-Cells to Resting and Cytokine-Activated High Endothelial Cells[a]

	% Lymphocyte adhesion		Ratio separated: unseparated
	Unseparated TDL	Separated B-cells	
Control	6.53 + 0.27	10.67 + 0.21	1.63
TNF/IFN	23.84 + 1.40	25.12 + 0.66	1.05
Fold increase	3.65	2.35	

[a]Unseparated TDL and B-cell adhesion were measured as described in the legend to Table III.

control subset adhesion to HEC or these three subsets use different accessory molecules for adhesion to HEC. Although there is no experimental evidence supporting these proposals, it is clear that the distribution of B-cells, CD4+ T-cells, and CD8+ T-cells are all independently regulated in vivo (31–33). A final possibility to explain differential adhesion is that all lymphocytes use the same adhesion molecules to bind to HEC, but lymphocyte subsets are differentially regulated by inhibitors of adhesion. For example, in the model we have described CD4+ T-cells would be much more sensitive to inhibitors of adhesion secreted by HEC than either CD8+ T-cells or B-cells. Further experiments are required to differentiate between these possibilities. However, these results indicate that the migration of CD4+ T-cells may be regulated independently of other lymphocytes. Since this cell population is a prerequisite for the initiation of immune responses, it may be necessary to tightly regulate its migration pathways in vivo in order to avoid the potentially deleterious effects of initiating immune responses outside of organised lymphoid tissues.

Relative Migration of Lymphocyte Subsets

Since the adhesion of lymphocyte subsets to cultured HEC was nonrandom, it was possible to determine the relationship between type I, surface bound lymphocytes and type II, migrated lymphocytes in this assay. The distributions of lymphocyte subsets in these two populations were compared directly.

These experiments have been described in detail (28). Briefly, cervical lymph node cell suspensions were plated onto HEC in 8-well chamber slides and the adherent lymphocytes were analysed by indirect immunoperoxidase staining using mouse monoclonal antibodies against rat lymphocyte markers (OX12 for B-cells; W3/13 for T-cells; W3/25 for CD4+ cells). Positive cells for each of the lymphocyte markers were identified as either type I or type II by light microscope analysis. The percentage of positive cells in these two populations were compared with the total adherent population. Results from 3 separate experiments were pooled and are presented in Table VI.

There was an enrichment for B-cells over T-cells in the HEC-adherent fraction of lymph node cells as reported above for thoracic duct lymphocytes. B-cells were increased from 23% in the plated lymph node cell suspension to 54% in the adherent fraction. T-cells were decreased from 59% in the population plated to 21% in the adherent fraction. The distributions of T- and B-cells in the type I, surface bound fraction and the type II, migrated fraction were not statistically significantly different. Similarly, the distributions of CD4+ cells in the type I, surface bound fraction and in the type II, migrated fraction were identical.

These results demonstrate that type II, migrated lymphocytes are a random subpopulation of the total HEC-adherent lymphocytes. Since lymphocyte adhesion to cultured HEC was a nonrandom process, it is possible to conclude that lymphocyte migration is preceded by specific adhesion to the exposed surface of HEC in this assay. Thus, the site of selection of lymphocyte subsets for extravasation is at the exposed surface of HEC. Once bound to HEC, all lymphocytes have an equal chance of migrating across the endothelial layer.

TABLE VI. Distribution of Lymphocyte Subsets in the Type I, Surface Bound and Type II, Migrated Lymphocyte Populations[a]

	% of Total bound cells	% of Surface bound cells	% of Migrated cells
B	54 + 8	60 + 8	38 + 15
T	21 + 8	23 + 13	18 + 8
CD4+	13 + 6	13 + 7	17 + 5

[a]Lymph node cells were allowed to adhere for 60 min at 37°C to HEC in 8-well chamber slides. Adherent lymphocytes were analysed by indirect immunocytochemistry using subset-specific markers and identified as either type I, surface bound or type II, migrated lymphocytes. Results are mean percentage positive cells +SD (4–6) in the total bound, surface bound, and migrated lymphocyte fractions.

SUMMARY

The dynamic interactions between lymphocytes and vascular endothelial cells (EC) have been discussed. Although a receptor–ligand interaction between a homing receptor on the lymphocyte and a vascular addressin on the EC has been proposed to mediate adhesion of lymphocytes to the luminal surface of high endothelial venules (HEV) in lymph nodes, this interaction does not appear to be restricted to the lymphocyte among other leucocytes. Consideration of data from two experimental animal models suggests that lymphocyte migration across HEV in vivo is controlled independent of initial adhesion to the luminal surface. In order to explain the selective extravasation of lymphocytes over other leucocytes into lymph nodes, it is proposed that the selection of lymphocytes occurs not at the adhesion step but during the migration phase via a lymphocyte specific migration stimulus emanating either from HEV or it's immediate microenvironment.

A new in vitro model of lymphocyte migration into lymph nodes has been described using cultures of high endothelial cells (HEC). Under basal conditions, lymphocytes adhered to the exposed surfaces of HEC at 50-fold higher levels than to non-HEV or flat EC. This observation provides a basic assay of HEV function in cultured HEC. It also supports our previous proposal that HEC are a type of cytokine-activated EC (Chapter 21), since the expression of lymphocyte adhesion molecules appears to be constitutively upregulated in these cells.

It has been shown that the adhesion of each of the major lymphocyte subsets, CD4+ T-cells, CD8+ T-cells, and B-cells, was regulated independently via subset specific adhesion molecules expressed by cultured HEC. The identity of these adhesion molecules is unknown, but it should be possible to determine their relationship to the known vascular addressins. Following adhesion to the surface of HEC, a random sub-population of lymphocytes migrated to a position underneath the endothelial layer. This suggests that the selection of lymphocyte subsets for migration occurs at the exposed (luminal) surface of HEC in vivo.

Cultured HEC allows two stages in the process of lymphocyte extravasation to be studied in vitro: the adhesive event and the migration event. For the first time, the migration of lymphocytes can be studied independently of adhesion in vitro. Preliminary results suggest that the vascular endothelium can directly regulate the extent of lymphocyte migration in this model. Identification of the stimulus for lymphocyte migration in this assay may contribute to our understanding of the mechanisms underlying the selective extravasation of lymphocytes in vivo.

ACKNOWLEDGMENTS

I gratefully acknowledge the expert technical assistance of Cheryl Holt with endothelial cell culture, the secretarial assistance of Jackie Jolley, and the photographic skills of Jane Crosby. This work was supported by the Medical Research Council (U.K.)

REFERENCES

1. Ford WL Lymphocyte migration and immune responses. Prog Allergy 1975; 19:1–59.
2. Butcher EC, Scollay RG, Weissman IL. Organ specificity of lymphocyte migration: Mediation by highly selective lymphocyte interaction with organ-specific determinants on high endothelial venules. Eur J Immunol. 1980;10:556–561.
3. Scicchitano R, Stanicz A, Ernst P, Bienenstock J. A common mucosal immune system revisited. In: Husband AJ, ed. Migration and Homing of Lymphoid Cells. Vol. II. Boca Raton, Florida: CRC Press, 1988;1–34.
4. Smith ME, Martin AF, Ford WL. Migration of lymphoblasts in the rat. Monog Allergy 1986;16:203–232.
5. Cahill RNP, Heron I, Poskitt DC, Trnka Z. Lymphocyte recirculation in the sheep fetus. In: Blood Cells and Vessel Walls: Functional Interactions. Ciba Foundation Symposium No 71. Amsterdam: Excerpta Medica, 1980;145–166.
6. Mackay CR, Kimpton WG, Brandon MR, Cahill RNP. Lymphocyte subsets show marked differences in their distribution between blood and the afferent and efferent lymph of peripheral lymph nodes. J Exp Med 1988;167:1755–1765.
7. Mayrhofer G. Thymus-dependent and thymus-independent subpopulations of intestinal intraepithelial lymphocytes. Blood 1980;55:532–535.
8. Goodman T, Lefrancois L. Expression of the $\gamma\delta$-T cell receptor on intestinal CD8 + intraepithelial lymphocytes. Nature (Lond) 1988;333:855–858.
9. Kuziel WA, Takashima A, Bonyhadi M, Bergstresser PR, Allison, JP, Tregelaar RE, Tucker PW. Regulation of T-cell receptor γ-chain RNA expression in murine Thy-1 + dendritic epidermal cells. Nature (Lond) 1987;328:263–266.
10. Parrot DMV, Wilkinson PC. Lymphocyte locomotion and migration. Prog Allergy 1987;28:193–284.
11. Jalkanen S, Steere A, Fox R, Butcher EC. A distinct endothelial cell recognition system that controls lymphocyte traffic into inflamed synovium. Science 1986; 233:556–558.
12. Hamann A, Thiele H-G. Molecules and regulation in lymphocyte migration. Immunol Rev 1989;108:19–44.
13. Pals ST, Horst E, Scheper RJ, Meijer CJLM. Mechanisms of human lymphocyte migration and their role in the pathogenesis of disease. Immunol Rev 1989;108: 111–133.
14. Stoolman LM Adhesion molecules controlling lymphocyte migration. Cell 1989;56:907–910.
15. Berg EL, Goldstein LA, Jutila MA, Nakache M, Picker LJ, Streeter PR, Wu NW, Zhou D, Butcher EC. Homing receptors and vascular addressins: Cell adhesion molecules that direct lymphocyte traffic. Immunol Rev 1989;108: 5–18.
16. Tedder TF, Isaacs CM, Ernst TJ, Demetri GD, Adler DA, Disteche CM. Isolation and chromosomal localisation of cDNAs encoding a novel human lymphocyte cell surface molecule LAM-1. J Exp Med 1989;170:123–133.
17. Camerini D, James SP, Stamenkovic I, Seed B. Leu8/TQ1 is the human equivalent of the Mel-14 lymph node homing receptor. Nature (Lond) 1989;342; 78–82.

18. Lewinsohn DM, Bargatze RF, Butcher EC. Leucocyte–endothelial cell recognition: Evidence of a common molecular mechanism shared by neutrophils, lymphocytes and other leucocytes. J Immunol 1987;138:4313–4321.
19. Stamenkovic I, Amiot M, Pesando JM, Seed B. A lymphocyte molecule implicated in lymph node homing is a member of the cartilage link protein family. Cell 1989;56:1057–1062.
20. Schoefl GI. The migration of lymphocytes across the vascular endothelium in lymphoid tissue. A re-examination. J Exp Med 1972;136:568–584.
21. Hendriks HR, Eestermans IL. Disappearance and reappearance of high endothelial venules and immigrating lymphocytes in lymph nodes deprived of afferent lymphatics: A possible regulatory role of macrophages in lymphocyte migration. Eur J Immunol 1983;13:663–669.
22. Andrews P, Milsom DW, Ford WL. Migration of lymphocytes across specialised endothelium. V. Production of a sulphated macromolecule by high endothelial cells in lymph nodes. J Cell Sci 1982;57:277–292.
23. Larsen CG, Anderson AO, Appella E, Oppenheim JJ, Matsushima K. The neutrophil-activating protein (NAP-1) is also chemotactic for lymphocytes. Science 1989;243:1464–1466.
24. Bjerknes M, Cheng H, Ottoway CA. Dynamics of lymphocyte–endothelial interactions in vivo. Science 1986;231:402–405.
25. Drayson MT, Ford WL. Afferent lymph and lymph borne cells: Their influence on lymph node function. Immunobiology 1988;169:362–379.
26. Hendriks HR, Duivestijn AM, Kraal G. Rapid decrease in lymphocyte adherence to high endothelial venules in lymph nodes deprived of afferent lymphatic vessels. Eur J Immunol 1987;17:1691–1695.
27. Ager A. Isolation and culture of high endothelial cells from rat lymph nodes. J Cell Sci 1987;87:133–144.
28. Ager A, Mistry S. Interactions between lymphocytes and cultured high endothelial cells: An in vitro model of lymphocyte migration across high endothelial venule endothelium. Eur J Immunol 1988;18:1265–1274.
29. Haskard D, Cavender D, Beatty P, Springer T, Ziff M. T-lymphocyte adhesion to endothelial cells: Mechanisms demonstrated by anti-LFA-1 monoclonal antibodies. J Immunol 1986;1237:2901–2906.
30. Hughes CC, Male DK, Lantos PL. Adhesion of lymphocytes to cerebral microvascular cells: Effects of interferon-gamma, tumour necrosis factor and interleukin-1. Immunology 1988;64:677–681.
31. Stevens SK, Weissman IL, Butcher EC. Differences in the migration of B and T lymphocytes: Organ-selective localisation in vivo and the role of lymphocyte-endothelial cell recognition. J Immunol 1982;128:844–851.
32. Kraal G, Weissman IL, Butcher EC. Differences in in vivo distribution and homing of T cell subsets to mucosal *vs* non-mucosal lymphoid organs. J Immunol 1983;130:1097–1102.
33. Westermann J, Willfuhr KU, Rothkotter HJ, Fritz FJ, Pabst R. Migration pattern of lymphocyte subsets in the normal rat and the influence of splenic tissue. Scand J Immunol 1989;29:193–201.

The Endothelium: An Introduction to Current Research, pages 253–261

19
Microscopic Methods of Investigating Endothelium

JOHN WHARTON, LEE GORDON, ROBERT F. POWER, AND JULIA
M. POLAK
*Department of Histochemistry, Royal Postgraduate Medical School,
London W12 ONN, England*

INTRODUCTION

Vascular endothelium forms a continuous lining to the inner surface of
all blood vessels, separating circulating blood from vascular smooth muscle
and surrounding tissue. This strategic localisation gives the endothelium
a cardinal role in the regulation of vascular function and the development
of cardiovascular diseases such as atherosclerosis. The endothelium has
therefore become the focus of extensive research; this has largely been
undertaken since the development of cell culture techniques and microscopic methods for the identification of endothelial cells (1,2). This chapter
highlights some of the microscopic methods available to investigate the
endothelium and the value of the morphological information they provide.

ENDOTHELIAL CELL IDENTIFICATION AND STRUCTURE

The principal marker for identifying endothelium has been the glycoprotein von Willebrand (vWf) factor, which is synthesised in endothelial
cells and mediates the adhesion of platelets to the subendothelium following vascular injury. Immunohistochemical studies have used antisera to
von Willebrand factor to identify endothelial cells at the light and electron
microscopic levels in both normal and diseased tissues (3–5). Endothelial
cells lack the secretory granules found in peptide producing endocrine cells
and neurons, but possess rod-shaped Weibel–Palade bodies. These organelles represent the intracellular storage site of von Willebrand factor
(6,7), which is secreted both through a constitutive process and, in response
to specific stimuli, by regulated release from Weibel–Palade bodies (8,9).
Endothelial cells, however, display variable amounts of immunoreactivity
for this glycoprotein, and it may be lacking altogether in the endothelium
of blood vessels invading tumours and in endothelium-derived neoplasms
(10,11). Additional markers have therefore been sought and lectin binding

is now considered the most reliable means of identifying vascular endothelium. The lectin *Ulex europaeus* agglutinin I (UEA-I) in particular has been advocated as a sensitive marker for endothelium in human tissues and tumours, where it appears to be a more consistent marker than von Willebrand factor (11–13). This lectin recognises α-linked fucose containing glycoproteins and glycolipids and selectively binds to such residues in the plasma membrane of human endothelial cells, in sections of either frozen or paraffin-embedded tissues. Other lectins, such as *Bandeiraea (Griffonia) simplicifolia* isolectin B_4 and *Dolichos biflorus* agglutinin (14), have been found to display preferential binding for nonprimate and murine endothelial cells, respectively. Lectins are commercially available with either fluorochrome or biotin labels and can therefore be localised using a wide range of detection systems, including the avidin–biotin peroxidase complex (ABC) technique (15). Alternatively, the availability of specific antisera raised to different lectins allows for the sensitive immunohistochemical demonstration of endothelial binding (11–13). By contrast to the diffuse cytoplasmic immunostaining of human endothelial cells observed with antisera to von Willebrand factor, the immunohistochemical localisation of UEA-I binding produces a distinct membrane labelling of the endothelium (Fig.1). UEA-I binding can be demonstrated at different stages of human development and appears to occur in all blood vessels, irrespective of size. These two markers are complementary, however; and although UEA-I binding, for example, is generally a more sensitive means of identifying intramyocardial vessels in the human fetal heart, immunostaining for von Willebrand factor can provide a clearer visualisation of pulmonary vessels in the developing lung (Fig.1).

One of the ways in which endothelial cells modulate vascular smooth muscle tone is by metabolising vasoactive agents, such as angiotensin and bradykinin. This is mediated by the carboxypeptidase angiotensin-converting enzyme (ACE), which converts angiotensin I to the vasoconstrictor octapeptide angiotensin II and inactivates the vasodilator bradykinin. This enzyme represents a further marker of endothelial cells and antisera to ACE have been used to isolate endothelial cells by fluorescence-activated cell sorting (16). The results of immunofluorescence and electron microscopic studies demonstrate that ACE immunoreactivity is localised to vascular endothelium in man as well as other mammals and is associated with the luminal membrane of endothelial cells (17–19). Relatively little attention has been directed towards ACE as an immunohistochemical endothelial marker and this probably reflects the general lack of suitable antisera and the apparent immunological heterogeneity of the enzyme in different species (19). An alternative approach to the immunohistochemical localisation of ACE is the use of selective radiolabelled ACE inhibitors to identify endothelial cells by autoradiographic means (20). Other microscopic methods of visualising endothelium include the use of fluorescent-labelled acety-

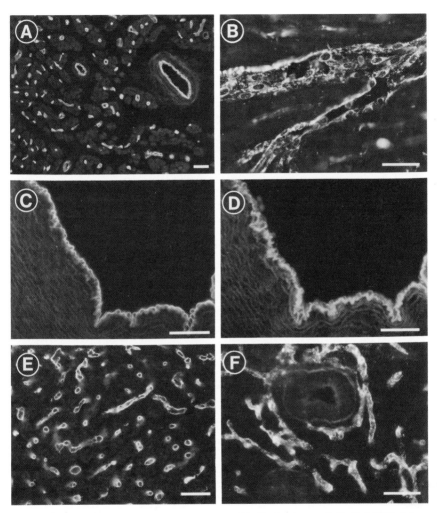

Fig. 1. Immunofluorescence photomicrographs displaying endothelial UEA-1 lectin binding (**A,C,E**) and von Willebrand factor immunoreactivity (**B,D,F**) in cryostat sections of human atrium (**A,B**); fetal aorta (**C,D**), right ventricle (**E**), and lung (**F**). The tissues were fixed in a modified Bouin's solution and cryostat sections (15 μm thick) immunostained using an indirect immunofluorescence technique. Bar: 50 μm.

lated low-density lipoprotein (LDL) to identify endothelial cells in tissue sections and cultures following receptor-mediated uptake and metabolism of the probe in vivo (21).

One of the main functions attributed to endothelial cells is the regulation of vascular permeability and transendothelial exchange of metabolites and gases. Attempts to relate these processes to the structure of the capillary wall have been hindered by the lack of suitable techniques. The structures involved, plasmalemmal vesicles and interendothelial channels, are dynamic in nature and affected by such factors as chemical fixation. Correlations between structure and function may now be feasible, however, with the use of cryofixation and freeze substitution methods to provide suitable fixation and the development of techniques for the ultrastructural analysis of the capillary wall (22). The limitations of conventional microscopic methods may also be overcome by the introduction of confocal microscopy, which facilitates the three-dimensional imaging of intact cells and permits direct visualisation of physiological parameters in living tissue.

ENDOTHELIAL RECEPTORS

Several substances are known to produce endothelium-dependent relaxation of blood vessels including acetylcholine (ACh), adenosine, substance P, bradykinin, histamine, and 5-hydroxytryptamine (23). These agents induce the release of an endothelium-derived relaxing factor, and it has been thought that the receptors mediating the response would be located on endothelial cells. Anatomical relationships of this type can be investigated microscopically using the technique of in vitro autoradiographic receptor labelling, which was originally described by Young and Kuhar (24). This is a more sensitive method than conventional techniques using tissue homogenates and provides receptor resolution and characterisation at the cellular level. Autoradiographic binding studies have, for example, been used to demonstrate that substance P receptors are located on vascular endothelium and exhibit a heterogeneous distribution that varies in different species and blood vessels (20,25). In marked contrast, radiolabelled ligands selective for muscarinic cholinoceptors and α_2-adrenoceptors display binding to the media rather than the endothelium, indicating that endothelial-dependent relaxation can also be induced indirectly through receptors on vascular smooth muscle (20,25). The localisation of ^{125}I-labelled calcitonin gene-related peptide (CGRP) binding sites to the endothelial and smooth muscle layers of mammalian blood vessels thus appears to be consistent with reports indicating that CGRP can induce a vasodilatory response by both a direct action on the media and via an endothelium-dependent mechanism (26). The situation is also further complicated by the proposal that in addition to responding to ACh and substance P, endothelial cells may be capable of producing such agents themselves (27,28). ACh for example may be synthesised in endothelial cells possessing choline acetyltransferase (ChAT) immunoreactivity and could be released following endothelial cell damage (27).

ENDOTHELIN

The endothelium contributes to the modulation of vascular smooth muscle tone by releasing endothelium-derived contracting as well as relaxing factors (23). These include the potent vasoconstrictor peptide endothelin, recently found to be produced by umbilical vein and aortic endothelial cells in culture (29,30). Three distinct 21-amino acid human endothelin sequences have now been identified, endothelin-1 and endothelin-3, possessing the same structures as porcine and rat endothelin respectively (31), but so far only the messenger RNA (mRNA) for endothelin-1 has been identified and its expression characterised in cultured endothelial cells. The isolation and sequencing of complementary DNA (cDNA) encoding human endothelin-1 has demonstrated that it is derived from a 212-amino acid precursor molecule transcribed from a gene containing five exons, located on chromosome 6 (32). In addition to its vasoconstrictor action, endothelin has a broad spectrum of pharmacological effects on the cardiovascular system as well as other tissues (33,34). These findings are consistent with those of autoradiographic studies, which have revealed a widespread distribution of ^{125}I-endothelin-1 binding sites in peripheral tissues. We have examined the localisation of endothelin-1 binding in cardiovascular and pulmonary tissues, from humans and other mammals, and demonstrated specific binding to the media of coronary arteries, myocardium, endocardium lining the surface of valve cusps, nerve trunks, airway smooth muscle, and alveolar walls (35,36). Quantitative analysis of the autoradiograms, using ^{125}I standards and computer-assisted densitometry, indicated that the binding was of a high density and affinity with a dissociation constant of 0.1–0.2nM and a maximum binding density of 0.25–0.41 fmol/mm^2. Similar endothelin-1 binding occurs in the rat kidney, where binding sites are localised to the glomeruli, vasa recta bundles, inner medulla, and smooth muscle of renal blood vessels (36,37). The existence of at least three endothelin peptides and the finding of binding sites exhibiting different molecular weights and affinities for endothelin isoforms indicates that there may be several receptor subtypes for endothelin in mammalian tissues (38–40). Quantitative in vitro receptor autoradiography will be an important tool for determining the differential distribution and relative affinities of these receptors.

The extent to which endothelin is expressed in endothelium in vivo has still to be resolved, but the level of expression could be much lower than that seen in cultured endothelial cells and may be related to endothelial cell damage (33,34). We have used polyclonal antisera raised against human endothelin-1 and immunohistochemical techniques to demonstrate endothelin immunoreactivity in human tissues. Umbilical cords were sampled at birth, following a normal delivery, and endothelin-like immunoreactivity localised to a subpopulation of endothelial cells in the umbilical vein (Fig. 2). A proportion of fetal and adult cardiac tissues, obtained at abortion and surgery, respectively, also displayed endothelin-like immunoreactivity; this appeared to be more prominent in the endothelial cells of microvessels ($\sim$3–40 μm in diameter) than in larger arterioles and arteries (Fig. 2). Labelled cRNA probes and in situ hybridisation techniques are now being employed to confirm the endothelial synthesis of endothelin in vivo and investigate which endothelin genes are expressed. It is known, however, that endothelin is also expressed in nonendothelial cells, recent studies having localised both endothelin immunoreactivity and mRNA to neuronal cell bodies in the human and porcine spinal cord and brain (41–43). The level of endothelin expression in cultured cells is modulated by several stimuli, including thrombin, adrenaline, Ca^{2+} ionophores, phorbol esters, transforming growth factor B, angiotensin II, vasopressin, and shear stress (29,33,34). Since endothelial cells lack the secretory granules, in which synthesised peptide is usually stored and its release regulated, it has been proposed that the secretion of endothelin from endothelial cells is a constitutive process with regulation occurring at the level of either transcription or translation, or both (33,34). As with the ultrastructural localisation of von Willebrand factor and other pep-

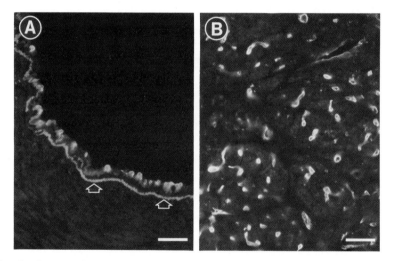

Fig. 2. Immunofluorescence photomicrographs showing the localisation of endothelin-like immunoreactivity to a subpopulation of endothelial cells in a section of human umbilical vein (**A**) and to the endothelium of microvessels in adult atrial myocardium (**B**). The internal elastic lamina (**A**, arrows) displays fluorescence due to the inclusion of Pontamine sky blue as a counterstain. Bar: 50 μm.

tides, the use of immunoelectron microscopy and region-specific antisera may help establish the intracellular processing of the endothelin precursor molecule and determine whether it is associated with organelles such as Weibel–Palade bodies in endothelial cells or secretory granules in neurons.

In view of the heterogeneous nature of endothelial cell responses and secretory products and the need to further our understanding of endothelial function, it is apparent that the microscopic methods alluded to here will have a significant role in endothelial research in the future.

ACKNOWLEDGMENTS

This work was supported by the Wellcome Trust and British Heart Foundation and was carried out in collaboration with Professor M.H. Yacoub, Professor K.M. Taylor, and Dr. G. Moscoso. We are grateful to Cambridge Research Biochemicals, Ltd., for providing antisera, and to Patricia Harley for technical assistance.

REFERENCES

1. Jaffe EA, Hoyer LW, Nachman L. Synthesis of antihemophilic factor antigen by cultured human endothelial cells. J Clin Invest 1973;52:2757–2764.
2. Gimbrone MA, Cotran RS, Folkman J. Human vascular endothelial cells in culture. Growth and DNA synthesis. J Cell Biol 1974;60:673–684.
3. Hoyer LW, De Los Santos RP, Hoyer JR. Antihemophilic factor antigen. Localization in endothelial cells by immunofluorescent microscopy. J Clin Invest 1973;52:2737–2744.
4. Piovella F, Nalli G, Malamani GD, Majolino I, Frassoni F, Sitar GM, Ruggeri A, Dell'Orbo C, Ascari E. The ultrastructural localization of factor VIII-Antigen in human platelets, megakaryocytes and endothelial cells utilizing a ferritin-labelled antibody. Br J Haematol 1978;39:209–213.
5. Burgdorf WHC, Mukai K, Rosai J. Immunohistochemical identification of factor VIII related antigen in endothelial cells of cutaneous lesions of alleged vascular nature. Am J Clin Pathol 1981;75:161–171.
6. Wagner DD, Olmsted JB, Marder VJ. Immunolocalization of von Willebrand protein in Weibel–Palade bodies of human endothelial cells. J Cell Biol 1982;95:355–360.
7. De Groot PG, Federici AB, De Boer HC, D'Alessio P, Mannucci PM, Sixma JJ. von Willebrand factor synthesized by endothelial cells from a patient with type IIB von Willebrand disease supports platelet adhesion normally but has an increased affinity for platelets. Proc Natl Acad Sci USA 1989;86:3793–3797.
8. Levine JD, Harlan JM, Harker JM, Joseph LA, Counts RB. Thrombin-mediated release of factor VIII antigen from human umbilical vein endothelial cells in culture. Blood 1982;60:531–533.
9. Loesberg C, Gonsalves MD, Zandbergn J, Willems C, Van Aken WG, Stel HV, Van Mourik JA, DeGroot PG. The effect of calcium on the secretion of factor VIII-related antigen by cultured human endothelial cells. Biochem Biophys 1983;763:160–168.
10. Sehested M, Hou-Jensen K. Factor VIII related antigen as an endothelial cell marker in benign and malignant diseases. Virchows Arch [A] 1981;391:217–225.

11. Stephenson TJ, Griffiths DWR, Mills PM. Comparison of ulex europaeus I lectin binding and factor VIII-related antigen as markers of vascular endothelium in follicular carcinoma of the thyroid. Histopathology 1986;10:251–260.
12. Holthofer H, Virtanen I, Kariniemi AL, Hormia M, Linder E, Miettinen A. Ulex europaeus I lectin as a marker for vascular endothelium in human tissues. Lab Invest 1982;47:60–66.
13. Ordonez NG, Batsakis JG. Comparison of ulex europaeus I lectin and factor VIII-related antigen in vascular lesions. Arch Pathol Lab Med 1984;108:129–132.
14. Rhodri J, Williams LL, Robertson D, Davies AJS. Identification of vascular endothelial cells in murine omentum using the lectin, Dolichos biflorus agglutinin: Possible applications in the study of angiogenesis. Histochemical J 1989; 21:271–278.
15. Hsu SM, Raind L, Fanger H. Use of avidin–biotin–peroxide complex (ABC) in immunoperoxidase technique. J Histochem Cytochem 1981;29:577–580.
16. Auerbach R, Alby L, Grieves J, Joseph J, Lindgren C, Morrissey LW, Sidky YA, Tu M, Watt SL. Monoclonal antibody against angiotensin-converting enzyme: Its use as a marker for murine, bovine, and human endothelial cells. Proc Natl Acad Sci USA 1982;79:7891–7895.
17. Ryan JW, Ryan US, Shultz DR, Whitaker C, Chung A. Subcellular localization of pulmonary angiotensin-converting enzyme (Kininase II). Biochem J 1975; 146:497–499.
18. Caldwell PRB, Seegel BC, Hsu KC. Angiotensin-converting enzyme: Vascular endothelial localization. Science 1976;191:1050–1051.
19. Seitz RJ, Neunen E, Henrich M, Schrader J, Wechsler W. Angiotensin I-Converting enzyme (ACE): A marker for vascular endothelium. In: Cervos-Navarro J, Ferszt R, eds. Stroke and Microcirculation. New York: Raven Press, 1987: 111–115.
20. Stephenson JA, Summers RJ. Autoradiographic analysis of receptors on vascular endothelium. Eur J Pharmacol 1987;134:35–43.
21. Netland PA, Zetter BR, Via DP, Voyta JC. In situ labelling of vascular endothelium with fluorescent acetylated low density lipoprotein. Histochem J. 1985;17: 1309–1320.
22. Wagner RC. Ultrastructural studies of capillary endothelium. In: Simionescu N, Simionescu M eds. Endothelial Cell Biology in Health and Disease. New York: Plenum Press, 1988:23–47.
23. Furchgott RF, Vanhoutte PM. Endothelium-derived relaxing and contracting factors. FASEB J 1989;3:2007–2018.
24. Young WS, Kuhar MJ. A new method for receptor autoradiography: [³H]opioid receptors in rat brain. Brain Res 1979;179:255–270.
25. Summers RJ, Molenaar P, Stephenson JA. Autoradiographic localization of receptors in the cardiovascular system. Trends Pharmacol Sci 1987;8:272–276.
26. Wharton J, Gulbenkian S. Peptides in the mammalian cardiovascular system. Experientia 1987;43:821–832.
27. Parnavelas JG, Kelly W, Burnstock G. Ultrastructural localization of choline acetyltransferase in vascular endothelial cells in rat brain. Nature (Lond) 1985; 316:724–725.
28. Burnstock G. Mechanisms of interaction of peptide and neuropeptide vascular neurotransmitter systems. J Cardiovasc Pharmacol 1987;10(suppl.12):S74–S81.

29. Yanagisawa M, Kurihara H, Kimura S, Tomobe Y, Kobayashi M, Mitsui Y, Yazaki Y, Goto K, Masaki T. A novel potent vasoconstrictor peptide produced by vascular endothelial cells. Nature (Lond) 1988;332:411–415.

30. Itoh Y, Yanagisawa M, Ohkubo S, Kimura C, Kosaka T, Inoue A, Ishida N, Mitsui Y, Onda H, Fujino M, Masaki T. Cloning and sequence analysis of cDNA encoding the precursor of a human endothelium-derived vasoconstrictor peptide, endothelin: Identity of human and porcine endothelin. FEBS Lett 1988; 231:440–444.

31. Inoue A, Yanagisawa M, Kimura S, Kasuya Y, Miyauchi T, Goto K, Masaki T. The human endothelin family: Three structurally and pharmacologically distinct isopeptides predicted by three separate genes. Proc Natl Acad Sci USA 1989;86:2863–2867.

32. Bloch KD, Friedrich SP, Lee M-E, Eddy RL, Shows TB, Quertermous T. Structural organization and chromosomal assignment of the gene encoding endothelin. J Biol Chem 1989;264:10851–10857.

33. Yanagisawa M, Masaki T. Endothelin, a novel endothelium-derived peptide. Pharmacological activities, regulation and possible roles in cardiovascular control. Biochem Pharmacol 1989;38:1877–1883.

34. Yanagisawa M, Masaki T. Molecular biology and biochemistry of the endothelins. Trends Pharmacol Sci 1989;10:374–378.

35. Power RF, Wharton J, Salas SP, Kanse S, Ghatei M, Bloom SR, Polak JM. Autoradiographic localisation of endothelin binding sites in human and porcine coronary arteries. Eur J Pharmacol 1989;160:199–200.

36. Power RF, Wharton J, Zhao Y, Bloom SR, Polak JM. Autoradiographic localization of endothelin-1 binding sites in the cardiovascular and respiratory systems. J Cardiovasc Pharmacol 1989;13(suppl 5):S50–S56.

37. Davenport AP, Nunez DJ, Brown MJ. Binding sites for ^{125}I-labelled endothelin-1 in the kidneys: Differential distribution in rat, pig and man demonstrated by using quantitative autoradiography. Clin Sci 1989;77:129–131.

38. Watanabe H, Miyazaki H, Kondoh M, Masuda Y, Kimura S, Yanagisawa M, Masaki T, Murakami K. Two distinct types of endothelin receptors are present on chick cardiac membranes. Biochem Biophys Res Commun 1989;161:1252–1259.

39. Sugiua M, Snajdar RM, Schwartzberg M, Badr KF, Inagami T. Identification of two types of specific endothelin receptors in rat mesangial cell. Biochem Biophys Res Commun 1989;162:1396–1401.

40. Kloog Y, Bousso-Mittler D, Bdolah A, Sokolovsky M. Three apparent receptors subtypes for the endothelin/sarafotoxin family. FEBS Lett 1989;253:199–202.

41. Yoshizawa T, Kimura S, Kanazawa I, Uchiyama Y, Yanagisawa M, Masaki T. Endothelin localizes in the dorsal horn and acts on the spinal neurons: Possible involvement of dihydropyridine-sensitive calcium channels and substance P release. Neurosci Lett 1989;102:179–184.

42. Giaid A, Gibson SJ, Nassif B, Ibrahim N, Legon S, Bloom SR, Yanagisawa M, Masaki T, Varndell IM, Polak JM. Endothelin 1, an endothelium-derived peptide, is expressed in neurons of the human spinal cord and dorsal root ganglia. Proc Natl Acad Sci USA 1989;86:7634–7638.

43. Shinmi O, Kimura S, Yoshizawa T, Sawamura T, Uchiyama Y, Sugita Y, Kanazawa I, Yanagisawa M, Goto K, Masaki T. Presence of endothelin-1 in porcine spinal cord: Isolation and sequence determination. Biochem Biophys Res Commun 1989;162:340–346.

The Endothelium: An Introduction to Current Research, pages 263–272
© 1990 Wiley-Liss, Inc.

20
Large Vessel Endothelial Isolation

J.B. WARREN
*Department of Clinical Pharmacology, Royal Postgraduate Medical
School, London W12 0NN, England*

INTRODUCTION

The first widely used successful method of isolating endothelial cells for culture involved instilling a solution containing proteolytic enzymes to dislodge the endothelium from the intima. This method can be applied to any sizable segment of artery or vein. Enthusiasm for enzymatic methods of isolating and propagating cultured cells has waned because of the accumulation of evidence demonstrating that exposure to proteolytic enzymes causes cell damage. This is particularly so for the cell surface, as it is composed of projections and caveolae of various sizes that, in vivo, increase the area in contact with the blood. Above this surface lies a thin, delicate layer of glycocalyx, and it is not surprising that this is particularly susceptible to damage. On exposure to a solution containing enzymes, the cells lose their normal cobblestone morphology, become rounded, and drift into suspension, but measures of function have been needed to document the more subtle detrimental effects that occur (1).

The use of trypsin to passage cells has been shown to cause the loss of lipid from the cell membrane (2), increase cellular aggregation (3), decrease receptor binding sites (4,5), and diminish the stimulatory effect of bradykinin on endothelium-derived relaxing factor (EDRF) release (5). The loss of bradykinin receptors induced by trypsin may be recovered in two cell passages, if mechanical methods of cell transfer are used (5). Endothelial cells in culture, even when mechanical methods are used, release EDRF to a much restricted list of stimulants when compared with endothelial cells in the intact vessel wall. This is usually quoted as evidence that cultured cells have differentiated in vitro. A more likely explanation is that some time is required to recover function fully after division. In support of this, the response to several agonists takes many months to return in vivo when endothelium has been denuded by angioplasty, even though the endothelium regrows within days (6). This has important implications for studies of receptor function in vitro.

The endothelium is the major source of angiotensin converting enzyme (ACE) or kininase II, and healthy cells rapidly convert angiotensin I to angiotensin II. This has been used as an assay of function to show that endothelium in culture takes about 7 days to recover ACE activity fully after a single exposure to proteolytic enzymes (7). Whereas ACE activity is suppressed by this exposure, complement receptors may become expressed on the cell surface (8). Healthy endothelium presents an inactive surface to the immune system, but mild proteolysis causes complement to bind to its surface. This has significant implications for any study of the interaction between the endothelium and the immune system, particularly the adhesion of leukocytes. Enzymatic damage is not confined to the surface of the cell, since exposure to collagenase solution is known to be capable of causing changes in intracellular DNA structure (9). Taking into account the limitations of enzymatic isolation, it is nonetheless the most convenient method of obtaining cells from the most reliable and plentiful human source, the umbilical vein.

ENZYMATIC ISOLATION OF HUMAN UMBILICAL VEIN ENDOTHELIUM

For any work with human tissue, it is sensible to first obtain vaccination against hepatitis B and also to assume that the source could be human immunodeficiency virus (HIV) positive. The cooperation of the local maternity unit is sought and it should be regularly explained to the staff that long pieces of cord with few clamp marks are preferred. Sterile disposal containers (150 ml) are half-filled with phosphate-buffered saline (PBS) containing penicillin 100,000 IU/L, streptomycin 100 mg/L, gentamicin 50 mg/L, and mycostatin 50,000 IU/L and left in the ward refrigerator. Cords may be used up to 72 hr after collection, provided they are kept in the container at 4°C.

Ideally, the cord is prepared in a horizontal laminar flow cabinet, although a clean bench is adequate. The cord is placed on a board covered with new aluminum foil. The longest length (minimum 10 cm) that is free of any trauma marks is selected and cut from the remainder with a sterile scalpel. If crushed areas of cord are used, this substantially increases the chances of fibroblast or smooth muscle contamination.

Collagenase solution is made by adding 250 mg collagenase to 500 ml plain medium containing 25 mM HEPES, aliquoting into 25-ml sterile tubes and freezing directly. After thorough washing, the plastic three-way taps can be sterilized in 70% alcohol and reused.

One end of the cord is examined and the umbilical vein identified, having the largest diameter of the three vessels. One arm of a plastic three-way tap with a luer lock fitting is inserted into the vein and tied in place with a length of suture. A 30-ml syringe full of sterile PBS is connected to the tap and the vein flushed through twice to remove red cells and debris. A second three-way tap is tied into the other end of the umbilical vein. The segment of vein is then filled with collagenase solution until it is distended. It is left for 15 min at 37°C either in an oven or beaker in a water bath. After this incubation period, the yield of cells is greatly increased if the cord is massaged by gently squeezing the whole length to loosen any endothelial cells still adherent to the vessel wall. The cord is held vertically, the bottom tap opened, and the contents allowed to drain into a 50-ml sterile centrifuge tube containing 10 ml of culture medium with 10% fetal calf serum (FCS), which neutralizes the proteolytic enzymes. Once empty it is flushed through with a further 20 ml of PBS into the centrifuge tube.

After centrifugation for 5 min at 500g, the supernatant is discarded and the cell pellet resuspended in 4 ml of culture medium. The pellet can be broken up by gently passing it up and down a 5-ml pipette 5 times and is then seeded into a T-25 flask, each flask requiring cells from 15–25 cm of cord. Flasks are left for 48 hr in an incubator at 37°C and a 5% CO_2 atmosphere, after which 3 ml of the medium may be aspirated and replaced with 4 ml fresh medium. The cells attach to the bottom of the flask within minutes of being seeded and migrate to spread evenly over the floor. The cells become confluent after 3–4 days.

MECHANICAL HARVESTING OF LARGE VESSEL ENDOTHELIUM

Mechanical harvesting is a simple method of obtaining large vessel endothelium for culture (10). This is particularly so for cow or pig aorta and pulmonary artery, but smaller vessels may also yield adequate primary cultures. Some vessels, such as the human umbilical vein, defy even the most determined efforts to obtain cells by mechanical scraping. Varicose veins removed at operation provide a useful source of human endothelium that can be isolated by scraping (11). For aortic cells, the heart and thoracic aorta are taken as one piece. For pulmonary artery cells, an intact heart and lung preparation is required. Fresh material should be placed directly on ice and the cells isolated within 12 hr.

Three sterile pots (150 ml) are each filled with 125 ml of sterile PBS containing calcium and magnesium with penicillin 200,000 IU/L, streptomycin 200 mg/L, and gentamicin 100 mg/L. The tissue is placed on a new piece of aluminium foil on a clean bench or preferably in a lamina flow cabinet. The surface is sprayed with 70% alcohol and excess fat trimmed. A 10-cm segment of thoracic aorta is cut with a sterile scalpel and placed into the first pot of buffer with antibiotics. The chance of subsequent microbial contamination is reduced if the tissue is left in this first pot for 1 hr at 4°C. The pulmonary artery is cut just above the pulmonary valve and at the distal ends of the two main branches and prepared in a similar fashion.

The next stage should be in a laminar flow cabinet with sterilised instruments. The vessel is removed from the first pot and rinsed in the second and third pots. It is then laid on a new piece of aluminum foil that has been cleaned with 70% alcohol. After the vessel is opened by cutting along its long axis, it is laid flat by pinning it to a small hard rubber board that has been previously autoclaved. The intimal surface is very gently scraped with a curved scalpel blade, and the endothelial cells that build up on the edge of the blade are rinsed into a centrifuge tube containing medium. Each area should only be scraped once, and it is important to avoid scraping close to any cut edge. The cell suspension is centrifuged at 500g for 5 min and the supernatant discarded. The cell pellet is resuspended in 3 ml medium and seeded into a T-25 flask. This is placed in an incubator at 37°C with a 5% CO_2 atmosphere. Significant growth should occur at 4–7 days when 2 ml of the medium may be removed and 3 ml added.

PASSAGING CELLS

Apart from causing less cell damage, mechanical methods of passaging are quicker and more economical on reagents. Confluent monolayers are usually passaged by splitting in a ratio of 1:3. The cells are dislodged by a rubber policeman that can be made from a 22-cm length of 2-mm-thick wire onto the end of which is threaded a semicircle of soft rubber, 2 cm in diameter, kept in place by burring the end of the wire. The other end of the handle should be taped to prevent it from perforating the autoclave bag. The half disk end of the rubber policeman is squeezed through the neck of the flask and its flat surface moved gently along the floor. Any remaining adherent cells can be identified as opaque areas on the floor of the flask when it is held up to the light, and these should be scraped again. The dislodged sheets of cells break up into small clumps if passed up and down a 10-ml pipette 20 times. The cells, suspended in their old medium, are seeded into new flasks in a ratio of 1:3. New medium is then added to correct to the original volume. Any spillage of medium in the neck of a flask must be immediately aspirated with a sterile disposable pipette.

Cells are usually passaged every 2 weeks, but this may be delayed to every 4 weeks or shortened to every 5 days, depending on demand. These guidelines will vary depending on the media and cell line. If a flask is left too long between passaging, the cells start to lose their normal morphology, fibroblast contamination may occur, there is an increase in the number of giant cells, and the edges of the monolayer begin to detach. Nearly all bovine cell lines will passage more than 20 times and retain their normal function; some may even passage more than 100 times.

IDENTIFICATION AND PURIFICATION OF CELL LINES

Before they reach confluence, endothelial cells with their pseudopodia look remarkably similar to fibroblast or smooth muscle cells. Once confluent, the cobblestone morphology is easily recognized by a trained observer. Small cells appearing as dots in the monolayer should not be mistaken for dead cells. Time-lapse photography has shown these mitosing cells lift off the plate as they divide. Giant cells may also be seen, particularly in mature cultures. These have transformed from normal endothelial cells and appear to be as active as surrounding cells, but what specialized functions they might possess is not known.

If the right combination of growth factors is present in the medium, mature cultures can organize to form cylinders, the preliminary step in angiogenesis. This first appears as straight lines of cells that grow to form tubes. These may lift off the plate, a phenomenon termed sprouting, but with passaging the cells revert to a monolayer.

Cell contamination is usually caused by fibroblasts. These are slower growing than endothelial cells and may take 2 weeks to appear. Contamination with smooth muscle cells is not usually seen, one reason being that they are slow growing and second, because this growth rate is further inhibited by the presence of endothelium. Gross fibroblast contamination is easily recognized on microscopy with spindly, thin-bodied cells piled in a criss-cross fashion. Single fibroblasts may also be identified in that they frequently lie on top of the monolayer, in contrast to endothelial cells, which never superimpose.

To obtain a pure culture, contaminating cells have to be removed during passaging. A fine-point indelible marker is used to draw a grid of 1-cm squares on the external surface of the floor of the flask. Each square is examined by phase-contrast microscopy, and any areas of definite or possible contamination are circled. Flasks with more than 10% contamination should be discarded, but lesser contamination can be separated by dislodging endothelial cells with a rubber policeman and carefully leaving behind the ringed areas of fibroblast contamination. Primary cultures should be grown in small T-25 flasks initially, to cut down on microscopy time, but four passages with selective scraping should be sufficient to yield a pure cell line.

To confirm that the cells obtained are endothelial, it is usual to stain for factor VIII activity. This has been shown to be present on all human and bovine cell lines, although porcine cells lose this property in culture after two passages. Smooth muscle cells and fibroblasts do not stain for factor VIII, whereas positive staining cells such as platelets and mast cells do not grow in culture. All staining is most easily done on endothelial cells grown on sterile glass coverslips placed at the bottom of 6 or 24 well plates. After washing with PBS and fixing for 1 min with 100% acetone, the cells are incubated with an antibody to factor VIII, 1:50 dilution, in 2 ml at room temperature for 30 min. After three washes with PBS (leave each wash for 5 min), the second antibody, immunoglobulin G (IgG) conjugated to fluorescein isothiocyanate, is added at 1:5 in 2 ml for 30 min. The coverslip is carefully dried, mounted with a drop of 9 parts glycine–1 part PBS, and examined by fluorescence microscopy. Similar staining techniques may be used to look for other endothelial cell markers such as angiotensin-converting enzyme, carboxypeptidase-N, and the polyvalent carbohydrate binding proteins, the lectins.

The function of endothelial cells may be assessed by measuring the response of prostacyclin to stimulation using a radioimmunoassay (RIA) for the hydrolysis product 6-oxo-$PG_{1\alpha}$, the production of EDRF using a bioassay or direct chemiluminescence, Factor VIII production by radioimmunoassay or the activity of ACE. For this last test, tritiated tripeptides such as ^{3}H-Hip-Gly-Gly (Ventrex Laboratories Inc, Portland, ME), can be used as substrates and the reaction rate measured as by the release of ^{3}H-hippuric acid (11). After the incubation phase, the mixture is acidified and toluene/Omnifluor (New England Nuclear, Boston, MA) scintillation cocktail added. The ^{3}H-hippuric acid enters the organic phase and is counted on a scintillation counter, whereas any remaining substrate remains in the aqueous phase and therefore does not contribute to the total count.

GROWING CELLS ON MICROCARRIER BEADS

Endothelial cells rapidly attach to suitable surfaces even when agitated in suspension and are well suited to growing on microcarrier beads. Shear stress is known to affect endothelial function with the increased synthesis of EDRF and prostacyclin. It is possible that cells grown in stirred medium are closer to conditions in vivo than are those grown in static flasks. To create even seeding and prevent the aggregation of beads, the cell–bead suspension is continuously mixed using either a magnetic stirrer or a bottle roller system. The roller system is more suitable if several bottles are being used.

Small volumes of cells may be grown in 150-ml glass bottles (reused buffer or serum containers). They should be of hard glass to prevent chemical leaching. After washing in phosphate-free soap and rinsing in tissue culture-grade water, the bottle is dried overnight and then siliconized. A few mls. of siliconizing fluid (Repelcote, Hopkin & Williams, Chadwell, Essex) is added to the bottle in a fume cupboard and rolled around to coat the entire internal surface. It is more economical to siliconize glassware in batches, the same siliconizing fluid being passed from one bottle to the next. The glassware is left to drain and dry in an oven. After washing, the bottle is autoclaved for 4 hr to be sure of removing any endotoxin.

To seed cells on beads a confluent T-75 flask is taken with medium that has been in contact with the cells for 24–72 hr. The cells are scraped with a rubber policeman and dispersed by passing up and down a 10-ml pipette 20 times. They are transferred to a siliconized sterile bottle together with the conditioned medium, 2 ml of microcarrier beads, and 10 ml of fresh medium. The bottle is gassed either by leaving it with a loose top in an incubator with a 5% CO_2 atmosphere or by gas that is first passed through a 0.2-μm filter from a cylinder of 95% air–5% CO_2. The top is sealed and the bottle rolled at 2–5 rpm in a 37°C incubator. New medium and beads are added and the bottle regassed every 2 days. An alternative to gassing with 5% CO_2 is to use HEPES buffer. The cells may be inspected without staining by direct phase-contrast microscopy of 100 μl of bead suspension on a glass slide.

An alternative method of seeding cells on beads is to introduce fresh beads into a confluent flask of cells. The cells migrate onto the beads, which can then be washed off into the medium using a pipette. In a similar fashion, cells can be seeded from confluent beads into a new flask.

Many different microcarriers are manufactured. Our laboratory uses Cytodex-3 microcarriers from Pharmacia AB, Uppsala, Sweden, who provide a useful booklet "Microcarrier Cell Culture." Beads are bought dry and are rehydrated in PBS (50 ml/g beads) for 4 hr, when they reach a diameter of 150 μm. After washing twice with sterile PBS, they are autoclaved in a siliconized bottle. Microcarriers stick to glassware; disposable plastic pipettes should therefore be used to handle bead suspensions.

For studies measuring the response of endothelial cells to various stimuli, it is useful to pack cells on beads into columns that can then be perfused and the effluent collected. The cells are trapped between two layers of filter paper and held in place with a rubber bung. The rubber bung from a 2-ml syringe is removed and a small hole made in the centre. Microbore plastic tubing is then threaded through using a 1-ml disposable pipette tip as a guide. The tip of the tubing should lie within the well, which formerly contained the end of the shaft of the plunger handle. The roof of the well is then covered with a layer of filter paper (large pore size and hardened such as Whatman 54, Whatman Paper Ltd, Maidstone) tied on the side of the bung with suture. A second bung may be threaded onto the tubing to provide an extra seal. A circle of filter paper of the same diameter as the inside of the syringe barrel is cut out and placed in the bottom of the syringe.

The syringe barrel is held upright in a 50-ml pot and, under sterile conditions, beads may be transferred from their container into the syringe. It is best to wet both pieces of filter paper with medium first. If the beads are confluent with 80–100 cells per bead then this will provide approximately 10^7 cells in 0.5 ml. The bungs with tubing are then inserted into the barrel and pushed down until the filter paper sieve rests on the top of the beads. The column needs to be perfused without delay with buffer at 37°C. This is most easily done if the apparatus is kept in a hot box maintained at 37°C. The effluent from the column may be bioassayed immediately, alternatively a fraction collector may be used to collect samples for later analysis. Glass wool plugs may be used as an alternative to filter paper as sieves at the top and bottom on the column. The flow of buffer is usually in the order of 0.2–2 ml/min, flows above 1 ml/min may provide sufficient shear stress to increase the release of products such as EDRF and prostacyclin.

MEDIUM

Tissue culture is dependent on a supply of sterile water that is organic, ion, and pyrogen free. Double-distilled water is adequate if hard glassware is used, but the most convenient method is to obtain a wall-mounted filter system connected either to a deionized or mains water supply. Examples of such systems are the Milli-Q Reagent Grade Water System (Millipore Corporation, Bedford, MA) or Fistreem Nanopure System, (Fisons plc, Loughborough).

The basic medium containing salt solution, amino acids, and vitamins made be bought as a powder or more conveniently as a solution. Suitable products include Medium 199 (with Earle's Salts and L-glutamine but without sodium bicarbonate) or Dulbecco's Modified Eagle's medium (with 4.5 g/L glucose but without sodium pyruvate) from Gibco Laboratories, Grand Island, New York.

Serum needs to be added to the medium and concentrations up to 10% markedly increase growth rate. Increasing the concentration up to 30% also stimulates growth further, but the effect is small, in part because of inhibitory factors present in the serum, and the cost considerable. An additional requirement is L-glutamine, which has a half-life in medium at 35°C of 9 days and a half-life of 22 days at 21°C. This should therefore be added fresh to each batch of medium. It is dissolved in sterile medium, filtered through a 0.2-μm filter and then added.

The constituents of different batches of serum show great variation (13). Ideally, batches should be bioassayed for their effect on cell growth and the most effective bought in bulk. This is not practical for most laboratories and it is easier to add important growth promoters such as insulin. The cost of FCS has risen considerably in recent years. Several synthetic alternatives have been marketed but none has yet replaced serum. Cost may be reduced by diluting the FCS with bovine serum.

Human cells have a limited life span of usually four passages. For this reason, growth factors are added to the medium, the most commonly used being endothelial cell-derived growth factor (ECGF). This is made more potent by the addition of heparin as a cofactor; heparin is not a growth promoter on its own and does not potentiate other growth factor such as fibroblast growth factor (14). ECGF is expensive to buy and, if human cells are grown in sufficient quantities, it is worth preparing a crude extract of ECGF from bovine brain (15). The growth of a difficult cell line can be further potentiated by the addition of fetuin, a purified fraction of FCS, (Sigma, St Louis, MO) and by growing cells in flasks with a specially modified surface (Primaria, Falcon Labware, Becton Dickinson, Oxford).

A commonly used recipe used in our laboratory for bovine endothelial cells and vascular smooth muscle cells is 500 ml DMEM, 50 ml FCS, 1 mg thymidine, 240 mg L-glutamine, $\frac{1}{10}$ vial ITS supplement (insulin, transferrin, and sodium selenite media supplement, Sigma Chemical Co, St Louis, MO), penicillin 25,000 units and streptomycin 25 mg. Mycostatin and gentamycin can both have a detrimental effect on cell function and are best avoided. The media pH should be corrected to pH 7.4, measured at 37°C, and in a 5% CO_2 atmosphere, using 1 M NaOH and 1 M HCl dissolved in tissue-grade water. This pH usually corresponds to a pH of 7.3 at room temperature in air. Great care should always be taken to keep media sterile. The outside of the bottle, particularly around the neck, should be sprayed with 70% alcohol before and after use, and the neck sealed with tape.

STORING CELLS

Once a cell line has been purified and characterised, it can be stored in liquid nitrogen. A freezing mixture is prepared under sterile conditions of 10-ml medium with 10% serum and 5% dimethysulfoxide. Neat dimethylsulfoxide is sterile because of its high toxicity. A confluent T-75 flask ($\sim 10^7$ cells) is scraped, and the dislodged cells spun down in a sterile centrifuge tube. The supernatant is discarded and 10 ml of freezing mixture added to the tube, which is kept on ice. This is then directly aliquoted in 1-ml fractions into freezing vials that are also kept on ice. The vials are clearly labeled, using a catalogue system and then cooled at approximately 1°C/min by placing them in a polystyrene box in a -70°C freezer overnight. The vials are then removed and placed directly in liquid nitrogen. Thawing of the vials must be done rapidly. The vial is pushed inside a thin polystyrene ring to make it buoyant and then floated in a 37°C waterbath. It is centrifuged at 500g for 3 min and the outside washed with 70% alcohol before it is opened under sterile conditions. The freezing mixture is aspirated and the pellet resuspended in 3 ml of medium and seeded into a T-25 flask.

CONCLUSION

The majority of endothelial cells reside in the microvasculature, and many sites such as the capillaries, arterioles, venules, and lymphatics are lined with highly specialized endothelium. We should aim to study these specialized cells, but to isolate, culture, and assess their function is both labour intensive and time consuming. Large vessel endothelium accounts for only a small proportion of the body's total endothelium, but it is relatively straightforward to isolate and propagate such cells to high standards in culture. It is therefore pragmatic to use large vessel cultured endothelium, which continues to provide many valuable insights into cell function, for most experiments.

ACKNOWLEDGMENT

I am most grateful to Professor U.S. Ryan for all her help and advice.

REFERENCES

1. Ryan US. The endothelial surface and response to injury. Fed Proc 1986;45:101–108.
2. Kirkpatrick CJ, Melzner I, Goller T. Comparative effects of trypsin, collagenase and mechanical harvesting on cell membrane lipids studied in monolayer-cultured endothelial cells and a green monkey kidney cell line. Biochim Biophys Acta 1985;846:120–126.
3. Brigham KL, Meyrick B, Ryan US. Trypsin induced aggregation of bovine pulmonary artery endothelial cells cultured on microcarrier. Tissue Cell 1984; 16:167–172.
4. Ryan US, Ryan JW. Vital and functional activities of endothelial cells. In: Nossel HL, Vogel HJ, eds. Pathobiology of the Endothelial Cell. Orlando, Florida: Academic Press, 1982:455–469.
5. Sung C-P, Arleth AJ, Shikano K, Zabko-Potapovich B, Berkowitz BA. Effects of trypsinization in cell culture on bradykinin receptors in vascular endothelial cells. Biochem Pharmacol 1989;38:696–699.
6. Shimokawa H, Aarhus LL, Vanhoutte PM. Porcine coronary arteries with regenerated endothelium have a reduced endothelium-dependent responsiveness to aggregating platelets and serotonin. Circ Res 1987;61:256–270.
7. Ryan US, Ryan JW. Vital and functional activities of endothelial cells. In: Pathobiology of the Endothelial Cell. Orlando, Florida: Academic Press, 1982.
8. Ryan US, Schultz DR, Ryan JW. Fc and C3b receptors on pulmonary endothelial cells; induction by injury. Science 1981;21:557–559.
9. Cesarone CF, Fugassa E, Gallo G, Voci A, Orunesu M. Collagenase perfusion of rat liver induces DNA damage and DNA repair in hepatocytes. Mutat Res 1984;141:113–116.
10. Ryan US, Clements E, Habliston D, Ryan JW. Isolation and culture of pulmonary artery endothelial cells. Tissue Cell 1978;10:535–554.
11. Ryan US, White LA. Varicose veins as a source of adult human endothelial cells. Tissue & Cell 1985;17:171–176.
12. Ryan JW, Chung A, Martin LC, et al. New substrates for the radioassay of angiotensin converting enzyme of endothelial cells in culture. Tissue Cell 1978; 10:555–562.
13. Freshney RI, ed. Animal Cell Culture. A Practical Approach. Oxford: IRL Press, 1986.
14. Maciag T, Burgess WH. The structural and functional properties of endothelial cell growth factor and its receptor. In: Ryan US, ed. Endothelial Cells. Vol. II. Boca Raton, Florida: CRC Press, 1988.
15. Macaig T, Cerundolo J, Ilsley S, Kelley PR, Forand R. An endothelial cell growth factor from bovine hypothalamus: Identification and partial characterization. Proc Natl Acad Sci USA 1979;76:5674–5678.

The Endothelium: An Introduction to Current Research, pages 273–293
© 1990 Wiley-Liss, Inc.

21
Isolation and Culture of High Endothelial Venule Endothelium From Rat Lymph Nodes

ANN AGER

Immunology Group, Department of Cell and Structural Biology, University of Manchester, Manchester M13 9PT, England

INTRODUCTION

Immune responses are normally initiated in lymphoid organs, such as the spleen and lymph nodes, in which antigen is sequestered. Lymphocytes in these organs are nomadic cells that migrate from and return to the blood within a few hours. A large pool of lymphocytes is continuously recirculating via the bloodstream and lymphatics through lymphoid organs that are widely distributed throughout the body. Lymphocyte recirculation is fundamental for the initiation of immune responses, since it permits the full repertoire of antigenic specificities to be continuously represented throughout the entire immune system. In addition, it enables products of the immune response generated in one site, such as effector cells and memory cells, to be disseminated to other tissues (1).

The selective entry of lymphocytes into lymphoid tissues over other leucocytes is thought to be controlled by the expression of recognition molecules for lymphocytes on specialised vascular endothelial cells. These are located in the marginal sinus capillaries of the spleen and postcapillary venules in the paracortical region of lymph nodes (LN). In some species, such as rodents and man, the postcapillary venules of LN are histologically distinctive because the lining endothelial cells are plump or cuboidal; these vessels are normally restricted to LN and are commonly known as high endothelial venules (HEV) (2). However, blood vessels resembling HEV in morphology have been reported at sites of chronic inflammation (3), suggesting that lymphocyte recruitment to inflammatory sites may occur via an HEV-related mechanism. The distinctive appearance of HEV, their induction during chronic inflammation, and their central role in the recruitment of lymphocytes from the blood have made them a target for intensive study.

The first step in extravasation has been studied in vitro using the frozen section assay of Stamper and Woodruff (4), in which the adhesion of lymphocytes to HEV in sectioned LN is measured at low temperatures. Three separate families of lymphocyte surface molecule that mediate adhesion to HEV have been identified using this assay (5,6). Because of their apparent ability to direct the migration of lymphocytes into LN, these molecules have been called LN homing receptors. Vascular endothelium is inaccessible to direct experimentation in the frozen section assay, since the tissue is frozen and usually fixed; consequently, the endothelial ligands for LN homing receptors are poorly understood.

The success of the frozen section assay in identifying lymphocyte determinants involved in extravasation has led to the conclusion that endothelium plays a purely passive role in lymphocyte recognition, that of presenting ligand(s) for LN homing receptors. However, the results of numerous studies show HEV endothelium to be significantly more activated than endothelia lining other blood vessels either inside or outside LN. Endothelial cells lining HEV are large cells in which protein synthetic and secretory pathways are up-regulated. HEV endothelial cells have substantially higher levels of cytoplasmic nonspecific esterase than do other endothelia (7). The function of this enzyme in HEV is unknown. The metabolism of sodium sulphate by lymphoid tissue has identified a unique biosynthetic pathway in HEV endothelial cells, resulting in the continuous secretion of a sulphated glycolipid (8,9). Recently, the application of hybridoma technology to the study of HEV has identified several antigens that are uniquely expressed on HEV endothelium in the mouse (5,10). It is tempting to speculate that some of these HEV-associated properties may be actively involved in the extravasation of lymphocytes. In fact, two HEV-specific antigens identified so far have been shown to mediate lymphocyte adhesion in the frozen section assay; they are thought to be ligands for LN homing receptors (5).

The activated state of HEV endothelium described above is dependent on an intact LN microenvironment. Lymph nodes are served by two vascular supplies: the blood and lymphatic systems. The majority of lymphocytes in a LN (> 95%) gain access directly from the blood via HEV. Antigen, antigen presenting cells, and low numbers of lymphocytes drain into the node from surrounding tissues via afferent lymphatics. Permanent ligation of afferent lymphatics induces a dramatic change in the phenotype of HEV over the first 3 weeks following operation. There is a gradual reduction in the "height" of endothelial cells lining HEV, such that after 3 weeks these paracortical postcapillary venules are lined with flattened endothelium (11). Loss of activated phenotype in HEV is accompanied by loss of function in these blood vessels. There is a rapid fall in lymphocyte migration across HEV which is detectable within 24 hr of deafferentisation. In addition, the rate of sulphated glycolipid synthesis in HEV is significantly reduced 2 weeks after deafferentisation (12). In the absence of an intact lymphoid microenvironment, HEV endothelial cells adopt a resting, flattened phenotype in which HEV function is barely detectable 3 weeks after deafferentisation. Whether HEV in deafferentised LN revert to a type of non-HEV postcapillary venule such as that found in nonlymphoid tissue remains to be determined.

The component(s) in afferent lymph responsible for controlling HEV phenotype and function have not been identified, although cellular and/or soluble products of immune responses have been proposed to play active roles (11,12). However, these studies show that the phenotype and function of HEV endothelium in intact LN are not constitutively expressed but are dependent on external stimuli derived from the lymphoid microenvironment. To determine the signals responsible for the control of HEV phenotype, it is necessary to study HEV endothelium in isolation from its normal microenvironment. In order to perform these studies, techniques for the isolation and culture of HEV endothelium have been developed (13). The endothelial cells lining HEV, referred to as high endothelial cells (HEC), were isolated from rat LN using the selective uptake of radioactive sulphate by HEC to identify and distinguish these cells from all other stromal cells in lymphoid tissues. Enriched populations of HEC ($\geq 70\%$) were obtained by limited digestion of lymphoid tissue. HEC underwent dramatic changes in morphology over the first 3 days following isolation, after which HEC readily proliferated and selectively outgrew the low numbers of contaminating stromal cells in primary LN cultures to give confluent cultures of $> 99\%$ purity. Serial subculture of primary LN cultures yielded stable lines of HEC that demonstrated several properties in common with other types of vascular endothelia. However, HEC were phenotypically distinguishable from non-HEV endothelial cells at all stages of culture. In the complete absence of a lymphoid microenvironment, in vitro cultured HEC lines adopted a resting phenotype that was significantly different from that of freshly isolated HEC. Prolonged co-culture with mitogen-pulsed lymph node cells induced the expression of an "activated" phenotype similar to that of HEC immediately after isolation from LN. It is proposed that cultured HEC constitutively express a resting phenotype such as that of HEV in deafferentised lymph nodes. However, under appropriate conditions HEC can be induced to express an "activated" phenotype such as that of HEV in intact LN. The transition between resting and "activated" phenotypes in cultured HEC provides a model in which to study the signals required for the control of phenotype and function in this type of specialised endothelium.

ISOLATION OF HIGH ENDOTHELIAL CELLS FROM RAT LYMPH NODES

Techniques for the isolation of HEC have been described in detail (13). Briefly, HEC in lymphoid tissue were selectively labelled by incubating LN slices with 50 μCi/ml sodium ^{35}S-sulphate in RPMI 1640 for 30 min at 37°C.

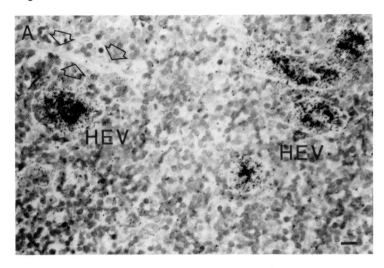

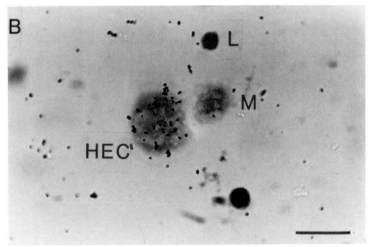

Fig. 1. **A:** Autoradiograph of radioactive sulphate-labelled LN showing numerous labelled HEV in paracortex. Note absence of label in venule lined with flat EC *(open arrows).* (Methyl green and pyronin.) Bar: 50 μm. ×100. **B:** Autoradiograph of cells isolated from LN (as in **A**) by collagenase digestion after 60 min in culture showing large labelled HEC, medium-sized unlabelled nonlymphoid cells (M), and unlabelled small lymphocytes (L). (Methyl green and pyronin.) Bar: 20 μm. ×1,000. **C:** Phase-contrast micrograph of parallel primary LN culture to **B** showing large vesiculated HEC, medium-sized phase-dark macrophages (M), and phase-light lymphocytes (L). Bar: 50 μm. ×325. **D:** Phase-contrat micrograph of microvascular EC colony occasionally found in primary LN cultures. Note different EC morphology. Bar: 50 μm. ×325.

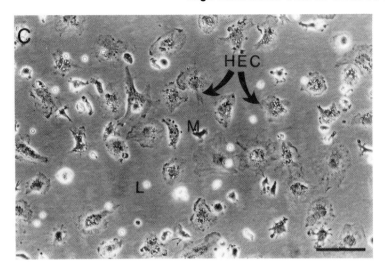

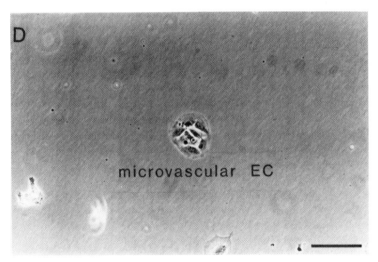

Autoradiographic analysis shows that the rapid localisation of sulfate in HEC can be used to distinguish these cells from all other stromal cells of lymphoid tissues (Fig. 1A). $^{35}SO_4$-labelled lymph node slices were digested with 0.5% type II collagenase in RPMI 1640 at 50 mg tissue/ml for 60 min at 37°C on a rotating table. Disaggregated cells were separated from undigested tissue by filtration through 100-μm nylon mesh. Isolated cells were resuspended in RPMI 1640 supplemented with 20% foetal calf serum (FCS)

(RPMI 20) to 50 mg tissue/ml and plated at either 0.2 ml (10 mg tissue)/ well onto 13-mm-diameter thermanox coverslips in 15-mm-diameter wells of tissue culture plates or at 4 ml (200 mg tissue)/flask in 25-cm^2 flasks (Nunclon). Nonadherent cells were removed after 60 min by vigorous washing, and adherent cells on coverslips were processed for autoradiography. Adherent cells in flasks were maintained in culture and analysed in parallel by phase-contrast microscopy.

Autoradiographic analysis of primary LN cultures showed that type II collagenase released three distinct populations of cells: (i) large, 20- to 30-μm-diameter, $^{35}SO_4$-labelled cells; (ii) medium-sized, 10- to 15-μm diameter unlabelled cells, and (iii) small lymphocytes that were unlabelled (Fig. 1B). Of the two populations of nonlymphoid cells (i + ii), 71.7 $\pm$ 4.9% ($\pm$SD, n=4) were labelled, large cells these were therefore HEC. The major population of ^{35}S-labelled HEC in autoradiographs were readily identified in parallel, primary LN cultures by phase-contrast microscopy. HEC were singly dispersed, large, (20–30-μm-diameter) cells that had numerous perinuclear vesicles and occasionally two or more lymphocytes attached. The minor population of unlabelled adherent cells seen in autoradiographs were small (<10-μm-diameter cells) with condensed cytoplasm and without clearly outlined nuclei. These cells were readily identified as lymph node macrophages by phase-contrast microscopy. There was surprisingly very little contamination of primary LN cultures by fibroblasts, non-HEV endothelium, or pericytes ($<1\%$). Primary LN cultures also contained numerous lymphocytes, but these were subsequently removed by vigorous washing (Fig. 1C). The morphology of freshly isolated HEC was readily distinguishable from that reported for other endothelial cells (EC). Occasionally, clumps of microvascular EC were seen in primary LN cultures; these consisted of aggregates of six to seven small (10-μm-diameter) condensed cells (Fig. 1D) as reported previously for bovine adrenal capillary EC (14).

CULTURE OF HIGH ENDOTHELIAL CELLS

Primary LN cultures enriched for HEC were maintained in RPMI 20 and monitored closely for cell type and morphology by phase-contrast microscopy. After 2–3 days, HEC had undergone dramatic changes in morphology. HEC flattened up to 50 μm in diameter and adopted an epithelial morphology. The perinuclear vesicular compartment in HEC was no longer visible. After 3 days, HEC started to proliferate with a doubling time of 1–2 days. Daughter cells adopted a migratory phenotype such that they became singly dispersed throughout the culture vessel (Fig. 2A). At confluence, HEC adopted a characteristic phenotype, that of closely apposed, bipolar cells that demonstrated a marked tendency to align in parallel arrays (Fig. 2B). HEC were subcultured using 0.1% trypsin–0.025% EDTA and plated at 50% confluent density. Subcultured HEC maintained an epithelial morphology at low density. At confluence, subcultured HEC adopted a bipolar, aligned morphology, although the tendency to align was never as great as in primary cultures. At all stages of culture, HEC grew in a monolayer configuration; although there was considerable cytoplasmic overlap between adjacent HEC, nuclear overlap was not seen. HEC were serially subcultured to 50% of confluent density and maintained in high concentrations of serum. In this way, lines of HEC have been generated from primary LN cultures. Individual HEC lines were stable in that there were no obvious changes in growth rate or morphology as the cells were passaged up to maximum of 25 times. Immediately after isolation, primary LN cultures were contaminated with $\leq 30\%$ macrophages and $< 1\%$ stromal cells. After 7–10 days, macrophages were no longer visible in these cultures. The colonies of non-HEV, microvascular EC, and fibroblasts occasionally seen in primary LN cultures did not proliferate (see under Selective Growth of High Endothelial Cells in Vitro). Thus, although no attempt was made to purify HEC further, the selective survival of HEC over macrophages and their selective outgrowth over other stromal cells yielded primary LN cultures of $> 99\%$ purity at first confluence.

IMPORTANT FACTORS FOR ESTABLISHING HIGH ENDOTHELIAL CELL LINES

We have been generating HEC lines since 1985 and over that time period, several crucial factors have emerged for the success of this work.

Batch of Collagenase

There is considerable batch variation in the ability of type II collagenase to release HEC. The variation appears to be restricted to the number of viable HEC released; it does not yield other stromal cell types from lymphoid tissue. Three batches are screened at a time and type II collagenase from Sigma Chemical Co. and Worthington Biochemical Co., both of specific activity 170 U/mg, have been used to isolate HEC. In order to measure the yield of HEC, the amount of $^{35}SO_4$-cell associated radioactivity released from prelabelled lymphoid tissue was expressed as a percentage of total labelled tissue. On average 12% of total labelled cells were released by type II collagenase; this corresponded to a yield of $1–5 \times 10^4$ HEC per 200 mg tissue. The yield of $^{35}SO_4$-cell associated radioactivity was increased to $> 50\%$ by including 0.5% Dispase (neutral protease; Boehringer-Mannheim) in the digestion mixture. However autoradiographic analysis showed that the number of $^{35}SO_4$-labelled HEC released was not increased (13). The difference in yield was accounted for by labelled cell debris resulting from the harsher enzyme treatment. Although digestion with type II collagenase was limited, the selective release of HEC yielded primary LN cultures enriched to $> 70\%$ purity. In addition, the number of HEC released per mg of tissue was sufficient to establish HEC lines; other studies have shown that a minimum of 10^4 HEC/25 cm^2 flask (400 cells/cm^2) is

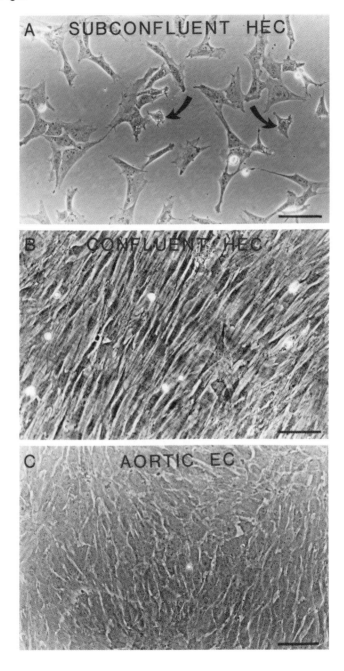

required for the maintenance of rapidly proliferating HEC (see under Serum-Dependent Proliferation).

Specific Biochemical/Immunological Markers for High Endothelial Cells

In order to identify microvascular EC after isolation from a solid organ, a range of specific markers is required to distinguish EC from other stromal cells which may be released. Routinely, EC have been identified by a combination of markers that include distinct morphology (15,16), localisation of vWF:Ag (16), growth factor dependency (17,18), uptake of acetylated low-density lipoproteins (LDL), lectin staining (20), and usually a functional assay that depends on the source of EC.

This list was of variable use when applied to the identification of rat HEC in culture. The morphology and growth factor dependency of cultured HEC could not be predicted in advance. Immunohistochemical staining of rat LN showed that the localisation of vWF:Ag was restricted to non-HEV blood vessels; HEV did not stain for vWF:Ag using immunohistochemical analysis (13). Rat HEC incorporated acetylated LDL for the first 2–3 days after isolation; uptake was localised to perinuclear vesicles in these cells. Incorporation of acetylated LDL was not detectable by fluorescence microscopy after 7–10 days of culture when perinuclear vesicles were no longer visible in rat HEC (Ager, unpublished observations). However, Ise et al. (21) reported uptake of acetylated LDL in a rat HEC line using FACS analysis. Recently, the application of hybridoma technology to the study of EC has generated monoclonal antibodies that detect endothelial cell-specific antigens. However, this approach is still in its infancy. In the absence of good phenotypic markers for rat HEC, we have concentrated on the use of functional assays to characterise these cells in culture. The rapid, selective uptake of sulphate by HEC has been used to identify these cells after isolation. In addition, we have found that cultured HEC constitutively express recognition molecules for recirculating lymphocytes. This observation forms the basic assay for HEV function in cultured HEC. The interactions between lymphocytes and cultured HEC are discussed in a separate chapter.

Proliferation of High Endothelial Cells In Vivo and In Vitro

To establish rapidly growing HEC lines, we have routinely used antigen activated LN in which HEC proliferation is elevated above its low basal

---

Fig. 2. Phase-contrast micrographs of endothelial cells in culture. **A:** Primary LN culture after 5 days showing numerous HEC with epithelial, nonvesiculated morphology. Note few remaining vesiculated HEC *(curved arrows)* and absence of macrophages and lymphocytes from these cultures (cf. Fig. 1C). **B:** Confluent primary LN culture showing distinct bipolar, aligned morphology of HEC. **C:** Confluent rat aortic EC showing polygonal or "cobblestone" morphology typical of vascular EC in culture. Bars: 50 μm. $\times$325.

level. Popliteal LN of F_1 hybrid rats were activated by administration of 10^7 parental lymphocytes into the footpad, which induces a local graft-versus-host response. After 4 days, nodes were collected from 4×250 g rats (200–250 mg total tissue) and pooled for HEC isolation. Alternatively, HEC lines have been established from cervical LN of rats kept under conventional animal house conditions. In the absence of a specific pathogen-free environment, these LN are sufficiently activated by environmental antigens to contain proliferating HEC.

Isolated HEC must be maintained in high concentrations of FCS to ensure rapid proliferation for the generation of cell lines. We have not found significant FCS batch dependency by HEC lines. However, we have found that the proliferative capacity of individual HEC lines can range from a minimum of three passages to a maximum of 25. HEC lines from AO or AO $\times$ DA rats have been maintained for longer periods than those from PVG rats. Ise *et al.* (21) reported the maintenance of HEC lines from PVG rat axillary LN in batch-tested FCS. In general, rat EC (aortic EC and HEC) proliferated more readily in either RPMI 1640 or MEM rather than in DMEM, MEM or M199 growth media (Ager, unpublished observations).

Selective Growth of High Endothelial Cells In Vitro

The conditions that supported the rapid proliferation of HEC in primary LN cultures did not support the growth of other stromal cells. This observation was tested directly by determining whether media conditioned by primary LN cultures supported the proliferation of either rat aortic EC (AEC) or rat aortic adventitial fibroblasts.

To measure proliferation, cells were plated in triplicate in 15-mm-diameter wells of Nunclon tissue culture plates (1–10 $\times$ 10^4 cells/well); the following day, growth was arrested by incubation for 24–48 hr in RPMI 1640 supplemented with 0.5% FCS. Cells were incubated in either test or control media for 3–5 days. The numbers of cells before and after incubation were measured by electronic particle counting after detachment using 0.1% trypsin–0.025% EDTA. Results were expressed as a percentage of final cell yield in control media.

Conditioned media were collected from primary LN cultures between the 2nd and 6th day after isolation and diluted 1:1 with RPMI 20. The effects of RPMI 20 (control) and primary LN culture conditioned media on the proliferation of HEC, AEC, and fibroblasts were measured in a 4-day assay. Following growth arrest, the recovery of HEC in RPMI 20 was much lower than the recovery of either AEC or fibroblasts. However, after 4 days in conditioned media, the yield of HEC was almost twice that in the control wells at 198%. The yield of AEC was considerably lower than in control wells at 36%. Similarly, the yield of fibroblasts was low at 24% of that in control wells (Fig. 3). Thus, primary LN culture-conditioned media supported the growth of HEC over and above that in its absence. At the same

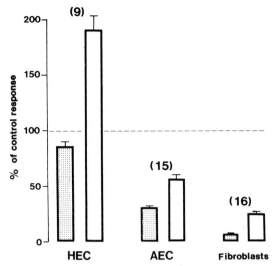

Fig. 3. Proliferation of HEC, AEC, and aortic fibroblasts in primary LN culture conditioned media. Following growth arrest cells were incubated for 4 days in either control or conditioned media. Results are expressed as percentages of growth in control wells to show the extent of proliferation following growth arrest and in the presence of conditioned media. Bars give cell numbers at the start (stippled bars) and end (open bars) of the incubation period. Results are average percentage of control $\pm$SD (n = 9–16).

time, the growth of AEC and fibroblasts were significantly inhibited by conditioned media. These results may explain the selective outgrowth of HEC over other stromal cells types that occurs in primary LN cultures.

GROWTH CHARACTERISTICS OF RAT HIGH ENDOTHELIAL CELLS

The growth of non-HEV EC demonstrates several distinctive properties such as contact inhibition of proliferation, serum dependency, and growth factor dependency. The growth characteristics of rat HEC were studied in order to compare this type of specialised microvascular EC with other types of EC.

Serum-Dependent Proliferation

HEC were plated at 5×10^4 cells per 25 cm^2 tissue culture flask (Nunclon) and grown in RPMI 1640 supplemented with either FCS, newborn calf serum (NBCS), or rat serum at 0.5, 5, 10, or 20% (v/v) concentration. Media were changed after 3 days; after a total of 7 days, cells were counted by electronic particle counting after detachment with trypsin/EDTA. HEC

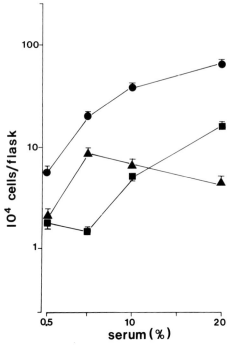

Fig. 4. Serum-dependent proliferation of HEC. Cells were plated at $5 \times 10^4/25$-cm^2 flask and grown for 7 days in increasing concentrations of foetal calf serum (FCS) (●), newborn calf serum (NBCS) (■), or rat serum (▲). Results are mean number of cells/flask $\pm$SD (n = 3).

proliferation increased in a dose-dependent manner in the presence of either FCS or NBCS. The plating efficiency of HEC in NBCS was low at 33% of that in FCS. After accounting for the lower plating efficiency, the yield of HEC in NBCS was only 60% of that in FCS. The plating efficiency of rat HEC in rat serum was also low at 35% of that in FCS. Rat serum was cytostatic for HEC at doses of 5% and above (Fig. 4). In a separate experiment, HEC were plated at 0.2, 1.0, 10.0, and 125.0 $\times$ 10^4 cells in replicate 25-cm^2 flasks and grown in RPMI 20 for $\leq$15 days. Media were changed every 3 or 4 days, and the cells were harvested for counting after 3, 7, 10, 13, or 15 days. When plated at $>10^4$ cells per flask (>400 cells/cm^2), HEC proliferated exponentially to a saturation density of 120–160 $\times$ 10^4 cells/flask. When HEC were plated within saturation density at 125 $\times$ 10^4 cells/flask, the cells did not proliferate further. At plating densities of less than 10^4/flask, there was a lag phase of 7 days before exponential growth was reached. The average doubling time of rat HEC during exponential growth was 1.2 days (Fig. 5).

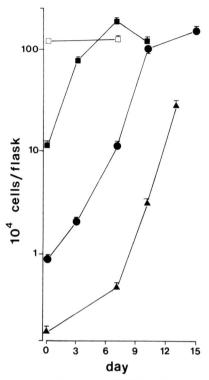

Fig. 5. Density-dependent proliferation of HEC. Cells were plated in replicate at $0.2, 1, 10$, and $125 \times 10^4/25\text{-cm}^2$ flask and grown in RPMI 1640 supplemented with 20% (v/v) foetal calf serum (FCS) for a total of 15 days. Flasks were harvested for cell counts after 3, 7, 10, and 13 days. Results are mean number of cells/flask $\pm$SD $(n = 3)$.

Thus, in order to maintain rapidly proliferating HEC lines, the cells must be seeded at a minimum density (equivalent to 400 cells/cm^2) in high concentrations of FCS. We have found that these two conditions were specifically required for the maintenance of proliferating HEC in primary LN cultures. In addition, these results show that HEC demonstrated saturation density-dependent inhibition of growth, a property in common with non-HEV endothelial cells in culture.

Immune Response-Dependent Proliferation

The turnover of non-HEV endothelia is tightly regulated in vivo. In the absence of neovascularisation, such as in endometriosis and tumour angiogenesis, labelling indices of large vessel and microvascular EC are low at 0.05–0.5% (22). In resting popliteal LN, the labelling index of HEC determined 4 hr after a single thymidine pulse was low at $< 0.4\%$. Following a single injection of antigen in the form of 0.1 ml of 10% sheep red blood cells into the footpad, the turnover of HEC increased by at least 19-fold to a peak of 7.6% after 4 days (23). This dramatically increased labelling index of HEC falls within the ranges reported for endothelial turnover during neovascularisation of tumours and placental tissues. Identification of a growth factor for HEC might permit the rescue of HEC lines with limited proliferative capacity in vitro, as well as cloning of HEC. A systematic study of the effects of soluble and/or cellular products of primary immune responses on the proliferation of HEC has therefore been undertaken.

Human recombinant interleukin 1α (IL-α; 20 U/ml; ref. standard, NIBSC), human IL-1β (20 U/ml; Genentech), rat IL-2 (0.5–50 half-maximal U/ml, Collaborative Research), and human recombinant tumour necrosis factor α (TNF-α; 200 U/ml, ref. standard, NIBSC) had no effect on HEC proliferation in a 4-day assay. Rat recombinant γ-interferon (IFNγ) at 100 U/ml had no effect on rat HEC growth in three experiments. In two further experiments, HEC growth was partially inhibited (yields of 24% and 32% of control). To accommodate species specificity of lymphokine action, mitogen-pulsed rat lymph node cells were used to prepare a mixture of rat lymphokines for analysis. Media were collected from rat lymph node cell (LNC) suspensions that had been incubated for 3 days in RPMI 1640 supplemented with 5% FCS (RPMI 5) at 5×10^6 cells/ml following a 4-hr pulse with or without 5 μg/ml concanavalin A (Con A) at 10^7 cells/ml. Conditioned media were dialysed against fresh RPMI 5 and tested in a 3-day assay in which HEC were plated at 3×10^4 cells per 15-mm-diameter well. In this series of experiments, HEC were not growth arrested prior to assay. In the presence of LNC-conditioned media, HEC growth was significantly inhibited in four experiments giving yields of 50–60% of those in control media. The inhibitory effects of LNC conditioned media were independent of mitogen activation, since media conditioned by unstimulated LNC inhibited HEC proliferation to a similar extent as media conditioned by Con A-activated LNC. In a further three experiments, LNC conditioned media had no significant effect on HEC growth.

In order to determine whether the variable effects of LNC conditioned media were due to short-lived mediators or to low-molecular-weight factors that were lost on dialysis, HEC proliferation was measured in the presence of either LNC or Con A-pulsed LNC. The results were compared directly with proliferation in the presence of media conditioned by either unstimulated or Con A-pulsed LNC. HEC growth was monitored for 3 days by electronic particle counting using a gate to exclude lymphocytes from the co-culture experiments. Triplicate wells were harvested for initial HEC counts, and the remaining cells were incubated with the following: control media, RPMI 5; LNC conditioned media; Con A-pulsed LNC conditioned media; LNC at 5×10^6/ml; and Con A-pulsed LNC at 5×10^6/ml (pulsed for 4 hr at 10^7 cells/ml with 5 μg/ml Con A and excess Con A removed by washing). After 5 washes to remove lymphocytes and/or incubation media, triplicate wells from each treatment were harvested daily for counting. As shown in Figure 6, HEC proliferated in the presence of RPMI 5 (media control) but with a slightly reduced doubling time of 2 days, presumably due to the low concentration of serum in this experiment. Proliferation of HEC in the presence of LNC conditioned media was significantly inhibited after 3 days. This effect was clearly visible after 48 hr, but not after 24-hr incubation, and was largely independent of prior activation of lymphocytes, since the yields were 61% in Con-A-LNC conditioned media and 69% in LNC conditioned media. This inhibitory activity is therefore unlikely to be due to carryover of Con A from the initial pulse period. The most dramatic effects on HEC growth were seen when LNC were co-cultured with HEC. In the presence of unstimulated LNC, the growth of HEC was stimulated over and above that in RPMI 5, such that the yield after 3 days was 127%. The stimulatory effect of LNC on HEC growth was detectable as early as 24 hr and was a consistent observation at 48 hr. Con A-pulsed LNC had an opposing effect on HEC proliferation. After 1, 2, and 3 days, the yields of HEC were consistently lower than those in control wells at 87%, 70%, and 31%, respectively. Between days 2 and 3, there was an absolute reduction in the number of HEC in wells containing Con A-pulsed LNC.

HEC growth-promoting activity has been identified during the co-culture of HEC with LNC. The relationship between this growth-promoting

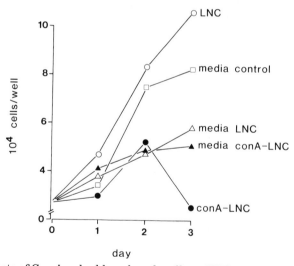

Fig. 6. Effects of Con A-pulsed lymph node cells on HEC proliferation. HEC were plated at 3×10^4/15-mm-diameter well and incubated in triplicate for 3 days with control media ($\square$), media conditioned by LNC ($\triangle$), media conditioned by Con A-pulsed LNC ($\blacktriangle$), LNC ($\bigcirc$), Con A-pulsed LNC ($\bullet$). See text for details. Results are average numbers of cells/well after 1, 2, and 3 days incubation.

activity and that seen in primary LN culture conditioned media remains to be determined. The apparent absence of HEC growth promoting activity from cell-free media conditioned by LNC suggests that this activity could be either short-lived or dialysable. Alternatively, the generation of this activity could depend on intimate contact between LNC and HEC. We have already shown that a fraction of LNC will adhere with high affinity to cultured HEC (24). For the first 48 hr, the inhibitory effects of Con A-pulsed LNC on HEC proliferation were indistinguishable from those of LNC conditioned media. It is not known whether the absolute reduction in HEC number after 2 days incubation was due to a cytotoxic effect or to physical detachment of HEC from tissue culture plastic. A parallel visual analysis of cultured HEC during this experiment demonstrated that prolonged co-culture with Con A-pulsed LNC induced substantial morphological changes in HEC that were not induced by unstimulated LNC or media conditioned by LNC. These phenotypic changes in HEC are described under Multiple Phenotype of Cultured HEC. The opposing effects of LNC and Con A-pulsed LNC on HEC growth were not simply dependent on soluble factors released by these cells, since media conditioned by either unstimulated or activated LNC were equally cytostatic for HEC. The factors responsible remain undetermined; however, the inhibitory effects of γ-interferon on HEC proliferation described above suggest that this is a possible candidate at least for the effects of mitogen-activated LNC.

Thus, the normal HEV microenvironment contains both growth promoting and growth arresting activities for HEC. It will be important to delineate these components in detail to understand the fine control of HEV development in vivo, which is crucial for the recruitment of lymphocytes from the blood into both normal and inflamed tissues.

HIGH ENDOTHELIAL VENULE ENDOTHELIUM REPRESENTS A DISTINCT TYPE OF VASCULAR ENDOTHELIUM

At all stages of culture, the morphology of rat HEC was markedly different from that of either rat microvascular EC or rat aortic EC. HEC were isolated as 20- to 30-μm-diameter single cells that were heavily vesiculated. Microvascular EC were isolated as colonies of six to seven small (10-μm-diameter) condensed cells (Fig. 1C, D). As HEC were maintained in culture, they lost their vesicular compartment, adopted a motile morphology, and proliferated in a serum-dependent manner. At confluence, HEC adopted a characteristic phenotype of bipolar cells that aligned in parallel arrays (Fig. 2B). In comparison, rat aortic EC demonstrated a polygonal cobblestone morphology at confluence (Fig. 2C) typical of other large vessel EC. Under the culture conditions used, the phenotype expressed by HEC lines was stable for up to 25 passages, referred to as resting phenotype. At no time did HEC lines demonstrate a morphology typical of non-HEV endothelial cells in culture.

The cobblestone morphology typical of non-HEV endothelial cells in culture is not a permanent feature of these cells. After prolonged incubation with immune mediators, such as IFNγ, TNF, or supernatants from mitogen-pulsed lymphocytes, human umbilical vein EC undergo a reversible reorganisation in that the cells adopt a bipolar morphology and align in parallel arrays (25,26). Cytokine-activated umbilical vein EC layers were more disorganised than were those of untreated cells. This altered morphology was associated with an increase in cell size (27) and redistribution of fibronectin (26) and proteoglycan (28) deposition in the extracellular matrix. The morphology of cytokine-activated umbilical vein EC was similar to that constitutively expressed by HEC lines. Thus, it is possible that cultured HEC represent a type of cytokine-activated non-HEV endothelium. Since HEC were originally isolated from antigen-activated LN, these cells would be exposed to factors such as IFNγ and TNF. However, in culture the supply of these factors has been removed. In fact, we have been unable to detect significant levels of IL-1, IFNγ, or TNF activity in media conditioned by either primary LN cultures or HEC lines. Thus, it would appear that HEC constitutively express the morphology of cytokine-activated non-HEV endothelia in a cytokine-independent manner. These results suggest that HEV endothelium is a distinct type of vascular endothelium that is irreversibly committed to its specialised phenotype and function in lymphoid tissue.

MULTIPLE PHENOTYPE OF CULTURED HEC: TRANSITION FROM RESTING TO ACTIVATED PHENOTYPE IN VITRO

Cultured HEC were incubated with either Con A-pulsed LNC or unstimulated LNC as described earlier. Phase-contrast microscopy showed that HEC morphology was dramatically altered by the 2nd day of incubation with Con A-pulsed LNC. There was a contraction of HEC into discrete aggregates of 5–10 cells. Within these clumps, individual HEC were small, condensed cells in which perinuclear vesiculation was visible (Fig. 7D). The condensed, vesiculated morphology of these activated HEC was similar to that of freshly isolated HEC (cf. Fig. 1C), referred to as "activated" phenotype. Co-culture with unstimulated LNC had no effect on HEC morphology (Fig. 7C). The reorganisation of HEC during co-culture with Con A-pulsed LNC did not appear to be due to the production of soluble factors, such as IFNγ or TNF, by activated lymphocytes. Prolonged incubation of HEC for up to 3 days with 200 U/ml of either IFNγ or TNF had no significant effect on the resting phenotype constitutively expressed by HEC lines (results not shown). The morphology of HEC was slightly altered following incubation with media conditioned by Con A-pulsed LNC. There was some condensation of HEC within discrete areas. However, a vesicular compartment was not seen in these cells (Fig. 7A,B).

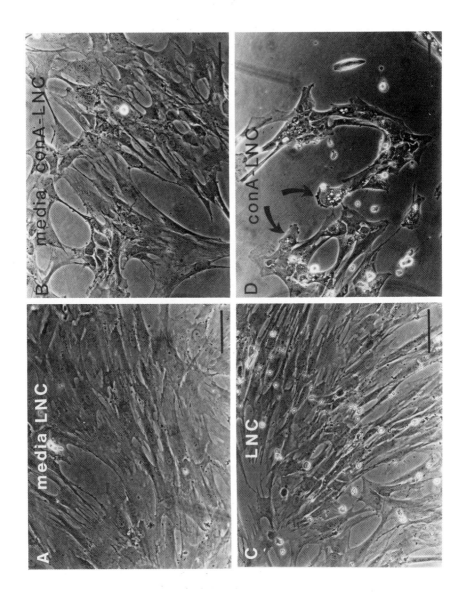

SUMMARY

The generation of high endothelial cell (HEC) lines from rat lymph nodes has been described in detail. A combination of selective release and selective outgrowth of HEC over other stromal cells yielded confluent primary LN cultures enriched for HEC to greater than 95% purity. Rapidly proliferating HEC lines were generated from primary LN cultures by serial subculture using trypsin/EDTA and maintenance in high concentrations of foetal calf serum. HEC demonstrated some properties in common with other types of vascular endothelia, such as monolayer configuration, contact inhibition of growth, and uptake of acetylated LDL. However other endothelial specific markers, such as vWF:Ag, were not detectable in HEC either *in situ* or in culture. HEC lines constitutively expressed a resting phenotype distinct from that of other types of endothelia at all stages of culture, suggesting that HEC are a distinct type of vascular endothelial cell. Following co-culture with mitogen-activated lymph node cells, HEC expressed an activated phenotype, which was similar to that seen in cells immediately after isolation from lymphoid tissue.

It is proposed that in the absence of a lymphoid microenvironment in vitro cultured HEC constitutively express a resting phenotype such as that of HEV in deafferentised LN. However, following co-culture with lymph node components, cultured HEC express an activated phenotype, such as that of HEV seen in intact LN. The use of cultured HEC lines provides a new approach with which to study the control of phenotype and function in this type of specialised postcapillary venule endothelium.

ACKNOWLEDGMENTS

I gratefully acknowledge the expert technical assistance of Cheryl Holt with endothelial cell culture and Pamela Walker with proliferation assays, the photographic skills of Jane Crosby and the secretarial assistance of Jackie Jolley. This work was supported by the Medical Research Council (UK).

Fig. 7. Phase-contrast micrographs of HEC following culture with Con A-pulsed lymph node cells. HEC were incubated for 2 days with media or lymph node cells as given in the legend to Figure 6 and washed vigorously to remove incubation media. **A:** Incubation with media conditioned by LNC. HEC adopt a bipolar, aligned morphology similar to that constitutively expressed by HEC in primary LN cultures (see Fig. 2C for comparison). **B:** Incubation with media conditioned by Con A-pulsed LNC. Note some condensation of HEC in a single area. **C:** Incubation with LNC. HEC morphology is indistinguishable from that in **A**. Note few phase light LNC that remain attached to HEC after washing. **D:** Incubation with Con A-pulsed LNC. HEC monolayer shows marked reorganisation into clumps of condensed, phase-dark cells. Perinuclear vesicles are seen in individual HEC within clumps *(curved arrows)*. Bars: 50 μm. ×325.

REFERENCES

1. Ford WL. Lymphocyte migration and immune responses. Prog Allergy 1975; 19:1–59.
2. Marchesi VT, Gowans JL. The migration of lymphocytes through the endothelium of venules in lymph nodes: An electron microscope study. Proc R Soc B 1964;159:283–290.
3. Freemont AJ, Jones CJP, Bromley M, Andrews P. Changes in vascular endothelium related to lymphocyte collections in diseased synovia. Arthritis Rheum 1983;26:313–319.
4. Stamper HB, Woodruff JJ. Lymphocyte homing into lymph nodes: In vitro demonstration of the selective affinity of recirculating lymphocytes for high endothelial venules. J Exp Med 1976;144:828–833.
5. Berg EL, Goldstein LA, Jutila MA, Natache M, Picker LJ, Streeter PR, Wu NW, Zhou D, Butcher EC. Homing receptors and vascular addressins: Cell adhesion molecules that direct lymphocyte traffic. Immunol Rev 1989;108:5–18.
6. Holzmann B, Weissman IL. Integrin molecules involved in lymphocyte homing to Peyer's patches. Immunol Rev 1989;108:45–61.
7. Anderson ND, Anderson AO, Wyllie RG. Specialised structure and metabolic activities of high endothelial venules in rat lymphatic tissues. Immunology 1976;31:455–473.
8. Andrews P, Milsom DW, Ford WL. Migration of lymphocytes across specialised vascular endothelium. J Cell Sci 1982;57:277–292.
9. Andrews P, Milsom DW, Stoddart RW. Glycoconjugates from high endothelial cells. I. Partial characterisation of a sulphated glycoconjugate from the high endothelial cells of rat lymph nodes. J Cell Sci 1983;59:231–244.
10. Duivestijn AM, Kerkhove M, Bargatze RF, Butcher EC. Lymphoid tissue- and inflammation-specific endothelial differentiation defined monoclonal antibodies. J Immunol 1987;138:713–719.
11. Hendriks HR, Eestermans IL. Disappearance and reappearance of high endothelial venules and immigrating lymphocytes in lymph nodes deprived of afferent lymphatic vessels: A possible regulatory role of macrophages in lymphocyte migration. Eur J Immunol 1983;13:663–669.
12. Drayson MT, Ford WL. Afferent lymph and lymph borne cells: Their influence on lymph node function. Immunobiology 1984;169:362–379.
13. Ager A. Isolation and culture of high endothelial cells from rat lymph nodes. J Cell Sci 1987;87:133–144.
14. Folkman J, Haudenschild CC, Zetter BR. Long term culture of capillary endothelial cells. Proc Natl Acad Sci USA 1979;10;5217–5221.
15. Gimbrone MA, Cotran RS, Folkman J. Human vascular endothelial cells in culture. J Cell Biol 1974;60:673–684.
16. Jaffe EA, Nachman RL, Becker CG, Minick CR. Culture of human endothelial cells derived from umbilical veins. Identification by morphologic and immunologic criteria. J Clin Invest 1973;52:2745–2756.
17. Jaye M, Houk R, Burgess W, Ricca GA, Chiu I-M, Ravera MW, O'Brien SJ, Modi WS, Maciag T, Drohan WN. Human endothelial cell growth factor: Cloning, nucleotide sequence and chromosome localisation. Science 1986;233:541–545.
18. Abraham JA, Mergia A, Wheng JL, Thomas A, Friedman J, Hierrild KA, Gospodarowicz D, Fiddes JC. Nucleotide sequence of a bovine clone encoding the angiogenic protein, basic fibroblast growth factor. Science 1986;233:545–548.

19. Vohta JC, Via DP, Butterfield CE, Zetter BR. Identification and isolation of endothelial cells based on their increased uptake of acetylated low-density lipoprotein. J Cell Biol 1984;99:2034–2040.
20. Miehinen M, Holthofer H, Lehto V, Miehinen A, Virtanen I. Ulex Europaeus I lectin as a marker for tumours derived from endothelial cells. Am J Clin Pathol 1983;79:32–36.
21. Ise Y, Yamaguchi K, Sato K, Yamamura Y, Kitamura F, Tamatanl T, Miyasaka M. Molecular mechanisms underlying lymphocyte recirculation. Eur J Immunol 1988;18:1235–1244.
22. Hobson B, Denekamp J. Endothelial proliferation in tumours and normal tissues. Continuous labelling studies. Br J Cancer 1984;49:405–413.
23. Ager A, Drayson MT. Lymphocyte migration in the rat. In: Husband AJ, ed. Migration and Homing of Lymphoid Cells Vol I. Boca Raton, Florida: CRC Press, 1988;19–50.
24. Ager A, Mistry S. Interactions between lymphocytes and cultured high endothelial cells: An in vitro model of lymphocyte migration across high endothelial venule endothelium. Eur J Immunol 1988;18:1265–1274.
25. Montesano R, Orci L, Vassalli P. Human endothelial cell cultures: Phenotypic modulation by leucocyte interleukins. J Cell Physiol 1985;122:4124–4134.
26. Stolpen AH, Guinan EC, Fiers W, Pober JS. Recombinant tumour necrosis factor and immune interferon act singly and in combination to reorganise human vascular endothelial cell monolayers. Am J Pathol 1986;123:16–24.
27. Cavender DE, Edelbaum D, Ziff M. Endothelial cell activation induced by tumour necrosis factor and lymphotoxin. Am J Pathol 1989;134:551–560.
28. Montesano R, Mossaz A, Ryser JE, Orci L, Vassalli P. Leucocyte interleukins induce cultured endothelial cells to produce a highly organised, glycosaminoglycan-rich pericellular matrix. J Cell Biol 1984;99:1706–1715.

The Endothelium: An Introduction to Current Research, pages 295–305
© 1990 Wiley-Liss, Inc.

22
Isolation and Culture of Microvascular Endothelium

J.D. PEARSON

Section of Vascular Biology, MRC Clinical Research Centre, Harrow, Middlesex HA1 3UJ, England

INTRODUCTION

Although scattered reports of the isolation and culture of endothelial cells from the microvasculature date back to the earliest days of tissue culture, it is only with the publication in 1979 by Folkman and Haudenschild (1) that long-term serial culture of homogeneous populations of microvascular endothelial cells was achieved. During the subsequent decade, there has been a steadily increasing publication rate in this field, but it is still true that culture of microvascular endothelium is far from routine and has yet to be satisfactorily demonstrated from several organs of particular interest (e.g., bone marrow). The difficulties are twofold. First, the methods used to obtain pure cell populations have often been quite different and depend on the anatomy of the particular vascular bed and the composition of the surrounding tissue. Second, it seems that microvascular endothelial cells from different sites express markedly heterogeneous properties in vitro, making it more difficult to characterise the cells as endothelial and in particular requiring the provision of quite different conditions for successful growth.

This chapter reviews briefly the advances that have been made in the culture of microvascular endothelium from a variety of tissues. Although it is not concerned primarily with the nature of endothelial cell heterogeneity, as recently reviewed by Zetter (2), several examples of different behaviour, some of which can be altered by changing the cellular environment and others of which seem to reflect invariant site-specific phenotypic expression, are apparent.

ADRENAL GLAND

Microvascular endothelial cells from bovine adrenal cortex were those studied in most detail in the original report by Folkman and Haudenschild (1). These investigators achieved serial culture by a technique involving tissue dissociation, first mechanical and then with collagenase, plating out small tissue fragments on gelatin-coated dishes, and then the patient and skillful isolation of individual colonies of endothelium by a combination of physical removal of contaminating cell types ("weeding") and addition of mitomycin-treated feeder cells to condition the medium. Serial culture was possible on gelatin-coated plates in the presence of tumour-conditioned medium. The endothelial nature of the cells was confirmed by immunolocalisation of von Willebrand factor (vWf) and angiotensin converting enzyme (ACE). It was subsequently shown that after growth to confluence in tumour-conditioned medium or medium containing endothelial cell growth supplement (ECGS), a crude preparation of bovine fibroblast growth factor (bFGF), the cells could be propagated in simple media containing serum but no extra source of growth factors (3).

Folkman and Haudenschild (4) first noted that these cells, unlike large vessel endothelial cells, tended to remodel to form capillary-like tubes when left in confluent culture; subsequently, Montesano et al. (5) demonstrated that tube formation could be induced rapidly by seeding cells within collagen gels. It has also been shown that the presence of fenestrae, a feature of adrenocortical microvascular endothelium in vivo, can be markedly enhanced by growing the cells on biologically derived extracellular matrices (6). Most recently, adrenal microvascular endothelial cells have been used by Ingber and Folkman (7) as a model system with which to analyse how the matrix on which the cells are grown modulates their responsiveness, so that either growth or differentiation and tube formation, can be promoted by the addition of bFGF. The demonstration that endothelial cells selectively take up acetylated low-density lipoprotein (LDL) also enabled Voyta et al. (8) to isolate pure cultures of adrenal microvascular endothelial cells from mixed primary cultures without weeding, by using for the first time fluorescence-activated cell sorting to select endothelial cells that had internalised fluorescently tagged acetylated LDL.

BRAIN

Primary culture of cerebral microvascular endothelial cells, from murine brain, was first reported in 1979 by De Bault et al. (9), who used the capillary isolation technique of Brendel et al. (10), that is, homogenisation and selective retention of microvessel fragments on 150-μm mesh filters. Spatz et al. (11), who cultured similar cells from rat brain after homogenisation and separation of capillary fragments by sucrose-gradient sedimentation, another method previously used to obtain isolated brain capillaries for biochemical studies (12), were able to passage the cells once and maintain them in a medium supplemented with peptone.

Subsequent adaptations to the isolation procedure have included trapping of microvessels on glass beads in addition to filters (13), again derived from earlier methods used for purification of brain capillaries for biochemical studies, as well as brief or overnight treatment with collagenase and/or dispase to disperse individual cells and promote adhesion (13–15). Removal of contaminating cells (mainly pericytes) in primary culture has also been done in several ways: weeding and cloning (16); selective cell suspension with pancreatin and the use of endothelial cell conditioned medium or bFGF (as retinal extract) to encourage endothelial cell growth (15); or purification by fluorescence-activated cell sorting after selective binding of *Griffonia* lectin (17).

Serial subcultivation of cerebral microvascular endothelial cells in conventional media seems straightforward for cells of bovine or human origin but has not been accomplished with cells from rat brain. In addition to standard markers for endothelial cells including vWf and binding of *Ulex* lectin (18), cerebral cells in culture can be induced to express γ-glutamyl-transpeptidase activity (a feature of these cells in vivo) by co-culture with glial cells or astrocyte conditioned medium (19,20). Carson and Haudenschild (15) found uptake of acetylated LDL, a general marker for endothelium (8), in bovine cells, but Vinters et al. (16) noted that human or mouse cerebral microvascular cell cultures failed to take up acetylated LDL.

RETINA

The major problem encountered with culture of retinal microvascular endothelial cells has been to separate these cells from accompanying pericytes, present in high abundance in vivo, and now known to exert powerful negative growth regulatory effects on endothelial cells (21). Purification was first successful in primary cultures, after homogenisation of retinas and serial sieving to collect capillary fragments, by mechanical weeding (22). Bowman et al. (23) treated fragments overnight with collagenase and dispase and then used a Percoll gradient to isolate clumps of endothelial cells before plating out on fibronectin-coated wells. Subsequent studies have all noted the poor growth of retinal endothelial cells (unlike pericytes) on uncoated plastic. Gitlin and D'Amore (24) successfully subcultured bovine retinal capillary endothelial cells in medium supplemented with retinal extract. They used brief collagenase treatment before cell plating, rinsing after 1–3hr to reduce selectively the proportion of pericytes and then weeding to eliminate these cells. Schor and Schor (25) used a similar method but treated with collagenase for several hours before serial sieving to collect microvessels. McIntosh et al. (26) treated vessels with collagenase after purification and used medium supplemented with tryptose and endothelial cell conditioned medium.

Despite the obvious desire to grow these cells in culture to study mechanisms involved in retinal vascular disease, it is clear from the small number of published papers that no simplistic method will work. In general, the use of selective media, to encourage endothelial cell growth and to discourage pericyte growth (stimulated by PDGF and thus reduced in plasma-derived serum), has had to be coupled with mechanical weeding and cloning procedures to obtain pure endothelial cell cultures. Indeed, the difficulty is apparent from the fact that one of the leading groups has used capillary endothelial cells from adrenal cortex, rather than from retina, to study the regulatory effects of retinal pericytes on endothelial cell growth (21).

DERMIS

Culture of dermal microvascular endothelial cells was first attempted by collecting cells in the effluent perfusate emerging from the rabbit central ear artery during slow retrograde infusion of trypsin solution (27), although it is not clear that the cells obtained were from microvessels. The same group has subsequently developed a successful technique for the isolation and culture of endothelial cells from dermal microvessels obtained from human neonatal foreskin or adult skin. The isolation procedure relies upon the dissection and removal of epidermis, incubation of 5-mm squares with trypsin + EDTA for 10–40 min, and "expression" of endothelial cells from the tissue by pressure from a straight scalpel blade (28,29).

A remarkable feature of these cells is their apparently unique growth requirements. Like other endothelial cells, they attach to, and grow much better on, fibronectin or other matrix components than plastic, but even in primary culture in otherwise unsupplemented medium they require very high (40–50%) serum concentrations, with a distinct preference for human serum. Thereafter, subculture was at first successful only on further addition of high concentrations of dibutyryl cyclic adenosine monophosphate (cAMP) or of agents such as cholera toxin, which elevated cellular cAMP levels (30). High doses of ECGS had slight effects, most tumour conditioned media were ineffective, and the growth-promoting effect of human serum was not attributable to heparin-binding factors. Currently, satisfactory growth and subculture of these cells is carried out in medium supplemented with thymidine, hypoxanthine, isobutylmethylxanthine, and dibutyryl cAMP and containing 8% newborn calf serum + 2% prepartum maternal serum (29).

ADIPOSE TISSUE

Primary culture of capillary endothelial cells from adipose tissue was first reported in 1975 by Wagner and Matthews (31). These workers treated rat epididymal fat pads with collagenase, separated adipocytes from vessel fragments by flotation, and single cells from the latter by filtration on 200-μm mesh. Contaminating cells, detected visually, were removed from the cultures by growth in the presence of thimerosal, which perhaps selectively kills rapidly dividing cells. A similar isolation procedure was used by Björntorp et al. (32), who demonstrated that the endothelial cells, as in vivo, bound lipoprotein lipase. Kocher and Madri (33) have used these cells to examine their phenotypic modulation by different extracellular matrix components and have described alterations in actin gene expression in response to TGFβ dependent on whether the cells are growing as monolayers or in capillary tubes.

Several groups have now reported on the isolation and serial subculture of cells derived from human omental fat (34–36), using an isolation procedure similar to that devised from the rat fat pad. Although the endothelial nature of these cells has been identified by a variety of procedures, including synthesis of prostacyclin and tissue plasminogen activator (tPA), the presence of vWf, thrombomodulin, ACE, and uptake of acetylated LDL, there is still considerable uncertainty as to whether subcultured cell populations (if not derived by cloning) remain endothelial or are overgrown by mesothelial cells. This cell type is a likely contaminant in the initial isolate and is detectable by the presence of cytokeratins (37) and, like endothelium, synthesises prostacyclin and tPA.

One major impetus for the isolation of omental cells is their suitability as a readily available source of autologous cells to coat synthetic vascular grafts; in this particular instance, since mesothelial cells also provide a non- or antithrombogenic monolayer, it may not be a practical concern. Nonetheless, further work is needed to clarify whether properties ascribed to omental endothelial cells in such cultures, e.g., insulin-like growth factor synthesis (38), actually reflect mesothelial cell properties.

HEART

Simionescu and Simionescu (39) first devised a procedure for the isolation of microvascular endothelial cells from rabbit hearts. The initial step of fine mincing was designed to break the majority of large cells (cardiac myocytes), while leaving most of the smaller endothelial cells intact. After collagenase digestion, the tissue was homogenised; capillary fragments were collected by centrifuging at low gravity force through 6% albumin. Cells isolated by this procedure were successfully grown and subcultured in a simple medium without added growth factors by Gerritsen and Cheli (40).

Two groups have used an alternative strategy to isolate and culture coronary endothelial cells. Nees et al. (41) obtained cells from guinea pig hearts by infusing collagenase and leaving it in the vascular bed for 15 min before reperfusing and collecting detached cells. Diglio et al. (42) used a similar approach in the rat heart, but with recirculation of collagenase. The drawback to this method is the inability to know from which parts of the coronary bed, almost certainly including large vessels, the endothelial cells derive, even if isolated cells are cloned; it is therefore difficult in the absence of any selective marker to attribute the properties of cells obtained in this way specifically to the microvascular endothelium.

Schelling et al. (43) refined the ingenious and potentially highly selective technique invented by Ryan. This involves infusing polystyrene beads of a known diameter, at 4°C in the presence of EDTA; when recovered by back-perfusion, they bring with them endothelial cells from the portion of the vascular bed where the beads were lodged. First used with 60-μm diameter beads to isolate pulmonary arteriolar endothelial cells (44), Schelling et al. (43) used retrograde infusion of 15-μm beads to obtain bovine coronary venular endothelial cells, which were cloned and subcultured in the presence of ECGS. Endocardial endothelium has also been isolated and cultured recently from rabbit heart, by filling the right ventricle with EDTA and shaking for 10 min (45).

LUNG

Habliston et al. (46) cultured endothelial cells obtained by retrograde collagenase perfusion of guinea pig, rat, or rabbit lungs. These cells were serially subcultured on plastic in simple media with no added growth factor. As in other perfusion techniques, although morphological examination of the perfused lungs revealed large-scale destruction or removal of capillary endothelial cells, there was no guarantee that the cultured cells did not derive from larger vessels.

Davies et al. (47) adopted methods analogous to those used in the retina, including the use of gelatin-coated plates and selective growth media, in order to obtain apparently homogeneous cultures of microvascular endothelial cells or pericytes from adult rat lung. Chung-Welch et al. (48) used a similar procedure for bovine peripheral lung parenchymal vessels but also employed the selective cell suspension technique (pancreatin followed by trypsin) of Carson and Haudenschild (15) to remove contaminating cells and were then able to passage serially pure cultures in nonsupplemented medium. Alternatively, endothelial cells were cloned from small islands in mixed initial cultures, without the use of selective media, by weeding nearby cells, isolating an island of endothelium within a cloning cylinder and adding microcarrier beads to the cylinder, which were colonised by the endothelium and then transferred to new dishes. Meyrick et al. (49) cloned microvascular endothelial cells from bovine or sheep lungs, selectively trypsinising endothelial cell islands from similar mixed primary cultures by isolating them in cloning rings.

KIDNEY

Outgrowth of endothelial cells from tissue explants, a procedure that has rarely been used to isolate microvascular endothelium from other tissues, though it has, surprisingly, proved successful where conventional collagenase treatment has failed in obtaining endothelial cells from rat aorta (50), has been the only method reported for the isolation of glomerular microvascular endothelium. These cells were first grown from explanted isolated human glomeruli and were cloned from single cells after trypsinisation (51). Remarkably, the cells required PDGF in addition to foetal bovine serum for growth, unlike other endothelial cells from large or small vessels, with the possible exception of dermal microvascular cells. The reason for this is not clear, since in more recent studies of similar cells, grown from explants of human glomerular remnants obtained by Percoll sedimentation after collagenase treatment of minced renal cortex, primary cultures were grown in medium supplemented only with 5% bovine and 10% human serum, and subcultures were maintained and grown in the same medium with added ECGS (52,53). One distinctive feature of these cells was their capacity to produce almost exclusively single-chain urokinase (uPA), under conditions in which umbilical vein or omental cells produced only tPA (53).

Another novel technique has recently been described for the isolation of rabbit preglomerular microvascular endothelial cells. After infusion of magnetised iron oxide, which only filled the arterial, arteriolar, and glomerular circulation, kidneys were squashed in a tissue press. Microvessels were then dissected out, collected magnetically, rinsed, minced, and treated with collagenase before filtering (54). Primary cell cultures were purified by weeding and grown and subcultured in medium supplemented with fibronectin and ECGS.

LIVER

Hepatologists have used centrifugal elutriation for more than 10 years to isolate purified hepatic cell populations, so it is perhaps unsurprising that reports of successful isolation and culture of sinusoidal endothelial cells have all used this technique. De Leeuw (55) dispersed rat liver cells by recirculating pronase and collagenase before static incubation in the same enzymes and then passing tissue through a gauze filter. Endothelial cells were separated by elutriation and grown in primary culture on collagen coated dishes. Irving et al. (56) used a similar method and were able to subculture their cells, again plated on collagen, in medium supplemented with ECGS, FGF, or tumour-conditioned medium. Both groups, as well as Shaw et al. (57), who isolated sinusoidal endothelial cells from guinea pig liver by analogous methods and serially subcultured them using dispase rather than trypsin, noted the characteristic presence of fenestrae or "sieve plates" in their cultured cells.

CONCLUSION

This review has focused on the methodologies employed to isolate and culture pure populations of microvascular endothelium from a variety of tissues, concentrating on those for which several publications are available. I hope that it provides a useful introduction to the techniques, which could be applied to new tissues, although it is clear that very few (if any) methods are as straightforward or agreed upon as those for large vessel endothelial cell isolation and culture. Nonetheless, they provide a framework for the rational, albeit somewhat empirical, design of new approaches. In particular, the advent of increasing numbers of endothelial cell-specific monoclonal antibodies provides an as yet under used tool for the immunopurification of endothelial cells in mixed cultures, whether by fluorescence-activated or magnetic cell sorting.

REFERENCES

1. Folkman J, Haudenschild CC. Long-term culture of capillary endothelial cells. Proc Natl Acad Sci USA 1979;76:5217–5221.
2. Zetter BR. Endothelial heterogeneity: Influence of vessel size, organ localization, and species specificity on the properties of cultured endothelial cells. In: Ryan US, ed. Endothelial Cells. Vol. II. Boca Raton, Florida: CRC Press, 1988; 63–79.
3. Furie MB, Cramer EB, Naprstek BL, Silverstein S. Cultured endothelial cell monolayers that restrict the transendothelial passage of macromolecules and electrical current. J Cell Biol 1984;98:1033–1041.
4. Folkman J, Haudenschild C. Angiogenesis in vitro. Nature (Lond) 1980;288: 551–556.
5. Montesano R, Orci L, Vassalli P. In vitro rapid organization of endothelial cells into capillary-like networks is promoted by collagen matrices. J Cell Biol 1983; 97:1648–1652.
6. Carley WW, Milici AJ, Madri JA. Extracellular matrix specificity for the differentiation of capillary endothelial cells. Exp Cell Res 1988;178:426–434.
7. Ingber DE, Folkman J. Mechanochemical switching growth and differentiation during fibroblast growth factor-stimulated angiogenesis in vitro: role of extracellular matrix. J Cell Biol 1989;109:317–330.
8. Voyta JC, Via DP, Butterfield CE, Zetter BR. Identification and isolation of endothelial cells based on their increased uptake of acetylated-low density lipoprotein. J Cell Biol 1984;99:2034–2040.
9. De Bault LE, Kahn LE, Frommes SP, Cancilla PA. Cerebral microvessels and derived cells in tissue culture: Isolation and preliminary characterization. In Vitro 1979;15:473–487.
10. Brendel K, Meezan E, Carlson EC. Isolated brain microvessels: A purified, metabolically active preparation from bovine cerebral cortex. Science 1974; 185:953–955.
11. Spatz M, Bembry J, Dodson RF, Hervonen H, Murray MR. Endothelial cell cultures derived from isolated cerebral microvessels. Brain Res 1980;191:577–582.
12. Mršulja BB, Mršulja BJ, Fujimoto T, Klatzo I, Spatz M. Isolation of brain capillaries: A simplified technique. Brain Res 1976;110:361–365.
13. Bowman PD, Betz AL, Ar D, Wolinsky JS, Penney JB. Shivers RR, Goldstein GW. Primary culture of capillary endothelium from rat brain. In Vitro 1981;17: 353–362.

14. Goetz IE, Warren J, Estrada C, Roberts E, Krause DN. Long-term serial cultivation of arterial and capillary endothelium from adult bovine brain. In Vitro 1985;21:172–180.
15. Carson MP, Haudenschild CC. Microvascular endothelium and pericytes: High yield, low passage cultures. In Vitro 1986;22:344–354.
16. Vinters HV, Reave S, Costello P, Girvin JP, Moore SA. Isolation and culture of cells derived from human cerebral microvessels. Cell Tissue Res 1987;249: 657–667.
17. Sahagun G, Moore SA, Fabry Z, Schelpher RL, Hart MJ. Purification of murine endothelial cell cultures by flow cytometry using fluorescein-labelled *Griffonia simplificolia* agglutinin. Am J Pathol 1989;134:1227–1232.
18. Miettinen M, Holthöfer H, Lehto V-P, Miettinen A, Virtanen I. *Ulex europaeus* I lectin as a marker for tumors derived from endothelial cells. Am J Clin Pathol 1983;79:32–36.
19. De Bault LE, Cancilla PA. γ-Glutamyl transpeptidase in isolated brain endothelial cells: Induction by glial cells in vitro. Science 1980;207:653–655.
20. Maxwell K, Berliner JA, Cancilla PA. Induction of gamma-glutamyl transpeptidase in cultured cerebral endothelial cells by a product released by astrocytes. Brain Res 1987;410:309–314.
21. Orlidge A, D'Amore PA. Inhibition of capillary endothelial cell growth by pericytes and smooth muscle cells. J Cell Biol 1987;105:1455–1462.
22. Buzney SM, Massicotti SJ. Retinal vessel; proliferation of endothelium in vitro. Invest Ophthalmol Visual Sci 1979;18:1191–1195.
23. Bowman PD, Betz AL, Goldstein GW. Primary culture of microvascular endothelial cells from bovine retina: Selective growth using fibronectin-coated substance and plasma-derived serum. In Vitro 1982;18:1191–1195.
24. Gitlin JD, D'Amore PA. Culture of retinal capillary cells using selective growth media. Microvasc Res 1983;26:74–80.
25. Schor AM, Schor SL. The isolation and culture of endothelial cells and pericytes from the bovine retinal microvasculature: A comparative study with large vessel vascular cells. Microvasc Res 1986;32:21–28.
26. McIntosh LC, Muckersie L, Forrester JV. Retinal capillary endothelial cells prefer different substrates for growth and migration. Tissue Cell 1988;20:193–209.
27. Davison PM, Bensch K, Karasek MA. Growth and morphology of rabbit marginal vessel endothelium in cell culture. J Cell Biol 1980;85:187–198.
28. Davison PM, Bensch K, Karasek MA. Isolation and growth of endothelial cells from the microvessels of the newborn human foreskin in cell culture. J Invest Dermatol 1980;75:316–321.
29. Karasek MA. Microvascular endothelial cell culture. J Invest Dermatol 1989;93:33S–38S.
30. Davison PM, Karasek MA. Human dermal microvascular endothelial cells in vitro: effect of cyclic AMP on cellular morphology and proliferation rate. J Cell Physiol 1981;106:253–258.
31. Wagner RC, Matthews MA. The isolation and culture of capillary endothelium from epididymal fat. Microvasc Res 1975;10:286–297.
32. Björntorp P, Hansson GK, Jonasson L, Pettersson P, Sypniewska G. Isolation and characterization of endothelial cells from the epididymal fat pad of the rat. J Lipid Res 1983;24:105–112.

33. Kocher O, Madri JA. Modulation of actin mRNAs in cultured vascular cells by matrix components and TGFβ. In Vitro 1989;25:424–434.
34. Kern PA, Knedler A, Eckel RH. Isolation and culture of microvascular endothelium from human adipose tissue. J Clin Invest 1983;71:1822–1829.
35. Jarrels BE, Williams SK, Stokes G, et al. Use of freshly isolated capillary endothelial cells for the immediate establishment of a monolayer or a vascular graft at surgery. Surgery 1986;100:392–399.
36. Anders E, Alles J-V, Delvos V, Pötzch B, Priessner KT, Müller-Berghaus G. Microvascular endothelial cells from human omental tissue: Modified method for long-term cultivation and new aspects of characterization. Microvasc Res 1987;34:239–249.
37. Van Hinsbergh VWM, Kooistra T, Scheffer MA, van Bockel JH, van Muijen GNP. Characterization and fibrinolytic properties of human omental tissue mesothelial cells. Comparison with endothelial cells. Blood 1990;75:1490–1497.
38. Kern PA, Svoboda ME, Eckel RH, Van Wyck JJ. Insulin-like growth factor action and production in adipocytes and endothelial cells from human adipose tissue. Diabetes 1989;38:710–717.
39. Simionescu M, Simionescu N. Isolation and characterization of endothelial cells from the heart microvasculature. Microvasc Res 1978;16:426–452.
40. Gerritsen ME, Cheli CD. Arachidonic acid and prostaglandin endoperoxide metabolism in isolated rabbit coronary microvessels and isolated and cultivated coronary microvessel endothelial cells. J Clin Invest 1983;72:1658–1671.
41. Nees S, Gerbes Al, Gerlach E. Isolation, identification and continuous culture of coronary endothelial cells from guinea pig hearts. Eur J Cell Biol 1981;24:287–297.
42. Diglio CA, Grammas P, Giacomelli F, Wiener J. Rat heart-derived endothelial and smooth muscle cell cultures: Isolation, cloning and characterization. Tissue Cell 1988;20:477–492.
43. Schelling ME, Meininger CJ, Hawker JRJr, Grainger HJ. Venular endothelial cells from bovine heart. Am J Physiol 1988;254:H1211–1217.
44. Ryan US, White LA, Lopez M, Ryan JW. Use of microcarriers to isolate and culture pulmonary microvascular endothelium. Tissue Cell 1982;14:597–605.
45. Manduteanu I, Radu A, Simionescu M. Isolation and cultivation of rabbit endocardial endothelial cells. Preliminary data. Morphol Embryol 1988;34:165–169.
46. Habliston DL, Whitaker C, Hart MA, Ryan US, Ryan JW. Isolation and culture of endothelial cells from lungs of small animals. Am Rev Respir Dis 1979;119:853–868.
47. Davies P, Smith BT, Maddalo FB, et al. Characterization of lung pericytes in culture including their growth inhibition by endothelial substrate. Microvasc Res 1987;33:300–314.
48. Chung-Welch N, Shepro D, Dunham B, Hechtman HB. Prostacyclin and prostaglandin E_2 secretions by bovine pulmonary microvessel endothelial cells are altered by changes in culture conditions. J Cell Physiol 1988;135:224–234.
49. Meyrick B, Hoover R, Jones MR, Berry LC Jr, Brigham KL. In vitro effects of endotoxin on bovine and sheep lung microvascular and pulmonary artery endothelial cells. J Cell Physiol 1989;138:165–174.
50. McGuire PG, Orkin RW. Isolation of rat aortic endothelial cells by primary explant techniques and their phenotypic modulation by defined substrata. Lab Invest 1987;57:94–105.

51. Striker GE, Soderland C, Bowen-Pope DF et al. Isolation, characterization, and propagation in vitro of human glomerular endothelial cells. J Exp Med 1984; 160:323–328.
52. Gibbs VC, Wood DM, Garovoy MR. The response of cultured human kidney capillary endothelium to immunologic stimuli. Hum Immunol 1985;14:259–269.
53. Wojta J, Hoover RL, Daniel TO. Vascular origin determines plasminogen activator expression in human endothelial cells. J Biol Chem 1989;264:2846–2852.
54. Chaudhari A, Pedram A, Kirshenbaum MA. PGI$_2$ is not a major prostanoid produced by cultured rabbit renal microvascular endothelial cells. Am J Physiol 1989;256:F261–F273.
55. De Leeuw AM, Barelds RJ, De Zanger R, Knook DL. Primary cultures of endothelial cells of the rat liver. Cell Tissue Res 1982;223:201–215.
56. Irving MG, Roll FJ, Huang S, Bissell DM. Characterization and culture of sinusoidal endothelium from normal rat liver lipoprotein uptake and collagen phenotype. Gastroenterology 1984;87:1233–1247.
57. Shaw RG, Johnson AR, Schulz WW, Zahlten RN, Combes B. Sinusoidal endothelial cells from normal guinea pig liver: Isolation, culture and characterization. Hepatology 1984;4:591–602.

Index